Denial

A Clarification of
Concepts and Research

Denial

A Clarification of
Concepts and Research

Edited by

E. L. Edelstein
The Hebrew University
Jerusalem, Israel

Donald L. Nathanson
The Institute of Pennsylvania Hospital
and Hahnemann University
Philadelphia, Pennsylvania

and

Andrew M. Stone
University of Pennsylvania
Philadelphia, Pennsylvania

Plenum Press • New York and London

Library of Congress Cataloging in Publication Data

Denial: a clarification of concepts and research.

Based on the International Symposium on Denial, held Jan. 26–31, 1985, in
Jerusalem.
  Includes bibliographies and index.
    1. Denial (Psychology)—Congresses. I. Edelstein, E. L. (Elieser Ludwig), 1922–
  . II. Nathanson, Donald L. III. Stone, Andrew M. IV. International Symposium
on Denial (1985: Jerusalem) [DNLM: 1. Denial (Psychology)—congresses. WM
193.5.D3 D3939 1985]
RC455.4.D45D46   1989   616.89   /   88-35671
ISBN 0-306-43058-4

© 1989 Plenum Press, New York
A Division of Plenum Publishing Corporation
233 Spring Street, New York, N.Y. 10013

Printed in the United States of America

To The Israel Psychoanalytic Society

Contributors

LEA BAIDER, Department of Clinical Oncology and Radiology, Hadassah University Hospital, Ein Karen, Jerusalem, Israel

RAMI A. BAR GIORA, ILAN Child Guidance Clinic, P.O. Box 8125, Jerusalem, Israel

MICHAEL FREDERIC CHAYES, Private Practice, Burmanstraat 9 hs., Amsterdam, The Netherlands

SHAMAI DAVIDSON, Late of the Shalvata Mental Health Center, Hod HaSharon, Israel

THEODORE L. DORPAT, Departments of Psychiatry and Behavioral Medicine, University of Washington School of Medicine, Seattle, Washington

E. L. EDELSTEIN, Department of Psychiatry, Hadassah University Hospital, Ein Karen, Jerusalem, Israel

RIVKA R. EIFERMANN, Department of Psychology, The Hebrew University of Jerusalem, Jerusalem, Israel

H. SHMUEL ERLICH, Department of Psychology, The Hebrew University of Jerusalem, Jerusalem, Israel

RICHARD C. FRIEDMAN, Private Practice, 225 Central Park West, New York, New York

GEMMA JAPPE, Private Practice, Riesstrasse 21, Bonn, Germany

HILLEL KLEIN, Private Practice, 14 Tchernichovsky Street, Jerusalem, Israel

ILANY KOGAN, Private Practice, 2 Mohaliver Street, Rehovot, Israel

RAFAEL MOSES, Sigmund Freud Center for Study and Research in Psychoanalysis, The Hebrew University of Jerusalem, Jerusalem, Israel, and Austen Riggs Center, Stockbridge, Massachusetts

HERMAN MUSAPH, Private Practice, C. van Renesstraat 30, Amsterdam, The Netherlands

DONALD L. NATHANSON, The Institute of Pennsylvania Hospital and Hahnemann University, Philadelphia, Pennsylvania

DIETER OHLMEIER, Sigmund Freud Institute, Myliusstraase 20, Frankfurt, Federal Republic of Germany

GIORGIO SACERDOTI, Private Practice, Rio de la Crose 149, Giudecca, Venice, Italy

ANTONIO SEMI, Private Practice, Rio de la Crose 149, Giudecca, Venice, Italy

RUTH S. SHALEV, Neuropediatric Diagnostic Unit, Bikur Cholim Hospital, Jerusalem, Israel

JOEL SHANAN, Department of Psychology, The Hebrew University of Jerusalem, Jerusalem, Israel

ANDREW M. STONE, Department of Psychiatry, Philadelphia Veterans Administration Medical Center, and University of Pennsylvania, Philadelphia, Pennsylvania

MICHAEL H. STONE, Beth Israel Medical Center/Mt. Sinai Medical School, New York, New York

MARTIN WANGH, Private Practice, 20 Neve Sha'anan, Jerusalem, Israel

AVERY DANTO WEISMAN, Department of Psychiatry, Massachusetts General Hospital, Boston, Massachusetts

LÉON WURMSER, Private Practice, 904 Crestwick Road, Towson, Maryland

Preface

We do not think about everything at once all the time. Various mechanisms allow us to choose from among the themes, issues, topics, feelings, ideas, and memories that might occupy consciousness. One can focus selectively on anything deemed important; yet the methods by which this is accomplished vary greatly. We clinicians assign to these various mechanisms names that fit whatever theoretical system is central to our work—the healthy *suppression* of "background noise" allows us to pay attention to certain matters; the *repression* of unconscious conflict may assist our functioning in one moment despite its later cost; whereas *denial* and *disavowal* are used as general and fairly nonspecific terms for matters that are left out of awareness in order to avoid the noxious emotions specific to the personal significance of such awareness. Despite the attitude of scientific objectivity characterizing Freud's introduction of psychoanalysis, an aura of morality clings to certain of these mechanisms, for we tend to judge people by their use of them. We are a society of doers, people of action and accomplishment who look with disrespect at the avoidance of any responsibility or task. Thus denial has taken on a negative connotation, and those who use this avoidance system are seen as the lesser among us.

Yet, in the clinical practice of psychotherapy, we see denial in so many ways that suggest its relationship to courage, bravery, and creativity that it seems almost irrational and perhaps unfair to use so negative a label for the underlying process. In a single day, a therapist might work with a patient riddled with metastatic carcinoma, able to accept the dehumanization and disfigurement of antineoplastic treatment only by disavowal of the ominous progression of the illness; a barely functioning patient reeking of alcohol, who claims "I can stop any time I want"; a physician drenched with sweat and shivering with chills,

ignoring fever as she continues to work in the hospital; and a war veteran discussing a moment when, in a fine disregard of what appeared to
others as certain death, he pulled a companion to safety. It may well be
that in some of these instances what has been disavowed might usefully
be recognized and discussed, whereas in others, what is denied cannot be
solved and is best left unanswered. This is a book as much about the skill
of denial as it is about denial as a defense.

The problem for us is one of language, not of action. A map is not
the territory it depicts but rather a description of a territory. The words
used to describe entities and events are not the things themselves but
complex forms by which we attempt to structure those portions of reality
amenable to such manipulation. Nowhere is this expressed more poi-
gnantly and simply than by Wittgenstein, who described his monu-
mental *Tractatus Logico-Philosophicus* as consisting of two parts, the one
resting in the hands of the reader and called a book, and another, to him
even more important but *inexpressible.* "Wovon man nicht sprechen
kann, daruber muss man schweigen." (Whereof one cannot speak,
thereof one must remain silent.) Yet here the not-saying is not denial but
rather a recognition of the limitations of language.

As psychoanalysis approaches its second century, some of its language requires refinement. The symposium "Denial: A Clarification of
Theoretical Issues and Research" was organized by Eli Edelstein for
precisely this purpose. A word with too many meanings ceases to be
useful; a concept limited too narrowly loses significance. Intended was a
broad-based, comprehensive review in which each participant would be
encouraged to discuss the idea of denial from a personal vantage point.
From the start, it was understood that some scholars would discuss theoretical issues, others a wide range of practical applications of the concept. We were unprepared for the intensity of interest created by this
request or for the excitement generated at the meeting itself. So complex was the resulting gestalt, so intriguing the data presented that week
in Jerusalem, that the task of turning this group of papers into a coherent book proved correspondingly complex. As a participant in the
symposium, Donald Nathanson has joined its organizer to complete the
conversion of the original symposium into the current volume; toward
this end we have enlisted as co-editor Andrew Stone, whose assistance
has been invaluable.

All of us know the experience of first recognizing, then learning a
new word that becomes part of our vocabulary. Not infrequently, just as
we come to recognize this word, it begins to appear everywhere we turn.
For Nathanson, this visit to Jerusalem was an introduction to the Middle
East—rather than return directly to Philadelphia, he and his wife lin-

gered as tourists in Israel for a few days, visiting Egypt as well. Clambering wide-eyed through the tomb of Rameses VI, they were asked by their Egyptian guide to pause before a wall painting depicting pharaoh in the act of being interrogated. The guide explained that this was The Hall of Negative Confession, an intriguing if perplexing description. "It is important that the wrong man not become Ra," continued the guide. "There are many things a real pharaoh would not have done. If the man who has died and has traveled the great river to get to this point is successful in his journey, he will become Ra, the sun god. It cannot be allowed for the wrong man to be made Ra. So he is asked a great many questions: 'Did you do this?' or 'Did you do that.' And to each question he must answer, 'I did not do it.' Only after he has made negative confession to all of the questions is he allowed to pass on to the final portion of his journey." Travelers from the International Symposium on Denial had journeyed from Mount Scopus to the Hall of Denial.

It is our hope that, in breaking through the limits of tradition, we have collected new material useful both within the professional disciplines of the healing arts and well beyond into other areas.

E.L.E.
D.L.N.
A.M.S.

Acknowledgments

Professor R. Rachamimoff, dean of the Medical School and rector of the Hebrew University at the time of its 60th anniversary, ensured the cooperation of the University for the International Symposium on Denial, the meeting on which this volume is based. To the many scholars and clinicians in Jerusalem who opened their homes to visitors from all over the world, we give our thanks for their hospitality. It was W. Doyle Gentry who forged the link to Plenum Press that made possible publication of the papers presented at that meeting; without his efforts the work of so many might have been ephemeral rather than enduring. There have been many at Plenum who worked hard to help us cope with the difficult task of editing papers written in several different national styles. Prime among these have been senior editor Eliot Werner, production editor Robert Jystad and a veritable army of copyeditors. Their patience and skill have been essential to the final product. Special thanks must also be given to Rosalind Nathanson for her support during the editorial phases of this project. Most of all we wish to thank the participants in the International Symposium on Denial for the quality of their presentations, the energy they brought to the resulting colloquium, and their remarkable tolerance for the editorial process.

Contents

I

Theoretical Issues

The very disparity of approaches seen in these first three chapters may be viewed as a microcosm of the history of psychoanalysis, as well as an indication of the problems inherent in any attempt to assign a specific meaning to the term *denial*. These chapters call attention not just to the matter of denial as a defense against the personal significance of a percept but illuminate as well a major shift in focus on the part of our field. Where Wangh discusses denial from the standpoint of the drives and their relationship to the intrapsychic representations of the object, Dorpat sees denial as an unconscious mechanism achieving great importance in its interactional mode, whereas Nathanson focuses on the affective life of the infant and defines denial in terms of interaffectivity and the modulation of affect.

Drawing most of his examples from the work of Freud, Wangh concentrates on the various ways of saying "No" within the confines of the intrapsychic domain. He defines negation, repression, denial, disavowal, refusal, isolation, the use of hypnotic trance to produce negative hallucination, and the intrapsychic representation of death (the final negation of life) as methods of handling drives and perception. In his schema, all defense mechanisms utilize denial; all defenses start with denial, making it as much the cornerstone of psychoanalysis as repression.

Dorpat, whose description of the cognitive arrest inherent in denial remains a major contribution to our field, points out that denial usually occurs in the context of an interpersonal relationship and that all defenses can be evaluated on the basis of their interactional significance. He brings to this work his knowledge of families in conflict, demonstrating how denial works to support family myths and systems. Describing projective identification as the quintessential example of the interactional nature of the defenses, he asserts that the mechanism of projective identification is called into operation only when some mental content is denied, after which the projection of that idea or feeling into another person serves to remove the offending ideo-affective complex from the intrapsychic realm. Thus denial is a method by which the individual evades, suspends or avoids knowledge of some part of the self (what may be called internal awareness) as well as a way of diminishing the effects of external perception.

But what is it that has been avoided in both examples? Nathanson reminds us that cognitions and perceptions are rendered problematic for the individual only when they are accompanied by unwanted or unacceptable emotion. The final chapter in this section focuses on what has been described as the weakest area in psychoanalytic theory, the nature of emotion. As Nathanson points out, Tomkins has suggested that the affects represent a system quite separate from the drives, a group of neurophysiologic mechanisms that work to amplify the drives, as well as cognition and any other brain function, thus providing the basic source of human motivation. What Kohut called *mirroring* and what Stern referred to as *interaffectivity* represent initially the interplay of facial affect mechanisms and later the sharing of emotion. Nathanson suggests that "the most mature among us do not live in a world of shared emotion" and that there must be some healthy ego mechanism allowing us to maintain a sense of ourselves in the face of powerful emotion broadcast by another. He postulates that such a defensive operation of the ego, which he calls the *empathic wall*, represents the earliest method by which the child wards off the experience of broadcast affect and is the prototype of what later come to be called *denial* and *projection*.

Perhaps this latter chapter serves as an indication of another important shift in psychoanalytic thinking, one central to the theme of this volume. It has been taken for granted since Freud that the mental mechanisms are methods of avoidance; ours is a culture that celebrates confrontation and looks down on evasion. Yet there are circumstances when pain cannot be relieved and when distress cannot be alleviated. In such situations, continued attention to pain and distress renders the organism dysfunctional; where denial can be used to foster a focus on the possible, to further the cause of life, then denial is a healthy mechanism. Wangh, however, cites evidence that the 400,000 Jews confined in the Warsaw Ghetto perished at the hands of their captors because they chose massive denial rather than experience the terror that might have led them to a different fate. Later, of course, the rebellion of the Warsaw Ghetto may indicate the operation of other, reparative mental mechanisms. But

Wangh's point is clear: "Denial of death may be a stabilizer of action for life's sake, but seduced by it, we may also be brought closer to the death we wish to evade." Much of our work as therapists involves the need to determine when denial should be allowed to provide a reasonable degree of protection from distress and when anxiety must be faced lest even worse danger threaten the organism. These opening chapters lay the groundwork for the clinical applications that form the remainder of the book.

The Evolution of Psychoanalytic Thought on Negation and Denial

MARTIN WANGH

Biblical, religious, philosophical and metaphysical ideas are surprisingly in unison in assigning priority or ultimate victory to "nothingness" over "being." Thus, in the Bible *tohoo-wabohoo,* that is, chaos, was *before* creation; as Abraham Ibn Ezra (ca 1200 A.D.) tersely states: *"yesh meayin"* (יש מאין), that is "something from nothing." Heidegger (1971) postulates that anxiety of "nothingness" fills "being" and Freud (1920) speaks of the great strength of *thanatos* that strives toward maximum entropy, that is, toward disorder, the negative of biological existence. Freud concludes in his exposition on "Negation" (1925) that the death drive is the source of all "No," of the negative in general, of repression and denial, disavowal, and refusal. On the other hand, he declares, all affirmation and assertion stem from *eros,* the uniting force of the life drive.[1]

---

[1] In what follows, I shall preferentially use the term *negation* to cover the subject at hand as a comprehensive abstract conception of all conscious or *un*conscious negating, refuting or refusing. *Denial* and *disavowal* will be used in more specific clinical context, whereby the term *disavowal* is thought of as being somewhat closer to consciousness than the warding off by denial. *Negativism* will be used to describe an either maturational phase-determined, thereby temporary, attitude, or a more permanent character stance.

MARTIN WANGH • Private Practice, 20 Neve Sha'anan, Jerusalem 93707, Israel.

In terms of logical thinking, there remains, of course, an unsolvable paradox: If a destructive drive exists, it exists within an *existing* subject. Drive *is* inherently an affirmation, even though its aim may be nothingness. Freud avoids this dilemma as long as he remains within the framework of the topographic theory. At the very end of his paper, "On Negation" (1925, p. 239), he asserts: "In analysis we never discover a 'no' in the unconscious." He (1923) had expressed this previously, as follows: "Death is an abstract concept with a negative content for which no unconscious correlative can be found" (p. 58).

A quasiclinical illustration of how troublesome this capability to conceive of death is for human beings can be found in the very person of Freud. Whenever Freud discusses this topic, he alternatively asserts and negates. As he admits death to his consciousness, he expresses doubt or he purely intellectually theorizes on and simultaneously neutralizes the concept. When he gives us a description of *thanatos* as the source of all negation, he immediately couples it with that of its opposite, *eros*, the acme of self- and species preservation.

Early on, in his "Interpretation of Dreams," Freud (1900) supports W. Steckel's (1911) demonstration of death symbolization in dreams. He even adds such an illustration himself: "Departing on a journey" (1900, p. 385) stands in for dying (v. also 9). Yet later, in 1923, he denounces (1923)[2] Steckel's (1911) declaration that "fear of death underlies all fear," most vigorously—too vigorously. In fact, 1923 is the year in which Freud had the first operation (April 20) for his oral cancer (Jones, 1957; Schur, 1972).[3]

Max Schur (1972), Freud's trusted physician, describes how Freud was convinced that he would die an early death. Yet Schur also directs our attention to the many places in Freud's writing and letters where such fears are omitted, when one could expect their expression, or where recognition is acknowledged, but only in projected form, or where a question mark makes for doubt.

Let me cite some examples of Freud's attempt to admit and yet also

---

[2]Here are the words of his condemnation: "Steckel's statement 'every fear is ultimately a fear of death' is a high sounding phrase, [it] has hardly any meaning and, at any rate, cannot be justified" (p. 57). In the German original (1923): "'*Das Ich und das Es*,' this denounciation sounds even more hyperbolic and its phrasing is even more awkward: *Der volltoenende Satz: Jede Angst sei eigentlich Todesangst schliesst kaum einen Sinn ein, ist jedenfalls nicht zu rechtfertigen*" (p. 288).

[3]Schur writes: "During the second half of 1922 Freud . . . also attempted to formulate his views on the psychological meaning of the fear of death in metapsychological terms. The book [*The Ego and the Id*] was published in April 1923, that fateful month when Freud's cancer was discovered" (p. 347).

to obscure from himself, or from whom he addresses, his fear of disease or death. In a footnote added in 1919 to his "Interpretation of Dreams" (1900), he speaks of his fear for the life of his son, who had been at the war front. The dream says: "[The son's] face or forehead was bandaged. He was adjusting something in his mouth, pushing something into it. . . . Has he got false teeth?" (p. 560). Freud's associations were to an accident of his own at the age of 2 or 3, when he had fallen and had injured his own mouth. Freud makes no reference at this time to his then-already present fear of oral cancer. A similar inference of omitting his concern about his own physical condition, we can make from the Irma dream (1900). Was he not, when he had this dream, already concerned about leucoplakias in his own mouth? We find an ambiguous confession of such fears in a 1917 letter to Ferenczi (reported by Schur, 1972, p. 347): "Yesterday I smoked my last cigar . . . palpitations appeared and a worsening of a painful swelling in the palate . . . [cancer?]."

From 1923 on, after his first operation for removal of an oral cancer, Freud's private comments change in character, though they still always show a libidinal input. (The quotes that follow are all taken from J. Cremerius's, 1983, interesting article, "Freud's *Sterben—Die Identität von Denken, Leben und Sterben.*") In 1931, Freud writes to his brother Samuel that he is losing the *"überlegene Indifferenz"* (the superior indifference) toward his suffering that he had been able to maintain earlier. Yet the libidinal admixture is still there in his comment to Arnold Zweig that he is fighting *"mein liebes altes Karzinom"* (my dear old cancer) (letter of March 5, 1939). His affirmation of life, beyond life, does not only get expressed via his concerned references for his family but also by his conviction that some *future* humanity will come to appreciate his discoveries; and so he continues to write almost to his last moment.

The need to deny death or at least to blunt consciousness of it is shared by everyone. We could not live with a persistent awareness of death. To do so would prevent all future-directed action. Any planned "next" moment implies future. Negation of death seems to keep us "alive" into eternity. (At the end of this exposition, I will, however, speak of nefarious results of this very need for denial).

Let us not turn to examine in greater detail Freud's (1925) paper, "Negation" (*Verneinung*). The editors of the *Standard Edition* call it "one of Freud's . . . most succinct" (1925, p. 234). The paper is very brief, barely five printed pages long. It is Freud's most comprehensive statement on this subject matter. Its very condensation asks for clarification. I hope that what follows will respond to this need to some extent. The paper begins with what one might consider a bit of treatment advice. I paraphrase: Ignore the negative preface in your patient's report. It aims at annulling the full consciousness of what cannot be held in repression. The patient's "No" separates intellect from affect (not unlike isolation). By holding back the recognition by consciousness of the affective portion of thought, a measure of repression still remains in force. Freud (1925, p. 236) formulates this as follows: "A negative judgement [i.e., a statement "this is not so"] is an intellectual substitute for repression." The effect of it is almost equivalent to repression. Thus far, Freud argues in terms of the topographic theory. He scrutinizes the conscious versus the unconscious quality of a matter. But when Freud switches to a genetic, economic question: How does the first repudiation, the first "No" come about? "The Pleasure-Principle demands it," is Freud's answer. What is pleasurable belongs to "Me"; what is not pleasure-bringing is "Not Me," is "outside." Once such an "outside" is discerned, its acknowledgment can be wholly withdrawn. Also what has been ejected can become affixed to it as a quality. This we call a projection. It firms up the first "No."

This first "No," the ejection itself, spares the organism from an inner, self-mortifying, reflexive reaction. Its immediate fixation by projection allows time for an outer-directed counteraction. The negativism inherent in this projection is thus a *second-phase negation*. These first two phases occur automatically and unconsciously under the dictate of the pleasure principle.

Projection can take place, of course, only after introjections have occurred, that is, when "psychic representations" of what has actually been perceived have established themselves. Thereafter every perception of an outside object is a "refinding" of it; then, however, every such "refound object" has inevitably some subjective qualities attached to it. Reality testing is what we call the comparison of these observations with the more pure memory of the original one. Should these reobservations be stimulative of impulses, that is, instinctual discharges that may endanger the organism, the whole complex—observation of what is on the outside, its significance for the organism and the arousal itself—*may become totally ignored*, that is, totally unknowable. This we call successful repression. It represents a *third phase of negation*. It is initiated by a judgment, a judgment of what is endangering, of what is good or bad for the organism. However, repression is often not totally successful. Repressed contents reveal themselves through displacements, in condensation, and symbols, that is, through derivatives. Repression may be only partial. The impulse itself may be ignored, or the stimulating object may become unseeable, or its sight is actively avoided (phobias), or what is seen or felt is plainly declared as *not being meaningful*. All these can be comprised under the terms *denial, disavowal,* or *negation*.

Each of them serves to plug leaks of what was to stay repressed. The subject who uses these auxiliary methods is never spontaneously aware that he or she "denies." Almost always an outside observer is required to notice the phenomenon. Usually only after the subject's attention has been called to it may he or she be prepared to uncover to her- or himself his or her tendency to say "no." It is not quite the same with repression. Here the subject *may* have an inkling that something is missing in his or her mind. Often enough he or she will try to grope for it, for something that he or she has forgotten.

Denial is truly thus a *fourth* phase of negation; it is mobilized against the leakages of repression. Freud (1925, p. 235) puts it this way:

> Negation is a way of taking cognizance of what is repressed; indeed, it is already a lifting of the repression, though not of course an acceptance of what is repressed. . . . We can see how in this the intellectual function is separated from the affective process. . . . In the course of analysis . . . we succeed in conquering the negation and [bring] about a full acceptance of the repressed; but the repressive process is not yet removed by this.

Freud's statement that "No" is the hallmark of repression can be reversed into saying that "Repression is the hallmark of 'No' "—however, if leakage occurs, it can be reinforced by a conscious statement of "No," which Freud then calls *denial* or *disavowal*.[4]

Yet the leakage that is to be stemmed by denial, that is, by preceding a statement with a negative proposition, may itself need some further plugging against the normal propulsion toward acknowledgment of reality. The negative declaration itself has to be bolstered through affirmations furnished by religious beliefs, that is, beliefs shared with others, by private *positive* fantasies, by ascribing victory over negative elements to mythical figures—which are then taken as ideals—or via lies. Fenichel (1945)[5] makes this last point so clearly; I paraphrase: "The liar, by convincing us, his listeners, can reinforce his own denial of real facts or situations" (pp. 528–529).

By turning to issues of reality testing and judgment, Freud's thinking runs now along the lines of the so-called "structural theory." Yet, as a

---

[4]Freud clinically takes notice for the first time of what he is later going to call repression and/or negation when he recalls a "negative hallucination" that Bernheim imposed upon a patient. Bernheim had commanded a patient in a hypnotic trance not to take any notice of him, the hypnotist, no matter what he did to her. She indeed could not do so while in trance (p. 109).

[5]Fenichel (1945) writes: "Making use of the infantile defense mechanism of denial constitutes the first lie. 'Absolute denial' is soon replaced by 'denial in fantasy,' and the denying effect is intensified if other persons (as 'witnesses') can be made to believe in the truth of the denying fantasy" (pp. 528–529).

next step, Freud, in his search *for the source of energy* of the phenomenon of negation, switches to the dualistic "instinct theory." The energy of the "No" and "Yes" alternative, he declares, is derived from the instinctual pair: *thanatos* and *eros*. (I have spoken of this at the very beginning of this exposition). Finally, in his very last paragraph (1925, p. 239), Freud once more thinks in topographic terms when he states that there cannot be any *psychic representation* of death in the unconscious of the human mind.

It is on this matter of "psychic representation" of an *outside* object that our attention must be focussed in the first place in our scrutiny of the concept *denial*.

A brief clinical vignette may illustrate what we mean by "psychic representation and its denial":

When I, as a young resident psychiatrist in a mental hospital, once tried to intrude into the hallucinated world of a chronically ill, paranoid, schizophrenic patient, I was "appropriately" rebuffed by her. She would stand arguing intensely before an imagined judge in an imaginary courtroom, uttering her accusations and defenses. I tried to interrupt her flow of speech by saying something that fitted in with the context of her hallucinations. She pointed to me and demanded loudly of the judge to "remove this court attendant from the courtroom." Obviously, she had taken notice of my presence—I was however not her psychiatrist (at that time I was still clothed *de rigeur* in a white coat)—but the "psychic representation" of me was that of a "court aide." (In measure, I had, of course, collaborated in this "misrepresentation" and hence deserved her indignation and rebuke). To come back to the essential point: *Denial does not actually change an outside object. Only its "psychic representation" gets modified.* Only its "meaning" has changed. Such a change of meaning of the stimulus object can entail, however, changes in attitude toward the object, changes in affects aroused by it, and of moods lingering on beyond the encounter. The "reality of the object persists," although psychoanalysts in their shorthand way speak of "denial of reality."

Freud's (1927, 1940) prime clinical example for the process of denial is the set of mind of the fetishist. During his search for a sexually exciting object, the fetishist behaves as though the female possessed a phallus, although he well knows that she is not possessed of this anatomical structure. When the fetishist chooses a body part or any other object for the stimulus point for his sexual excitement, he does not have any awareness that he is thereby substituting a *present* item in lieu of the one, the sight of which is unconsciously objectionable to him: The *absence* of the penis is replaced in his mind by some item that can serve as a symbol for a phallus.

Freud calls this process within the fetishist's mind "a splitting of his ego." We must be aware that, at this point, Freud's meaning of the ego is not the early one, in which only conscious and unconscious were contrasted, but more the ego of the structural hypothesis. But, as in this conception, in each "split-off" sector, id—ego—superego participation is involved, we might just as well speak of a "splitting of the personality" or of the self.

To come back to the main issue: What matters in denial and negation is the effect upon the "psychic representation" of what is out there in reality, or in there, in the subject. Cathexis of these psychic representations may arouse instinctual impulses and concomitantly evoke mnemonic images of previously received punishment, or of previously encountered dangers, which had prevented discharge and thereby caused frustration. To prevent repetition of such sequences, and in the service of self-preservation, "denial" may intersect the arc from arousal to discharge at any of its points. Thus, first of all, the presence of the stimulating image may be negated, or, whereas the stimulus object is perceived, it may be considered meaningless, or the *image of the danger* conjured up by its sight can be declared unimportant, or any other appropriate affect may become "unfelt."

Otto Fenichel (1945) has made a particular issue about the idea that the arc of reaction can be interrupted by means of denial at any point. He believes that Freud overemphasized that "denial" is outward directed, that only "ideas" or "actual views" of outer objects are negatable. He, Fenichel, places under the potential aegis of denial affects such as anxiety and/or guilt. The controversy on this score has continued over the years. Anna Freud (1936) prefers to limit denial to the negation of reality, or of ideas. Others, like Helene Deutsch (1933), Bertram D. Lewin (1932, 1940), and Edith Jacobson (1964) stand on Fenichel's side. Brenner (1982), in his latest book, *The Mind in Conflict*, says that in the technical psychoanalytic context, he holds to the Sigmund Freud–Anna Freud side:

> [In a] . . . strictly psychoanalytic . . . *technical* . . . sense the word denial refers to the defensive distortion of one's perception of some aspect of one's environment, of what is usually called external reality. (A. Freud, 1936)

Brenner holds that it is "midleading to extend the term as Lewin, Jacobson, and others have done, to include defensive distortion or disavowal of one's own wishes, affects, memories, etc" (p. 76). Because, as we have seen, "every defense denies something," Brenner (1982) argues that anything can be used in the service of defense, and, therfore, in the *ordinary* sense of the word, denial or negation is ubiquitous.

Technical or ordinary, as everything can be said to have a "psychic representation" and denial affects these psychic representations, the arc of perception–apperception–emotion–reactive action can be interrupted by denial of any of these points. The basic stimulus for it always stems from the need to ward off an unconscious danger.[6]

Negating the existence of an object—meaning by this of course, its psychic representation—or disavowing a feeling are akin to having a "negative hallucination." Where there should be something, there is nothing. Such a perceptual vacuum is, however, not easily tolerated under the growing pressure of the sense of reality and the hunger for percepts.

Just as the hull of a Gothic church is held up by buttresses, so denial in order to be sustainable is often buttressed by means of positive, substitutive images, by "dreams of glory," self-invented or gleaned from the mythologies of the peoples, by dreams of the might of, and identification with, fairy-tale figures, and more often than not, by solid appearing rationalizations, or by religious consolations of afterlife. One might call all these "positive hallucinations," filling the space left free by "negative" ones. Just as "denial" comes to the aid of the loosened grip of "repression," so do these scaffoldings support failing denial. They are mostly pleasure bearing and therefore almost always ego syntonic. They are stabilizers, if only momentarily so. The déjà-vu phenomenon, as Arlow (1959) describes it, together with similar phenomena, belongs here too.

I mentioned Freud's postulation that the signal of negation derives its energy from the death drive, yet as a defense it clearly serves the purposes of the life drive. The listening psychoanalyst will stay alert to both directions of what a negation, or more broadly, negativism might communicate in a primary order at a given time.

The developmental path of this ambiguity has been brought out by the researches of Rene Spitz (1957). In his book, *No and Yes,* Spitz asks himself a series of questions: (1) When in the infant's life do we first observe "No" gestures?; (2) from which kinetic source do they spring?; (3) when do they become movements that definitely signal opposition to

---

[6]Fenichel (1954, p. 220) states: "We cannot differentiate so exactly between defensive attitudes directed toward without and within, between denial and repression, for . . . every known mechanism is also employed against affects." (See also Fenichel, p. 130: "The tendentious forgetting of external experiences . . . [allows for] . . . no rigorous distinction between denial directed outward and 'repression directed inward.'")

Fenichel (1945) also gives an impressive example of the difference between blocking the whole of external perception and the blocking of an introjected image or better its representation. *Fainting* causes the stopping of all perception coming from the outside, even more so than sleep. In the neuroses (and psychoses), only the "representations" of the external world may be forgotten, misinterpreted, or their existence denied.

the environment?; (4) what is their developmental purpose?; and (5) during which phases of life are they particularly marked?

According to Spitz, what appears to be a "No" gesture—the turning of the head from side to side—of the very young infant is, to the contrary, a "rooting" movement, a reflexive searching for the nipple, that is, a life-affirming effort. Then, by a change of function, around 3 months, these movements appear to become "satiated avoidance behavior." Out of that a headshaking refusal signal evolves. This grows into a semantic, object-related motion in the second part of the first year of life. Thus, for the biological researcher Spitz, *affirmation* clearly precedes *negation*.

Spitz (1957) enthusiastically proclaims:

> The volitional use of the ideational content of negation in the semantic 'No' gesture is beyond doubt the most spectacular, intellectual semantic achievement in childhood. (p. 98)

Spitz puts the matter this way:

> The acquisition of the "No" is the indicator of a new level of autonomy, of the awareness of the "other" and of the awareness of the "self." . . . The dominance of the reality principle over the pleasure principle becomes [then] increasingly established. (p. 125)

The toddler's hiding himself by covering his head or closing his eyes or hiding behind his mother's skirt—the so-called manifestations of the 8 months' anxiety, are all signs of this active refusal to make contact. To be able to say "no" is to be able to dissent and to stay independent (at least for a given measure of time). The normal infant and toddler in the anal phase most energetically practices his or her assertiveness in this way, and so does the adolescent when he or she climbs up the ladder toward "independent adulthood." But what may be normal and necessary for growth in infancy or adolescence may be, if indiscriminately practiced in adulthood, pathological.

Negation, Spitz states, is a first abstraction—because it leads away from immediate action toward a "nonaction," particularly once identification with the functioning, care-taking, adult "no-sayer" has occurred. One may put it this way: The "no," this refusal to act/react in a purely reflex manner toward a stimulating object, inserts a time lag into automatic reaction—just as does thought, a trial action, according to Freud. Such pauses may often be as life preserving as they can be destructive.

This brings us back to Brenner's (1982) formulation: Anything may be used for defense, just as anything may be used for drive satisfaction. It all depends on the perspective to be applied. In the end, it is a teleological issue.

Please forgive me if I end this exposition on the concept of denial on a somber note. I am moved to do so by the very name of the building, Research Institute for the Advancement of Peace, in which the meeting was held on which this volume is based, by the past and present experiences of many of the inhabitants of this country and by the issue of the threat of nuclear war that hangs over humankind.[7] The choice of our subject itself may have been dictated by these very societal factors. In considering denial, we must stay aware of its Janus face. Denial of death may be a stabilizer of action for life's sake, but seduced by it, we may also be brought closer to the death we wish to evade. The fate of the 400,000 Jews, who were jammed by the Nazis into the Ghetto of Warsaw remains a warning pillar of fire for all of us. In his book, *The Terrible Secret* (the German title of which is *Was Niemand Wissen Wollte*), Walter Laqueur (1980, 1981) gives us a most painful example of denial's nefarious results. The 400,000 Jews compressed into the Warsaw Ghetto, although warned of their peril by the news of the death of thousands of Jews in Vilna and subsequently of still more in the still nearer Chelmno, denied that there was mortal danger to them. They convinced themselves that only those Jews who had been communists were murdered in revenge by the Nazies. "This is Warsaw," they reasoned, "in the center of Europe; there are 400,000 Jews in the Ghetto; a liquidation on this scale is surely impossible" (Laqueur, 1980, p. 127). Laqueur believes were it not for the depth and extent of such denial, a good many of the Warsaw Ghetto inhabitants might have had a chance to save themselves—although, I would add, they might also have committed suicide as the chairman of the Judenrat (Jewish Council), Adam Cherniakow had done.

With such precedents in mind, we psychoanalysts must make a paradoxical demand of ourselves and our fellow humans. Although we know that denial serves to relieve us of anxiety, and such relief is necessary for living, we must renounce its comfort to remain alert to the danger to our whole biosphere that a "nuclear winter" brought about by a nuclear war holds out for our planet Earth.

REFERENCES

Adler-Vonessen. (1971). Angst in der Sicht von S. Kierkegaard, S. Freud, und M. Heidegger. *Psyche*, 25, 696.
Altman, L. (1975). *The dream in psychoanalysis*. New York: International Universities Press.

---

[7]The grave danger brought about by the impairment of reality testing linked to the defense by denial has recently been particularly pointed out by Becker and Nedelmann (1983).

Arlow, J. A. (1959). The structure of the déjà-vu experience. *Journal of the American Psychoanalytic Association, 7,* 611–633.

Becker, H., & Nedelmann, C. (1983). *Psychoanalyse und Politik.* Frankfurt: Suhrkamp.

Brenner, C. (1982). *The mind in conflict.* New York: International Universities Press.

Cremerius, J. (1983). Freud's Sterben. Die Identitat von Denken, Leben, und Sterben. *Psychotherapie, Psychosomatik, Medizinische Psychologie, 33,* 163–166.

Deutsch, H. (1933). Zur psychologie der manisch—Depressiven zustande, insbesondere der chronischen hypomania. *1933,* 19.

Ezra, Abraham Ibn. (ca. 1200 a.d.). *Commentary to Genesis.*

Fenichel, O. (1945). *The psychoanalytic theory of the neurosis.* New York: Norton.

Fenichel, O. (1954). *The ego and the affects: Collected papers.* New York: Norton.

Freud, A. (1936). *The ego and the mechanisms of defence.*

Freud, S. (1900). *The interpretation of dreams.*

Freud, S. (1920). *Beyond the pleasure prinicple.*

Freud, S. (1923). *The ego and the id.* [In German, *Das ich und das es.*]

Freud, S. (1925). *Negation.*

Freud, S. (1937). *Fetishism.*

Freud, S. (1940). *Splitting the ego in the process of defense.*

Jacobson, E. (1964). *The self and the object world.* New York: International Universities Press.

Jones, E. (1957). *The life and work of Sigmund Freud* (Vol. 3). New York: Basic.

Laqueur, W. (1980). *The terrible secret.* London: Penguin.

Laqueur, W. (1981). *Was niemand wissen wollte. unterdruckung der nachrichten uber Hitler's endlosung.* Frankfurt: Ullstein.

Lewin, B. D. (1932). Analysis and structure of a transient hypomania. *Psychological Quarterly.*

Lewin, B. D. (1950). The psychoanalysis of elation. *Psychological Quarterly.*

Schur, M. (1972). *Freud, living, and dying.* New York: International Universities Press.

Spitz, R. (1957). *No and yes.* New York: International Universities Press.

Steckel, W. (1911). *Die sprache des traumes.* Weisbaden.

2

Interactional Perspectives on Denial and Defense

Theodore L. Dorpat

In this chapter, my aim is to provide an overview and discussion of the literature on the interactional aspects of denial and defense. Psychiatrists and psychoanalysts often speak or write about defense mechanisms as independent mental operations dissociated from the ebb and flow of interpersonal events. This review will show defense as an important aspect of communication between individuals and how they relate to each other. Until recently, classical psychoanalytic literature contained few studies of the influence of interpersonal relations on the formation or maintenance of defensive operations. The investigations summarized later reveal how both the form and the content of a person's denials and defensive functioning throughout life are influenced and even partly shaped by interactions with other individuals operating out of their awareness.

STUDIES OF DENIAL IN DISABLED AND SERIOUSLY ILL PATIENTS

Several investigations of seriously ill and/or disabled patients have revealed that interactional factors profoundly influence patients' denials

THEODORE L. DORPAT • Departments of Psychiatry and Behavioral Medicine, University of Washington School of Medicine, Seattle, Washington 98105.

of their illnesses. Weinstein and Kahn (1955) observed that denial was by
no means restricted to the patient and that many relatives, nurses, and
physicians showed varying degrees of denial of the illness or disability
found in these hospitalized patients. In nurses, for instance, denial could
be seen in the forms of ignoring, minimizing, or excusing behavior
changes. Weinstein (1980) underscores the importance of interpersonal
factors in the denials of brain-damaged persons, and he indicates that
the denial syndromes served an adaptive function in dyadic interactions
and would not exist unless created or solicited by the hospital situation.

In his study of denial reactions of seriously ill and terminal patients,
Weisman (1972) notes that one danger likely to evoke denial is jeopardy
to a relationship with a key person:

> The distinctive quality of denying and denial is that it occurs only in relation
> to certain people, not to all, and has the primary purpose of protecting a
> significant relationship. (pp. 75–76)

This explains why patients tend to deny more to certain people than to
others. Weisman tells of a patient with an inoperable carcinoma who, in
conversation with various hospital personnel (physicians, nurses, social
workers) showed considerable denial of her impending death. Only with
the consulting psychiatrist was the patient able to speak openly and
frankly of her illness and steadily approaching death. Many severely ill
patients, according to Weisman, have an overriding need to preserve
contact and to stabilize their relationship with someone essential to their
well-being. To these people they deny their illness because they assume
that such an admission would jeopardize their relationship.

Weisman (1972) observes that seriously ill patients can venture to
speak with individuals who do not have authority over them because,
with such individuals, they do not risk the rupture of a significant relationship. His conclusion about the role of denial in interpersonal relations is similar to Rubinfine's (1962) formulation that denial in young
children is needed to preserve object relations when aggression threatens object loss.

According to Weisman (1972), clinicians tend to ignore the significance of the external observer or participant when making the diagnosis
of denial. Equivocation on the part of physicians produces uncertainty in
patients that creates an excess of denial. Patients in the studies by
Weisman (1972) and Kubler-Ross (1969) used denial when the doctor or
family member expected denial.

Kubler-Ross (1969) investigated psychological reactions to impending death among 200 hospitalized patients with known terminal illnesses. She notes that doctors who themselves needed denial also found

it in their patients. Physicians capable of discussing terminal illness created conditions in which patients could address their concerns about death and dying. The patient's need for denial, she concluded, was in direct proportion to the doctor's need for denial.

Studies by Rothenberg (1961) and Waxenberg (1966) show that physicians commonly facilitate denial in cancer patients by their tendency to discourage such patients' communication about themselves, their illness, and its consequences. They found that many doctors, when dealing with cancer patients, tend to support denial by encouraging social isolation and by underestimating their patients' capacities for understanding. Communication under these circumstances is always discouraged, and, as a result, little information is sought or exchanged.

There exists a consensus among the previously cited investigators and others who have studied denial reactions in seriously ill and terminally ill patients that both the extent and frequency with which they deny is affected significantly by the attitudes and communications of the physicians and other medical personnel in attendance. All of these studies emphasize the importance of free and open communication, on the part of medical personnel, for the minimizing of pathological denial reactions in patients.

DENIAL OF PARENTAL SUICIDE IN SUICIDE SURVIVORS

A number of studies of the traumatic effects of parental suicide on surviving children reveal that the child's denial of the parental suicide is facilitated and supported by similar denials and evasions used (by the adult surviving relatives) to hide from themselves and others both the facts and the affective significance of the suicide (Cain, 1972; Dorpat, 1972; Rosen, 1955; Wallerstein, 1967). The inability to talk with others about the parental suicide deprives surviving children of opportunities for appropriate mourning and for testing and comparing the reality of the traumatic events with their fantasy distortions and fabrications about the suicide (Dorpat, 1972). Cain (1972) notes that surviving parents, to an extent difficult to imagine, avoid communicating directly with their children about the suicide. Distortions of communication between surviving parents and children are even more profound.

Rosen (1955) describes an analytic patient with severe disturbances in reality testing and derealization symptoms who struggled since childhood to carry out the command of his father (and later of his superego) to deny his mother's suicide attempt, witnessed by him when he was 3½ years old. His father had denied the traumatic episode and had treated any mention of the event on the part of the patient as something he had imagined or as a "bad dream." The patient's derealization symptom could be traced back to the trauma of witnessing his mother hanging, and his use of denial was supported and sustained by his father's deceptions and denials of the mother's suicide attempt.

These investigations of suicide survivors revealed that the patients' denial of the parental suicide was a prominent and long-lasting defense that was associated with arrested mourning reactions and developmental fixations. Clinical studies of these survivors, including the psychoanalysis of some of them, agree on the central importance of interactional factors in the formation and maintenance of the patients' denials. When the surviving parent, by evasion and distorted communication, prevented the surviving children from dealing with the parental suicide, this played a critical role in causing, supporting, and perpetuating the surviving children's denial of the parental suicide.

THEORIES OF INTERACTIONAL DEFENSES: TRANSACTIONAL DEFENSE MECHANISMS

Räkkölainer and Alanen (1982) propose that defensive processes that cannot be properly understood outside of their current interpersonal context should be called "transactional defense mechanisms." The authors comment on the contradiction between the strictly intrapsychic nature of the basic theory of psychoanalysis and the interactional nature of the psychoanalytic situation itself. They observe accurately that most definitions of defensive functions limit the scope of inquiry to the intrapsychic world of the individual. Their paper deals with "transactionality," that is, the mutual intertwining of defensive functions in lasting and intimate—though conflictual—dyads, groups, and families. From the individual point of view, the transactionality defense concept refers to the use of those defensive functions through which the person tries to protect against anxiety by drawing on other persons and/or fantasies about them. The authors describe families in which there was a lasting mutual state of projective identification, a concept that simultaneously conveys the complementary as well as the transactional nature of the phenomenon.

TRANSPERSONAL DEFENSES

Laing (1967) introduced the term *transpersonal defenses* in a paper entitled "Family and Individual Structure." He noted that the defenses described in psychoanalysis are intrapsychic defenses and refer to the ways a person processes his or her own experience. In actual families and in real life generally, people attempt to affect the experiences of other people in order to preserve their own inner worlds. He emphasizes the need for a systematic psychoanalytic theory for the transpersonal defenses, wherein one person attempts to regulate the inner world of the other in order to preserve the integrity of his or her own inner world.

According to Muir (1982), the so-called "primitive defenses" (e.g., denial, splitting, projective identification) are in fact the transpersonal defenses described by Laing (1967). Because these defenses require the active participation of other individuals for their successful operation, they may be described as shared or group defenses. The studies reviewed in this chapter and the investigations reported in my book on denial (Dorpat, 1985) agree with Muir's (1982) conclusion that the environment must go along with, if not actually share in, certain defensive processes, if these defenses are to be sustained.

LANGS'S VIEW ON INTERACTIONAL DEFENSES

Langs (1981, p. 467) criticizes the classical conception of defenses because it has ignored the interactional aspects of defensive functioning. The classical theory of defenses is essentially an intrapsychic conception, with an overriding emphasis on the individual's use of a variety of inner protective mechanisms that are mobilized to defend against instinctual drive wishes. The classical line of thought and its concentration on issues of intrapsychic conflict and unconscious fantasy—memory formations have been challenged by Kleinian analysts and others who have written from an object relations point of view. Writings on object relations present persuasive arguments for a conception of defense that would take into account both intrapsychic and interactional factors and processes. Langs argues for a revised theory of defenses that would recognize the role played by object relations in the development, maintenance, and internalization of defenses. This approach would expand the classical conception of defenses, which is so exclusively intrapsychic at the present time, to include interactional defenses such as projective identification. Langs (1982a) defines interactional defenses as:

> . . . intrapsychic protective mechanisms that are formed through vectors from both patients and therapist. This type of defense may exist in either participant to the therapeutic dyad, and has both intrapsychic and interpersonal (external) sources. (p. 729)

COMMUNICATIVE MODES AND DEFENSE

Langs (1978, 1981) describes three communicative modes and types of bipersonal field (Types A, B, and C) that are related to specific kinds of defensive interactions. Type A, characterized by the predominance of symbolic imagery, communicates the most meaning and facilitates insight. It is the optimal and constructive mode for both therapist and patient. In the Type A mode, defensive activity can be inferred from the manifest and latent content of the patient's verbal communications. This is not true of Type B and Type C communicative modes, where the patient's defensive activity is expressed mainly in the communicative mode itself rather than in the content. Defense in the Types B and C modes is expressed much more in *how* the individuals communicate than in *what* is communicated. The Type B communicative mode is one characterized by major efforts at projective identification and action discharge. This mode is basically designed not for insight but instead to facilitate the expulsion of unconscious conflicted and unpleasurable contents.

In the Type B field, either the patient, the therapist, or both make extensive use of projective identification and use the other member of the dyad as a container for disruptive projective identifications. Langs's (1976, 1978, 1979, 1980) psychotherapy seminars for psychiatric residents clearly demonstrate that major contributions to the development of a Type B field often come from *both* the therapist and the patient. My supervisory work with psychotherapy trainees and with analytic candidates indicates that a Type B field is a common one in both psychiatric and psychoanalytic practice and that often therapists and analysts unconsciously either initiate or sustain this pathologically symbiotic mode of communication and relatedness.

A primitive kind of denial is often operative in the Type C mode, where spoken language is used to erect barriers against the emergence of disturbing affects and ideas. In the Type C mode and field, the essential links between the patient and the therapist are broken, and verbal communications are designed to destroy meaning and relatedness. Communications involving the destruction of meaning and relatedness are described by Bion (1959) as "attacks on linking". Some of the narcissistic patients described by Kohut (1971, 1977) and Kernberg (1976) communicate in this way; they treat the analyst as nonexistent, and they often evoke intense feelings of boredom and deadness in the listener.

PROJECTIVE IDENTIFICATION

The most intensely studied kind of explicitly interactional defensive activity is projective identification. It was first described by Klein (1946), and Grotstein (1981) provides a comprehensive review and discussion of the subject. Langs (1976) holds that projective identification and introjective identification are the primary interactional mechanisms within the bipersonal field. Bion (1977) views projective identification as the single most important form of interaction between patient and therapist as well as in groups of all kinds.

Projective identification has been investigated in family relationships, in groups, and in individual and group psychotherapy sessions, and it has been described by diverse investigators with disparate theoretical perspectives. The following include some of the various labels attached to the different variants of a broadly defined concept of projective identification: *merging* (Boszormenyi-Nagy, 1967), *trading of dissociations* (Wynne, 1965), *irrational role assignments* (Framo, 1970), *symbiotic* (Mahler, 1952), *evocation of a proxy* (Wangh, 1962), *externalization* (Brodey, 1965), *scapegoating* (Vogel & Bell, 1960), *actualization of wished-for object relations* (Sandler, 1976), and *dumping* (Langs, 1982b).

Ogden (1982) describes projective identification as a psychological process that is simultaneously a type of defense, a mode of communication, and a primitive form of object relationship. He had made an important contribution through integrating object relations, defense, and communicative approaches. For him, projective identification is a type of defense in which one can distance himself from an unwanted or endangered part of the self while in unconscious fantasy keeping that aspect of oneself "alive" in another. As a mode of communication, projective identification is one in which the subject makes himself or herself understood by exerting pressure on another person to experience a set of feelings similar to his or her own. Projective identification is a primitive kind of object relatedness in which the subject experiences the object of the projection as separate enough to serve as a receptacle for parts of the self but sufficiently undifferentiated to maintain the illusion that one is literally sharing a given feeling with another person.

Sandler (1976) identifies one kind of transference reaction that involves the patient's unconscious manipulations of the therapist in order to actualize some wished-for relationship. Sandler reinforces the link between transference and countertransference from the standpoint of seeing transference as the patient's attempt to manipulate the analyst into reactions that represent for the patient a concealed repetition of old object relations. Countertransference is viewed as a compromise between the analyst's own tendencies and his or her response to the role that the patient attempts to force upon him or her. The relationship between transference and countertransference is conceptualized as a specific instance of the general phenomenon of *actualization*.

In psychotherapy as in everyday life, individuals attempt to actualize the particular object relationships inherent in their dominant unconscious wishes and fantasies. This striving toward actualization is explained by J. & A.-M. Sandler (1978) as part of the wish-fulfilling aspect of all object relationships.

EVOCATION OF A PROXY

Wangh (1962) discusses the manner in which individuals, for unconscious defensive motives, attempt to mobilize in other persons their own forbidden instinctual drive needs and a variety of ego experiences and functions. In these persons, there is an unresolved symbiotic tie to the mother that produces a deficit in the sense of identity and an inability to control their impulses. With them, there is a special sensitivity to separation from any object that has served as a narcissistic extension of the self (a self-object). The *evocation of a proxy* utilizes the symbiotic mode of relatedness for defensive purposes in which another person is mobilized to function as an alter ego.

Selected unconscious contents and functions are not only assigned to the partner but evoked in him or her instead of in oneself. Wangh emphasizes that there is something more than projection involved here. The subject's aim is to mobilize and activate the object's feelings and reactions, and it is therefore a manipulation by proxy evocation. The evocation of a proxy has the purpose of preserving a good relationship with a narcissistically cathected object (a self-object). Wangh underscores the importance of both denial and projection in the evocation of a proxy. Individuals use their perception of the activated emotional and instinctual manifestations in the proxy object to deny those impulses and contents in themselves. In an article on Shakespeare's *Othello*, Wangh (1950) underlines the point that Iago needs to rid himself of an intolerable jealousy and succeeds in doing so by arousing the selfsame emotion in Othello.

Anna Freud (1936) describes a form of projection, "altruistic surrender," in which an individual evades the pressures of his or her superego by participating through unconscious identification in the instinctual gratifications of another person. Anna Freud's patient found some proxy in the outside world to serve as a repository for her forbidden, unconscious impulses. Greene (1958, 1959) describes such proxy mechanisms in the context of vicarious object functioning. He explicates the need for the existence of the vicariously functioning object and observes that some patients became physically ill when the proxy mechanisms were no longer feasible. In a panel discussion reported by Kanzer (1957), Adelaide Johnson reviews her studies on the pathogenesis of acting out. She notes that ostensibly forbidden impulses in children are unwittingly sanctioned and induced by their parents, who then derive a vicarious gratification of their own unconscious impulses through the behaviors of their children.

PROJECTIVE IDENTIFICATION IN THE FAMILIES OF DISTURBED ADOLESCENTS

Zinner and Shapiro (1962) report on 45 emotionally disturbed adolescents and their families at the Clinical Center of the National Institute of Health. Their observations focus upon parental perceptions and behavior toward their children, and they introduce the term *delineations* to describe those acts and statements of the parents that communicate the parental image of the adolescent to him or her. Among parental delineations are those that more serve parental defensive needs than any realistic appraisal of the actual attributes of the adolescent. Defensive delineations are the expression, at an individual level, of family group behavior that is determined more by shared unconscious fantasies than by reality considerations. Family group behavior and subjective experience are all determined to varying degrees by shared unconscious fantasies and assumptions. Role allocations for the collusive living out of these unconscious fantasies and assumptions are communicated and evoked in family members by the mechanism of projective identification.

For projective identification to function effectively as a defense, the actual nature of the relationship between the self and its projected part in the object must remain unconscious, although the subject may feel an ill-defined bond or kinship with the recipient of his or her projections (Zinner & Shapiro, 1972). The disavowal of the projected part of the self is not so complete that the subject loses the capacity to experience the feelings that the subject has evoked in the object. These vicarious experiences may contain features of punishment, rejection, and deprivation as well as those of gratification.

DENIAL AND PROJECTIVE IDENTIFICATION

An *implicit denial* is an essential component of projective identification, and this denial profoundly affects the subject's self and object representations involved in the projective identification. What the subject denies as some part of the self, he or she projects onto the object. Also, in projective identification, the subject most often denies the meaning of any communication or behavior of the object that is not congruent with his or her projections onto the object.

What are the denied parts of the self that are projected in projective identification? Clinical reports in the literature reveal that a wide range of unconscious contents, conflicts, and affects may be denied and then projected. When the object is idealized, "good" parts of the self are projected, and when the object is denigrated, it "receives," as it were, the "bad" parts of the self. Thus whole objects, part-objects, self-objects, introjects, conflicts, affects, functioning, ego ideal, superego elements, drive representations, and many other contents have been identified as the projected elements of the personality. Often projection is used as a means of distancing conflicting parts of the self. For example, an individual may marry a person with the ego-dystonic aspects of the individual's unconscious psychic conflicts.

In projective identification, the object is perceived and related to as a distanced but not separate part of the self, and any behavior of the object that does not fit the subject's projection is frequently ignored or discounted. The reality of the object that cannot be used to verify the projection is not consciously perceived, and, according to Brodey (1965), the subject has a negative hallucination for whatever there is about the object that is discordant with his or her expectations and wishes.

STAGES OF PROJECTIVE IDENTIFICATION

The common threads that have been noted in the various studies may be summarized in terms of three stages of projective identification. In Stage 1, the subject perceives the object as if the object contained elements of the subject's self. This is usually explained on the basis of an unconscious fantasy in which the subject projects parts of the self onto an object. Most investigators of projective identification have given too much weight to the causal significance of unconscious fantasy and too little to that of unconscious interactional dynamics. As an interactional process, projective identification is unconsciously activated and sustained by the projector's communicative interactions with others. As I shall argue in a later section, unconscious processes of perception, memory, and introjection as well as fantasy often play important roles in projective identification.

In Stage 2, through any one or more of a wide variety of pressures (e.g., manipulation, persuasion, coercion, intimidation, idealization, and so on), the subject elicits or provokes conflicts and affects in the object that conform with the subject's unconscious projection. Through these pressures, the subject seeks to control the responses of the object and to actualize an unconsciously wished-for kind of symbiotic relationship. These pressures are transmitted by both conscious communications, and, more often, unconscious verbal and nonverbal communications.

In Stage 3, the object of the projective identification receives the subject's conscious and unconscious communications and responds to the pressures placed upon him or her. There is a wide range of both normal and pathological sorts of reactions to projective identification. When the object of a projective identification "contains" (Bion, 1967) and "processes" (Langs, 1978) the induced thoughts and feelings in a more mature way than did the projector, the recipient's methods of handling the projected thoughts and feelings become available for therapeutic internalization by the projector via introjection and/or identification. If, however, the recipient resorts to expulsion of the induced feelings, the projector's introjection of the recipient's rejecting and defensive attitude leads to augmentation of the projector's pathology.

The individual who receives the projective identification may identify himself or herself with what has been attributed to him or her. This reaction is called *projective counteridentification* by Grindberg (1962), and, depending on how much and how long the individual has identified with what has been projected onto him or her, it could have pathological effects.

MUTUAL PROJECTIVE IDENTIFICATION

The object of projective identification may respond by communicating with another projective identification. In so doing, he or she will be participating in what Langs (1978) calls a Type B communicative field and in what may also be called *mutual projective identification*. Relationships in which there is a mutual projective identification involve the enactment of pathological symbiotic (or self–object) modes of relatedness and communication. In such interactions, each party unconsciously colludes with the other in verifying and validating the other's projections.

In mutual projective identification, both parties unconsciously support and sustain the denials and other defensive activity of each other. How do we account for the fact that the object of projective identification may collude in this defensive activity, with the result that the subject's defensive projections become a self-fulfilling prophecy? There is a consensus in the literature that one of the most powerful unconscious motives for sustaining these shared denial systems and symbiotic patterns of relatedness is the participants' anxieties and fears over object loss.

Brodey (1965) notes that the terror of abandonment perpetuates these kinds of relationships. Adolescents studied by Zinner and Shapiro (1972) feared that object loss would ensue if they did not act in such a way as to verify their parents' defensive projections. These adolescents were afraid not to collude, not to comply, and not to identify with what had been projected upon them by their parents. Räkkölainer and Alanen (1982) found that the primary target of transactional defense mechanisms was separation anxiety. According to Wangh (1962), separation from objects experienced as part of the self was an important factor in both initiating and maintaining relationships based on the "evocation of a proxy."

UNCONSCIOUS COMMUNICATIONS AND PROCESSES IN MUTUAL PROJECTIVE IDENTIFICATION

As I noted earlier, most investigators on this subject give exclusive attention to the importance of unconscious fantasy, and they conceptualize projective identification as the enactment of an unconscious fantasy. Their view excludes the crucial role of unconscious perception, unconscious memory, and unconscious introjection. As it is commonly used, the concept of unconscious fantasy implies that the origins of the fantasy are wholly endogenous and isolated from the subject's current interactions with others. This exclusive focus on unconscious fantasy excludes the powerful effects and meanings of the subject's conscious and unconscious communications with other individuals in both the formation and the maintenance of projective identification.

In interactions marked by mutual projective identification, there exist complementary modes of communicating in which the subject evokes a complementary communication in the object. Compliant communications, for example, tend to elicit directive communications from the object. Similarly, in other interpersonal situations, masochistic and passive-dependent modes are apt to evoke, respectively, sadistic and active-independent modes of response. In pathological symbiotic relations, such complementary modes are used not only for their defensive and adaptive function but also for the sense of wholeness and integrity they provide for both partners of the relationship.

In order to demonstrate the significance of unconscious communications and processes in mutual projective identification, I shall present a schematized and sequential account of the interactional dynamics involved in a sadomasochistic type of interaction. For the purposes of this exposition, the terms *sadistic* and *masochistic* are used in a general sense to refer to a variety of related behaviors, affects, and ideas. Though this outline is about a hypothetical interaction, it is derived and abstracted from my psychoanalytic and supervisory experience, and it is consistent with reports in the literature on mutual projective identification.

What follows is a schematic and condensed outline of the important and typical interactions in the sadomasochistic type of mutual projective identification. The sadist unconsciously denies the masochistic part of her- or himself, projects the rejected part of her- or himself onto an object (hereinafter called the "masochist"), and by his or her sadistic mode of communicating manipulates the masochist to behave masochistically. Then the masochist introjects what has been projected onto him or her and acts out the masochistic role (e.g., he or she behaves or communicates in a weak, demeaned, submissive, or punished manner). At the same time, the masochist denies the sadistic part of her- or himself, projects it onto his or her representation of the object, and by his or her masochistic mode of communicating provokes the sadist to behave sadistically. By responding sadistically, the sadist completes and renews the vicious cycle of spiraling communication in mutual projective identification in which the communication of each party acts as a signal and a provocation for the complementary behavior of the other party.

Now we are in a position to outline the role of unconscious processes of perception, introjection, memory, and fantasy in the masochist's unconscious motives for projective identification. One motive is defensive: By behaving masochistically, the masochist can deny his or her sadism and attempt to actualize his or her wish to be rid of sadistic feelings by projecting his or her sadism onto the sadist. Other important unconscious motives are associated with his or her introjection of the sadist's projected masochism and his or her unconscious perceptions of the sadist's communications. He or she may, for various reasons, feel compelled to comply with the masochistic role ascribed to him or her, to introject and to identify with what has been projected onto him or her, and to gratify the sadist by behaving masochistically. The masochist's interactions with the sadist may activate the masochist's unconscious childhood memories that are then acted out in his or her masochistic behavior.

The masochist may unconsciously perceive, for example, that the sadist is attempting to intimidate and control him or her. By behaving masochistically, he or she also attempts to control and to shape the sadist's actions. Often, the masochist unconsciously perceives the sadist's underlying vulnerability and defensiveness, and, by behaving masochistically, he or she may be attempting unconsciously to support the sadist's denial and projection by acting out in his or her own behavior the rejected vulnerable part of the sadist's personality.

An additional powerful unconscious motive for the projective identifications of both participants is their wish to maintain the relationship and to avoid a rupture in their symbiotic bond. They unconsciously seek to carry out these aims by unconsciously supporting the defenses of the other. For example, by behaving masochistically the masochist verifies and confirms the sadist's denial and projection. The foregoing are only a few of the many possible unconscious motives for projective identification that are triggered and energized by the subject's communicative interactions with another individual.

To sum up, in mutual projective identification, unconscious wishful fantasies are only one aspect of a complex matrix of unconscious aims associated with the subject's unconscious introjection of what has been projected onto him or her, with his or her unconscious perceptions of the object, and with the activation of unconscious memories. These unconscious processes (i.e., projection, perception, memory, fantasy, and introjection) are strongly affected by the individual's conscious and unconscious communications with others. Unconscious wishes for maintaining symbiotic bonds, for supporting the defenses in the object that safeguard these bonds, are often potent underlying motives for both initiating and sustaining states of mutual projective identification.

SHARED DENIAL

In the hypothetical sadomasochistic interaction just described, *both* the masochist and the sadist deny aspects of the masochist's unconscious sadism and the sadist's unconscious masochism. Through their unconscious communications, each of the parties reinforces and contributes to the denials of the other party.

Both parties of mutual projective identification unconsciously participate in denying important aspects of their interactions, and they unconsciously support each other's defensive operations. For mutual projective identification to function effectively for both individuals, the actual nature of their communicative interaction must remain unconscious. An unconsciously collusive or shared denial is an integral element in mutual projective identification. Through the shared denial, both parties can disavow the dystonic aspects of their own unconscious conflicts and project them onto the other party. Their shared denial is the binding force that protects their symbiotic mode of relating and provides both individuals with a sense of illusory wholeness and freedom from anxieties over separation and object loss.

Although it is a common phenomenon, there are few reports in the literature on shared denial. The *folie-à-deux* syndrome is based on a shared denial of psychotic proportions in which a more disturbed and psychotic individual induces a less disturbed person to join him or her in believing some delusion. Silverblatt (1981) reports six cases of denial of pregnancy in which there was an unconscious collusion with the patient on the part of others, including physicians, in their shared denial of any awareness of the pregnancy. In a previous publication, I wrote about the relatives and physician of a young suicidal woman who unconsciously joined her in denying the seriousness and lethal meanings of her suicidal behaviors (Dorpat, 1974). Their shared denial kept them from taking the kinds of preventive and therapeutic actions that might have prevented her ultimate suicide.

CONCLUDING REMARKS

An individual's defensive functioning is influenced by many causes, including the status of one's ego and superego development, unconscious conflicts, and the psychic consequences of trauma and developmental deficits. The psychoanalytic literature has emphasized preexisting structural and developmental elements, but until recently it has paid scant attention to adaptive and interactional processes that affect how a person defends her- or himself, why he or she defends, and what he or she defends.

There exists a consensus among different investigators that anxiety over object loss, broadly defined, is the most important and powerful of the motives for denying in interpersonal situations. Under the category of anxiety over object loss, I would include the following specific unpleasurable contents: separation anxiety, separation guilt, fear of rejection, fear of abandonment, and anxieties over loss of love and narcissistic supplies. In short, individuals in interpersonal situations will deny something or other in order to maintain their relationship with the other person and to avoid a disruption of their relationship.

How people deny and what they deny is strongly influenced by the conscious and, more significantly, the unconscious communications of others. In the studies of seriously ill and disabled hospitalized patients, there was abundant evidence that the patients' denials of death and disability were profoundly affected by how the hospital staff communicated with them. The patients' denials were sharply reduced when staff members invited and participated in open, free communication. All of the studies reviewed on a child's denial reactions to the suicidal death of a parent revealed that these denials were shaped and maintained by the evasions, denials, and lack of open communication on the part of the surviving adult relatives.

The behavior and communications of groups of all kinds, including family groups and the therapist–patient dyad, are determined to varying degrees by shared unconscious fantasies and unconscious assumptions. Role allocations for the collusive enactment of these unconscious fantasies are communicated and evoked by the mechanism of projective identification. In such groups, individuals often unconsciously collude with each other in establishing and maintaining their mutual projective identifications. In mutual projective identification, there is a shared denial concerning the actualities of their interaction, and each participant's communications validate and verify the projections of the other participant. The important unconscious processes in mutual projective identification are those of projection, introjection, memory, perception, and fantasy.

Defensive operations affect the mode of communication as well as the content. Denial may be an aspect of *what* one communicates and *how* one communicates. In the Type B and C communicative modes, denial occurs in how one communicates. Projection of a denied part of the self is the central feature of projective identification of the Type B mode, and a primitive kind of denial of meaning and relatedness is an essential element of the Type C mode.

Several studies reviewed earlier testify to the inadequacy of the classical concept of defenses as isolated events occurring in a closed "intrapsychic" system. These investigators recommend establishing a revised theory that would conceptualize defensive operations as an aspect of how individuals relate and communicate with each other, a comprehensive theory that would account for the role of unconscious communications in initiating and sustaining defensive actions in individuals, dyads, and groups. Some analysts propose a special class of defenses involving the individual's interactions with others, and they label this category as *transpersonal* (Laing, 1967), *interactional* (Langs, 1982a), and *transactional* (Räkkölainen & Alanen, 1982). Though I agree with the criticisms made by the cited authors about the lack of attention to the interactional aspects of defenses in the psychoanalytic literature, I do not agree with their proposals for establishing two different categories of defensive activity with one category having to do with the intrapsychic or inner world and the other concerning the outer or interpersonal world.

As I argued in a previous paper (Dorpat, 1981), there is a fallacy in the concept of a dichotomy of "intrapsychic or intrapersonal (or interactional)." The word *intrapsychic* is a spatial metaphor that is commonly and incorrectly interpreted in a lateral sense to mean inside the psyche or mind. Using the word in this way, the subject commits the error of reification because he or she speaks of the mind as if it were a space. It does not make sense to speak of defenses or any other kind of human activity as taking place in two different worlds, an inner or intrapsychic world and an external physical or interpersonal world. Only in fantasy and not in actuality do humans exist in two worlds.

This is not to say that individuals defend themselves only in interpersonal situations because one may defend in one's thinking and imagination. Denial and defense are just as much a part of how individuals communicate and relate with each other as it is an aspect of how and what they think to themselves. A valid and meaningful distinction can be made between carrying out defensive activity *privately* and defending oneself *publicly* in one's transactions with others. The word *private,* as Schafer (1976, p. 160) usefully explains, is not just another word for *inner* because it expresses an entirely different way of conceptualizing psychic actions.

Even those defenses carried out privately do involve conscious or unconscious fantasies and memories of a person's feared or wished-for relationships with objects. Defensive activity is developed from the individual's relations with others. What is internalized and ultimately transformed into defenses and other psychic structures is interactions with objects (Loewald 1970). Therefore, an object relations element is an essential part of all defensive activity, whether that defensive activity is carried out privately in one's thinking and imagination or publicly in one's interactions with others. There is no need for a new and different category for interactional, transactional, or transpersonal defenses. What is needed is an expanded awareness of the interactional aspects of defensive activity and clinical research and developmental studies on the role of object relations in the development, maintenance, and internalization of defenses.

It is not possible to provide a comprehensive description or explanation of an individual's defensive actions without taking into account interactional dynamics, the mainly unconscious ways in which persons influence and contribute to both the conscious experience and the unconscious psychic functioning of other persons. The interactional point of view should be part of any systematic theory of defense. Studies reviewed in this chapter demonstrate that why people defend, how they defend, and what they defend are strongly influenced by their communicative interactions with other individuals.

REFERENCES

Bion, W. (1959). Attacks on linking. *International Journal of Psycho-Analysis, 40,* 308–315.

Bion, W. (1967). *Second thoughts.* New York: Jason Aronson.

Boszormenyi-Nagy, I. (1967). Relational modes and meaning. In G. H. Zuk & I. Boszormenyi-Nagy (Eds.), *Family Therapy and Disturbed Families* (pp. 71–89). Palo Alto: Science and Behavior Books.

Brodey, W. M. (1965). On the dynamics of narcissism: I. Externalization and early ego development. *Psychoanalytic Study of the Child, 20,* 165–193.

Cain, A. C. (1972). Children's disturbed reactions to parental suicide: Distortions of guilt, communication, and identification. In A. C. Cain (Ed.), *Survivors of Suicide,* (pp. 93–111). Springfield: Charles C Thomas.

Dorpat, T. L. (1972). Psychological effects of parental suicide on surviving children. In A. C. Cain (Ed.), *Survivors of suicide* (pp. 121–144). Springfield: Charles C Thomas.

Dorpat, T. L. (1974). Drug automatism, barbiturate poisoning and suicide behavior. *Archives of General Psychiatry, 31,* 216–220.

Dorpat, T. L. (1981). Basic concepts and terms in object relations theories. In S. Tuttman, C. Kaye, and M. Zimmerman (Eds.), *Object and self: A Developmental approach* (pp. 149–178). New York: International Universities Press.

Dorpat, T. L. (1985). *Denial and defense in the therapeutic situation.* New York: Jason Aronson.

Framo, J. L. (1970). Symptoms from a family transactional viewpoint. In N. W. Ackerman (Ed.), *Family therapy in transition* (pp. 48–62). Boston: Little Brown.

Freud, A. (1936). *The ego and the mechanisms of defense.* New York: International Universities Press.

Greene, W. A. (1958). Role of vicarious object in the adaptation to object loss: I. Use of a vicarious object as a means of adjustment to separation from a significant person. *Psychosomatic Medicine, 20,* 20–29.

Greene, W. A. (1959). Role of vicarious object in the adaptation to object loss: II. Vicissitudes in the role of the vicarious object. *Psychosomatic Medicine, 21,* 29–41.

Grindberg, L. (1962). On a specific aspect of countertransference due to the patient's projective identification. *International Journal of Psycho-Analysis, 43,* 436–440.

Grotstein, J. S. (1981). *Splitting and projective identification.* New York: Jason Aronson.

Kanzer, M. (1957). Panel Report. Acting out and its relation to impulse disorders. *Journal of the American Psychoanalytic Association, 5,* 136–145.

Kernberg, O. F. (1976). *Object relations theory and clinical psychoanalysis.* New York: Jason Aronson.

Klein, M. (1946). Notes on some schizoid mechanisms. *International Journal of Psycho-Analysis, 27,* 99–110.

Kohut, H. (1971). *The analysis of the self.* New York: International Universities Press.

Kohut, H. (1977). *The restoration of the self.* New York: International Universities Press.

Kubler-Ross, E. (1969). *On death and dying.* London: Macmillan.

Laing, R. D. (1967). Family and individual structure. In P. Lomax (Ed.), *The predicament of the family* (pp. 107–125). New York: International Universities Press.

Langs, R. (1976). *The bipersonal field*. New York: Jason Aronson.

Langs, R. (1978). *The listening process*. New York: Jason Aronson.

Langs, R. (1979). *The therapeutic environment*. New York: Jason Aronson.

Langs, R. (1980). *Interactions: The realm of transference and countertransference*. New York: Jason Aronson.

Langs, R. (1981). *Resistances and interventions*. New York: Jason Aronson.

Langs, R. (1982a). *Psychotherapy: A basic text*. New York: Jason Aronson.

Langs, R. (1982b). *The psychotherapeutic conspiracy*. New York: Jason Aronson.

Loewald, H. (1970). Psychoanalytic theory and the psychoanalytic process. *Psychoanalytic Study of the Child, 25*, 45–68.

Mahler, M. S. (1952). On child psychosis and schizophrenia: Autistic and symbiotic infantile psychoses. *Psychoanalytic Study of the Child, 7*, 286–294.

Muir, R. C. (1982). The family, the group, transpersonal processes and the individual. *International Review of Psycho-Analysis, 9*, 317–326.

Ogden, T. H. (1982). *Projective identification and psychotherapeutic technique*. New York: Jason Aronson.

Räkkölainen, V., & Alanen, Y. O. (1982). On the transactionality of defensive processes. *International Review of Psycho-Analysis, 9*, 263–272.

Rosen, V. H. (1955). The reconstruction of a traumatic childhood event in a case of derealization. *Journal of the American Psychoanalytic Association, 3*, 211–221.

Rothenberg, A. (1961). Psychological problems in terminal cancer patients. *Cancer, 14*, 1063–1073.

Sandler, J. (1976). Countertransference and role-responsiveness. *International Review of Psycho-Analysis, 3*, 43–47.

Sandler, J. & Sandler, A.-M. (1978). On the development of object relationships and affects. *International Journal of Psycho-Analysis, 59*, 285–296.

Schafer, R. (1976). *A new language for psychoanalysis*. New Haven: Yale University Press.

Silverblatt, H. (1981). Denial of pregnancies extended to physicians. *Psychiatric News, 16* (22).

Vogel, E. F., & Bell, N. W. (1960). The emotionally disturbed child as the family scapegoat. In N. W. Bell & E. F. Vogel (Eds.), *A modern introduction to the family* (pp. 28–41). Glencoe: Free Press.

Wallerstein, R. S. (1967). Reconstruction and mastery in the transference psychosis. *Journal of the American Psychoanalytic Association, 15*, 556–569.

Wangh, M. (1950). Othello: The tragedy of Iago. *Psychoanalytic Quarterly, 19*, 202–212.

Wangh, M. (1962). The evocation of a proxy: A psychological manoeuvre, its use as a defense, its purpose and genesis. *Psychoanalytic Study of the Child, 17*, 463–469.

Waxenberg, S. E. (1966). The importance of the communication of feelings about cancer. *Annals of the New York Academy of Science, 25*, 1000–1005.

Weinstein, E. A. (1980). Affects and neuropsychology. *The Academy Forum, 24*, 12.

Weinstein, E. A., & Kahn, R. L. (1955). *Denial of illness*. Springfield: Charles C Thomas.

Weisman, A. D. (1972). *On dying and denying: A psychiatric study of terminality*. New York: Behavioral Publications.

Wynne, L. C. (1965). Some indications and contraindications for exploratory family therapy. In I. Boxzormenyi-Nagy & J. L. Framo (Eds.), *Intensive Family Therapy* (pp. 81–99). New York: Hoeber.

Zinner, J., & Shapiro, R. (1972). Projective identification as a mode of perception and behavior in families of adolescents. *International Journal of Psycho-Analysis, 53*, 523–531.

3

Denial, Projection, and the Empathic Wall

Donald L. Nathanson

NEUROPHYSIOLOGY

To walk in Jerusalem is to learn the essence of archaeology. Any new structure must displace not just the old, but the archaic, for there is only a finite space that can be occupied by humans. The building stones of the biblical era are the pathstones of today; shards of our shared history are venerated in shrines at our museums or hawked by vendors in the marketplace. The evolution of a culture is vertical, the new built upon the rubble of the old, which itself was built on the rubble of that which died before, its predecessor. In such a world, one searches to learn the past, to learn from the past, to retrieve or recapture from the past.

Imagine another, hypothetical city, whose people never knew the dangers of war, a city built slowly in terrain and climate that supported growth in any direction. In this favored city, the dwelling places, shops, and schools of its earliest culture are kept in good repair, inhabited by a vital population that maintains the commerce, the transportation system, the educational system, and the science of its builders as if the river of time had never passed their way and nothing need ever change (Buck, 1984; Sagan, 1980).

DONALD L. NATHANSON • The Institute of Pennsylvania Hospital and Hahnemann University, Philadelphia, Pennsylvania 19103.

In and around this culture of its past, embracing it as might an oaken forest enfold a grove of ancient cypress trees, imagine a newer city with its own homes, business establishments, colleges, modern transportation systems, and its science; a thriving metropolis entirely accepting of its past, frequenting the shops of that earlier culture, using its produce without interference in its way of life. And further, imagine yet another more modern society, delicately arranged around and above and below the others, integrated with both, learning and taking from both, but with its own more advanced form of educational system based on its own science, which has spawned its own new modes of travel and industry. The air that circulates through this city is breathed equally by all citizens; birds in flight take no notice of the structures below.

Such is the city of the human brain, built first for the reptile, whose needs were served by what we preserve as the medulla and what we call the autonomic nervous system. Layered thereon in fold after fold of tissue evolved the subcortical, then the paleocortical, and now the neocortical structures, each bringing its own systems and science, each necessitating integration with those of the earlier, still functioning mechanisms. It is important for my thesis to hover lightly over the structure of the human brain so that, when we return to our consideration of "mind," we will be working from shared information.

By now it is well known that the left half of the neocortex is associated with the linear, sequential processing that finds expression as distinguishable concepts and articulated ideas, whereas the right hemisphere is associated with syncretic conceptualization, characterized by fusion of sensory and cognitive elements into analogs. Analysis is left neocortex, insight is right brain.

It has been suggested (Galin, 1974) that primary-process thinking is right hemisphere, whereas secondary process is a function of the left hemisphere. Psychodynamic demonstrations of primary-process thinking and contemporary neurologic investigation of the right hemisphere agree in their descriptions of nonverbal, image-dependent representations that are not ordered in time or sequence, connected by nonlogical association. Left hemisphere processing seems to be dominant in the human and to exert control over the right side. In an intriguing speculation, Galin offers the example of a paradoxical interaction in which the parent tells the child, "I love you," whereas communicating a quite contradictory negative message via emotional expression as perceived in tone of voice and facial display. Because the left hemisphere favors verbal information and will tend to ignore the nonverbal, whereas the right hemisphere will preferentially decode the nonverbal gestalten, conflict between the opposing views decoded by each may be diminished by a mechanism that reduces or shuts off the right-to-left flow of information. The child's positive-valued operational view of the parent will emanate from the left brain, whereas a quite different understanding will remain in the right brain in what may be the physiological definition of repression. The appearance in dreams of such repressed material may reflect relaxation of left hemisphere censoring. Other investigators (Tucker, 1981; Tucker & Williamson, 1984) postulate a continuous dialectic between the hemisphere allowing interchange of information.

Most of our work as healers involves the facilitation of such dialectic between logical and nonlogical systems of thinking—we are laborers in the newest city of the human brain. Although this recent neuropsychological research is fascinating, it confirms rather than advances our art. It is the interpretation of the phylogenetically earlier systems with the newest that will occupy our attention in this contribution, for although "emotion" plays some role in higher cortical function, it does not originate in the neocortex.

AFFECT THEORY

Modern affect theory begins with the work of Silvan Tomkins, whose major books (*Affect/Imagery/Consciousness*, Vols. I and II) were published in 1962 and 1963. Observing the face of his newborn son, Tomkins saw what looked like "emotion" displayed on the face of an organism with none of the history, none of the life experience we have always considered necessary for the development of emotion. "Certainly the infant who emits his birth cry upon exit from the birth canal has not 'appraised' the new environment as a vale of tears before s/he cries" (Tomkins, 1987, p. 141). Nonetheless, the crying infant looks quite like a crying adult—this cry of distress must have been *available* to the infant courtesy of some preexistent mechanism triggered by some stimulus acceptable to that mechanism.

Tomkins sees nine of these mechanisms, a group of primarily facial responses that he calls *innate affects*, as operating from birth. The positive affects are *interest–excitement* and *enjoyment–joy*. *Surprise–startle* acts to reset a central assembly system and is neutral with respect to both its stimulus and whatever follows. The negative innate affects, also present from birth and visible on the face of the newborn, are *distress–anguish*, *fear–terror*, *shame–humiliation*, *anger–rage dissmell* (literally turning one's nose away from something), *disgust* (similarly, turning away from something distasteful).

Each of these innate affects has its own subcortical "address," or

location in the brain that contains the affect "program." Each is triggered by discrete activators of affect. Tomkins postulates that the affects
are triggered by the way information comes into the brain through
neural pathways—it is variation in the number of neural firings per unit
time, what he calls the "density" of neural firing, that is responsible for
affect activation. Once activated, the subcortical program then begins to
produce affect, which itself is capable of triggering more affect. It does
not matter whether the stimulus comes in on the auditory, visual, or
kinesthetic track—in this theory, the affects are essentially neutral with
respect to their activators. Thus memory can trigger affect by the way it
produces stimuli.

Tomkins postulates that a stimulus that begins at a low level and
increases gradually produces the affect *interest,* which affect at higher
levels of intensity is experienced as *excitement. Distress* is activated by
stimuli that are relatively constant but higher than an optimal level, and
anger by stimuli that are constant but at a still higher nonoptimal level.
Tomkins suggests that *enjoyment* will result when any stimulus is suddenly decreased, by which he explains phenomena as varied as our
pleasure on vacation to the release from active involvement (the affect
interest) at the punch line of a joke. In this system, *surprise* will be activated when the stimulus gradient is sudden and upward, as with a pistol
shot. Babies are thus equipped from birth with perceptual and protective systems that allow them to react to stimuli that they will not "understand" for quite some time.

Affective behavior patterns are inherited programs available to the
infant, which may be combined with each other and with the experiences
that triggered them to form complex patterns just as the letters of our
alphabet may be combined to form words and words combined to form
sentences. Thus free association can produce a memory that causes the
shock of recognition and therefore cause an affective response to the
suddenness with which various higher cortical systems presented the
association. Affect programs involve a host of bodily systems, including
of course what we have always called the "muscles of expression" in the
face, but also the endocrine and exocrine glands and nearly any group
of odors, postures, and colors. Basch (1976, 1983) has suggested that we
use the term *affect* to refer to biological events, *feeling* to our awareness of
these events, and *emotion* to the complex interrelationships formed by
the experience of an affect and our associations to it. "Emotion," he
suggests, "when developed, is evidence of neocortical activity of a highly
sophisticated sort" (1976 p. 770).

Buck (1984) suggests that the emotions evolved in three phases.
Arising first as subcortical mechanisms concerned with bodily adapta-

tion and the maintenance of homeostasis, they operated completely out of awareness (Emotion I). In the second phase, the affects became expressed in externally accessible behaviors as spontaneous expressions of internal states, perhaps useful for the coordination of behavior in a species (Emotion II). The final phase of development (Emotion III) involves the direct subjective experience of the state of certain neurochemical systems. It is this last adaptation that has allowed the linkage of the phylogenetically earlier subcortical affect mechanisms with higher cortical function to form the type of emotion with which we are most familiar in psychoanalytic thinking.

PSYCHOANALYTIC CONCEPTS

The historic focus of psychoanalysis on drives and on cognitive, intrapsychic function has tended to obscure the importance of affect expression and affective communication. Yet, as Modell (1978) has said, "assuming that psychoanalysis is a study of meaning, meaning itself is determined by the communication of affects" (p. 170).

It is in the nature of evolution that already existing systems are recruited for new functions—we should not be surprised that the affects evolved into a quite sophisticated communication system. That the affects are displayed on the signboard of the face is not limited to man, as any dog owner can testify. Our pets convey messages of the most remarkable complexity by a combination of intentional gesture and affect display. Affective communication in the human is of greater complexity still, and nowhere is this of greater importance than in the relationship between mother and infant.

Although it suited the previous generations of theorists to view the infant as entirely self-involved, it has become clear that the baby spends a considerable portion of its time observing the mother with rapt attention. As Winnicott has said, there is no such thing as a baby—mother and infant are linked in a dyadic relationship. Lichtenberg (1981) states:

> The overwhelming weight of evidence from infant research indicates that the neonate begins life in an interactive dialogue with his mother. From the beginning, for both partners, this dialogue has modes of perceptual organization that activate the responsiveness of the other. Within this dyadic communicative exchange there is no distinction between affect response and perceptual-cognitive ordering. (p. 333)

From the moment of birth, the infant is delivered into the climate of the mother's affect. Any competent theory for the development of the infantile ego must include systems for the processing of affective communication.

Anna Freud (1946) may have alluded to this when she wrote that:

> The efforts of the infantile ego to avoid "pain" by directly resisting external impressions belong to the sphere of normal psychology. Their consequences may be momentous for the formation of the ego and of character, but they are not pathogenic. When this particular ego-function is referred to in clinical analytical writings, it is never treated as the main object of observation but merely as a by-product of observations. (p. 75)

In this communication, I wish to refocus our attention on such ego functions and to demonstrate their relevance to our clinical work.

AFFECTIVE TRANSMISSION

It is beyond the scope of this chapter to discuss in detail the full range of theories for the mechanism of affective transmission. Spitz (1965) likened it to telepathy and gave it the name *coenesthetic communication*. Freud (1921) postulated that this is accomplished by a subtle mimesis, an automatic imitation of the bodily position and facial expression of the other. Ekman, Levenson, and Friesen (1983) asked subjects to follow instructions that arranged their facial features: "raise your brows and pull them together"; "now raise your upper eyelid"; "now also stretch your lips horizontally, back towards your ears." These actors reported the subjective experience of fear, confirming Freud's much earlier hypothesis. The relationship between affect display as odor to the elaboration and reception of pheromones is poorly understood but may yet have clinical significance. That affect is transmitted seems beyond question.

I have been, for some time, interested in such phenomena as infectious laughter and gloom, by the flow of intrapsychic events in members of a crowd or a mob, by my understanding of the human as herd animal rather than merely as solitary thinker. So often we are taken over by the "emotion" in our milieu. The difference between reading a play and seeing it "live" in a theater is that we are exposed to the affect display of the performers and to the way that affect is received and rebroadcast by the audience both to itself and to the performers.

This responsivity is what actors and singers mean when they talk about "good" and "bad" audiences and what athletes call the "home team advantage." Affective interplay between performer and audience is a significant factor in the performer's choice of occupation—the roar of the crowd is an affective avalanche, not cognitive confirmation of personal adequacy. Part of the release provided by public entertainment, perhaps accounting for much of its importance in our lives, derives from the phenomenology of affect transmission. Among our social conventions is permission for a degree of affective resonance at public spectacles not permitted in ordinary interpersonal interaction.

EMPATHY

The term for such an affective linkage forged during psychotherapy is *empathy*. As Basch (1983a) has so convincingly demonstrated, whereas it is affect that is transmitted in empathy, we experience this empathic perception as emotion because of our associations to the particular affect transmitted. We never really share the other person's emotion because each of us has lived too complex a life, has formed associations to these innate affects based on experiences that are different despite their general similarity. Your experience of shame is not mine; your anger is not my anger. Yet through empathy, I may clench my jaw when you feel angry and look away in embarrassment when you are shamed. Many clinicians are loathe to diagnose depression in a patient who does not make them *feel* depressed; similarly, we accept without comment that mania is infectious.

The psychoanalyst is a paradigm of the "good" audience. Indeed, for many people, therapy provides the first life experience in which they feel heard, in which they feel real. So highly do both therapists and patients value this feeling of being known on an affective level, of being in contact at the level of the subcortical message centers, that a significant underlying truth has been obscured: We consider the absence of emapthy normal and the presence of it special. The most mature among us do not live in a world of unintentionally shared emotion. Maturity implies a certain degree of isolation from the emotions of others.

THE EMPATHIC WALL

It may be more central to our work to consider, rather than how the message of happiness, grief, resentment, anger, or distress is *transmitted,* how such transmission is *blocked.* How is it that we are not more often taken over by affect so broadcast? When infectious disease was the frontier of science, such transmission was called "contagion of affect." (Scheler, 1912; Sullivan, 1954) One has only to watch dispassionately the flow of laughter through an audience or the flow of anger through a mob to

wonder how does the normal human develop immunity to this contagion; how do we learn to remain self in the presence of the affect of
the other?

These and many other questions may be answered by the recognition of an ego mechanism to which I have given the intentionally paradoxical name *the empathic wall*. The empathic wall allows us to monitor
our affective experience and determine whether the affect of the moment is generated from within or without, thus defining the difference
between self and other—yet it must act like a gate to allow the child to
feel the love of the mother. It may be the root mechanism for a host of
normal and pathological defensive operations of the ego.

Rather than consider all experience of affective transmission to be
synomymous with empathy, I would agree with Basch (1983a) that *mature* empathy involves the intentional acceptance of such transmission. It
is my feeling that mature empathy can occur only in a person with a
healthy empathic wall mechanism, who is capable additionally of relax-
ing this ego function, opening an empathic gate in order to merge briefly with the affective broadcast of the other. In our analytic work, this
lapse into primary process, which is analogous to other examples of the
creative process, is followed by a return to secondary process accompanied by data about the other learned during the empathic link. In the
remainder of this chapter I will focus on the development of the empathic wall and its relationship to denial, projection, and the phenomenology of certain psychopathological conditions.

INFANT RESEARCH

That infants reward the smile of the mother with a smile of their
own is an indication of the relationship between mimesis and affective
transmission. Emde, Gaensbauer, and Harmon (1976) have written extensively about affect mutualization between mother and infant. The
infant's smile makes the mother feel good, which sense of pleasure may
be communicated to the child; conversely, the infant's cry of distress
activates distress in the mother. Demos (1982) describes the infant as
scanning its environment with interest, accepting it as a provider of
stimulation: "When this stimulation begins to produce distress, he attempts to decrease the level of stimulation by turning away from the
object" (p. 565). One form of stimulation is, of course, the affect available in his environment; I believe that such activity of turning away
represents the early beginnings of the empathic wall.

Beebe and Sloate (1982) describe the attempts of an infant to handle the affective onslaught of a psychotic, intrusive mother. By 3 to 4 months, the child had lost her fascination for mother's face and demonstrated extensive gaze aversion:

> It can be hypothesized that the pattern of extensive looking away was already being used by this infant to help modulate inappropriate stimulation that was experienced as aversive. [p. 606] [at 8 months] she tuned out and withdrew from mother's attempts to engage her in play, turning her back, looking out the window, behaving as if she did not hear her mother. (p. 616)

Adequate data are given in this case material to allow the conclusion that the infant was avoiding mother's affect, using what I believe to be the blocking function of the empathic wall mechanism. Beebe and Sloate explain this by reference to Rubenfine's (1962) comments "on the child's use of denial to conserve the object relation in situations where the mother has taken on the properties of an aversive stimulus" (p. 616).

Selma Kramer (personal communication, 1983) has suggested that, in the normal child, the appearance of stranger anxiety marks achievement of an ego mechanism that can allow him or her to recognize the difference between the affective transmission of mother and of anybody else. Awareness of the difference between such transmission sets may be one way the infant learns to recognize individuals; more important for our purposes here, it certainly may provide the anlage for recognizing the difference between self and other on the affective level. Emde *et al.* (1976) note that, by this time, the:

> Transactions between mother and infant have differentiated to the point where both are "tuned in" to a mutually specific attachment. As a stranger approaches [the infant] looks with an expression of interest which then becomes one of sober perplexity. This is followed by what is rated as a fearful expression, with frowning and then crying . . . accompanied by gaze aversion and a turning away of the head and body. (p. 145)

DENIAL AND PROJECTION

I have always been bothered by the fact that denial and projection are discussed as intrinsically pathological defense mechanisms and that they are supposed to arise *de novo* in the growing child. It does not seem logical to postulate that the organism is born with systems that are intrinsically pathological; everything that appears during development must have a demonstrable substratum.

More likely, both denial and projection involve application of skills learned in the formation and operation of the empathic wall mechanism.

The child has learned to evaluate intense experiences of affect by checking to see whether a feeling has arisen from within self or from other. In the face of intense, perhaps unacceptable affect broadcast by mother, the empathic wall allows the child to succeed in the struggle to maintain affectional ties while *separating from the feeling*. Proper use of the empathic wall allows the child to remain self while leaving broadcast feelings outside the self. The case of Beebe and Sloate (1982) cited above represents an extreme example of the affect blocking provided by the empathic wall mechanism, one in which the child was forced to keep closed the gate that might normally have allowed the affect of the mother to become that of the child.

Here then is a mechanism that allows the individual to sample his or her own affective state and determine its source, a mechanism valuable for an organism whose perceptual and communicative apparatuses are not developed adequately to allow symbolic communication. If such a mechanism can allow the child to wall off external affect, to decide that a certain affective state comes from outside the self and rightly should remain outside the self, then that mechanism is capable of being recruited for further use when unpleasant affect derives from *inner* conflict. The child can wall off the feeling, even to the extent that the feeling is viewed as an intrusion from the outside, the result of affective transmission. Denial utilizes the affect-blocking portion of the empathic wall, whereas projection makes use of its ability to perform a "vector analysis"—to determine from which direction a particular affect originated. When the gate has allowed in too much maternal affect, thus producing a noxious internal as well as external environment, the child strengthens the empathic wall and develops denial and projection to explain away that moiety of maternal affect that slips through. If we can understand Kohut's (1971) concept of *mirroring* as the process by which infant and mother reflect each other's facial (and bodily) expressions of innate affect, then the empathic wall may be defined as the mechanism of *not-mirroring*.

Useful as this mechanism may seem in allowing the individual to disavow some portion of the meaning of an event or a percept in order to reduce the associated painful affect (Weisman & Hackett, 1961), it alters rather than solves the problem. As Waelder (1951) said, even if projection shifts the focus from self to other, "the denied instinct remains in the limelight; he who projected his aggressiveness onto others has his mind occupied with aggressiveness, albeit somebody else's" (p. 224). The noxious affect is still being experienced, but it is attributed to the other.

INTERPERSONAL ASPECTS OF DENIAL

An often ignored yet supremely important matter is the interpersonal aspect of denial, what denial does in a relationship, what it does to a relationship. We take it for granted that in a good, healthy object relationship the participants share reality. But as Dorpat (1983) has said so well,

> The dynamic defensive function of denial is carried out by the active exclusion of information from focal attention, i.e., explicit conscious awareness. (p. 48)

What if, through denial, one member of a dyad acts as if some piece of information, taken for granted by the other, and the competent subject of focal attention by that other, does not exist?

Our observation is that each belief system produces its own characteristic affective display—that is, we wear on our faces the feeling state or mood that derives from the sum of our knowledge, whether conscious, preconscious, or unconscious. When the intimate other senses, by affective transmission, the disparity between the two belief systems, anxiety is produced. This anxiety causes interpersonal tension that must be resolved if the relationship is to endure at the previous level of intimacy. Each relationship has a characteristic mode of tension resolution, ranging from friendly inquiry to open hostility and fighting. Denial seems to work better in the privacy of one's defenses. Thus denial in the subject causes anxiety in the object, verifying again Waelder's (1951) observation that, at least in a relationship, there may be no such thing as "successful" denial.

PROJECTIVE IDENTIFICATION

Kernberg (1967) comes close to my understanding of the empathic wall mechanism in his discussion of projective identification, where he states that the patient's aggression, although projected onto the object, remains active:

> This leads such patients to feel that they can still identify themselves with the object onto whom aggression has been projected, and their ongoing "empathy" with the now threatening object maintains and increases the fear of their own projected aggression . . . . In summary, projective identification is characterized by the lack of differentiation between self and object in that particular area, by continuing to experience the *impulse* [italics mine] as well as the

fear of that impulse while the projection is active, and by the need to control the external object. (p. 669)

But it is affects, not impulses that are experienced during the period of resonance with the other person. Further, in the language developed here, it is through a defensive misuse of the empathic wall mechanism that one has attributed an affect to the object and decided that one is experiencing this noxious affect by affective transmission from the object. What Kernberg calls *empathy*, I see as *affective transmission*, which by its nature is a transient or reactive state; identification, which implies a move toward likeness to another person including the adoption of interests, ideals, or mannerisms of the other, is therefore a much more lasting phenomenon. It would appear, in view of our current understanding of affect, that the term *projective identification* is a misnomer at many levels.

Pulver's (1971, 1974) helpful observation that affect can be *unconscious* and that at other times it may be *potential* bears mention here. Unconscious affect, existing "in an activated or aroused state out of awareness" (1974, p. 78), would fit Buck's (1984) criteria for Emotion I—affect as a homeostatic mechanism remaining out of awareness—or those of Tomkins (1962, 1963) for affect that achieved its aim without emerging into consciousness. That affect can be potential is another matter. It is clear from this work of Tomkins (1983a,b) and of Basch (1976) cited earlier that affect is either triggered or not triggered; what is repressed is not affect but the conflict that acts as its activator. Thus, it is not repressed affect that is uncovered in analysis but repressed activators of affect, explaining perhaps why the affect associated with newly uncovered material always seems so "fresh." If inner conflict can be repressed, or perception of it denied, the affect becomes potential, achieving the status of a land mine from a forgotten war—of potential danger at all times but truly dangerous only when encountered.

CLINICAL ILLUSTRATIONS

Case 1

Perhaps a few clinical examples may demonstrate the usefulness of the empathic wall concept. Karen, a 24-year-old graduate student, entered therapy in an attempt to interrupt a recurring cycle of unhappy romantic liasons. Men flocked around her in bars and at parties; she was courted impulsively by suitors who responded to her with a degree of sexual intimacy and openness one might expect in a more developed relationship. She remarked, "They seem to be turned on, ready for sex when I am just getting to know them. The first couple of guys who said 'Come on, I know you want it too' made me furious. But enough men have said something like that, and I thought I should bring it up here."

What excited those men? Karen noted with some interest that, although in intercourse she experienced a considerable degree of vaginal anesthesia and that she did not look forward to intercourse, she was aware of nearly constant vaginal wetness unassociated with conscious sexual ideation. That she had disavowed sexual excitement as a compromise settlement of Oedipal conflicts became apparent to her much later; what helped her at this stage in treatment was the recognition that men were sexually aroused by her denied arousal. Knowing that her body was responding to unconscious forces with which she was not yet ready to deal, she was better able to integrate relationships with men now that she understood that portion of their behavior deriving from her denied arousal. Late in her fourth year of therapy, she was well on her way towards healthy object relatedness, beginning to be involved in genital sexuality with a loved and loving partner. She commented that occasionally, during sexual excitement, she was seized with the awareness that her face felt "strangely familiar" to her, that her facial expression was reminiscent of the facial set which, before therapy, she had displayed nearly constantly.

Sullivan (1954) commented that lust begins to drive the organism in early adolescence. It is during this period of development that sexual ideation becomes connected to excitement. Parents of adolescents know this best, for children previously unsuspected of sexual ideation "suddenly" are seen as being "sexy." "Sexiness" is an affective broadcast. I have confirmed this observation in clinical practice on countless occasions—men and women who are read by others as sexually exciting are themselves, at that moment, involved in their own sexual excitement. This is normal affective transmission, handled as Anna Freud said (in the passage quoted above) by the ego functions that monitor external impressions.

Such a hysteric is decidedly uncomfortable with the Oedipal ideation that has produced her sexual excitement and has used the affect blocking portion of the empathic wall mechanism to keep this complex of affects out of awareness. The fact that she is condemned by this defensive decision to be the object of sexual pursuit confirms Waelder's observation that denial is not freedom.

Finally, this case illustrated the relationship between denial, projection, and the empathic wall, for Karen's denial of sexual feeling does not eradicate her own genital excitement, which is still being triggered, but now by forces which have become unconscious. In this particular coassembly of lust and excitement, the resulting drive-affect complex remains in the interpersonal field, while neither party is certain of its origin. Both the hysteric and the paranoid see the disavowed, unacceptable affect as emanating from the object. The difference lies in the competence of the vector-analyzing portion of the empathic wall mechanism. The hysteric has blocked the feeling and remains relatively free of it—the sexual affect and ideation is attributed to the object through a defensive misuse of the empathic wall. The paranoid, whose empathic wall is weaker than the hysteric, continues to experience the affect but blames the object for "influenc-ing" him.

CASE 2

Any ego function can be eroded in the schizophrenic process—indeed, study of the schizophrenias has taught us much about the range of normal ego functions. If a breach in the empathic wall has been forced by illness, the patient may complain that the feelings of others are being experienced as an unwelcome intrusion. Wurmser (1981) reports the statement of Blanche, three years before an overt schizophrenic psychosis, trying to defend against terrible discomfort in the presence of others: "I try consciously to get to know them, but it's as if I lack empathy" (p. 140). Later, during the worst of her illness, she reported, "I'm so dependent on what other people think. I wanted to get away from people—to be myself, to feel my own feelings. Why do other people affect me that much?" (p. 140). This failure to block braodcast affect may be also interpreted by the patient as fantasies of telepathic power or delusions that one is the subject of messages broadcast from another's space ("outer space").

Failure of the empathic wall ego mechanism is seen in "psychotic insight," which involves involuntary empathic acceptance of affective and gestural com-munication otherwise denied by the sender. Such insight is considered psychotic because the patient either is unable to use the empathic wall to return to self or cannot use other ego mechanisms to integrate this new information about the other for the purposes of normal interpersonal relatedness.

CASE 3

Another patient, Jocelyn, complained bitterly that, when in the company of others, she was unable to maintain her own emotions. If a friend seemed upset about something Jocelyn had said, she too would begin to feel upset; if a com-panion were to be gleeful, she would feel inappropriately gleeful, then confused and angry as she felt a loss of her own identity. The experience of affective resonance was quite unpleasant for her. Concomitantly she was restricted to an extraordinary degree in the display of her own emotions. I will take up two facets of her relationship with her mother in an attempt to explain the develop-ment of what she regarded as her most uncomfortable symptoms.

Jocelyn avoids contact with her mother, whom she describes as an affective steamroller whose rages and sulks dominated the family. The family dog was severely beaten whenever it soiled a floor or rug, despite the fact that no attempt at house training was ever made. The patient was often awakened to hear her mother screaming at her father. In dreams, this mother is usually represented as a dark figure, frequently a witch, always an object of terror. Such a parent provides an environment overloaded with unmodulated affect, depriving the growing child of the opportunity to develop an adequate empathic wall, render-ing the child succeptible to external impression.

By age 11, Jocelyn had discovered lying, which gave her some sense of distance from her mother. Later she learned to control her own affective output around her mother, developing first a sort of facial flatness and then a number of elaborately conceived and practiced pseudoemotional behavioral entities that we came to call "affective modules." The face is the major display board of the affect system—by maintaining (initially consciously, later unconsciously) her facial musculature in a masklike state, she reduced the affective resonance which so upset her. This served another function, for as she described interactions with her mother, "Unless I am in complete control of my emotions when I am around her, she takes over my emotion. I can't be in a bad mood, or she will not only be in a bad mood, but it will be her bad mood, and she will tell me what I should do. After I am around her for a little while when one of these things is happening, I feel crazy because I can't even remember why I was in a bad mood to begin with, let alone what I was really feeling." I suspect that this mother's problems with affect modulation bear some relationship to a defect in her own empathic wall mechanism.

In treatment, Jocelyn gave up the defensive flatness only when she had thoroughly and repeatedly tested my ability to maintain a calm, warm manner despite her attempts within the transference to see me as volatile. A breakthrough of enormous importance came in the third year of therapy when she decided to stand before a mirror experimenting with facial expression. As she mimicked the expressions of anger, distress, shame, joy, surprise, and disgust, she felt herself flooded with feeling that she could now control by turning off the expression. Through a year-long series of exercises she worked through a wide range of affects, building her ability to tolerate emotion. Growth in therapy has strengthened her ability to handle her own affect as well as that broadcast by others. Now, in her fifth year of intensive psychodynamic psychotherapy, she has begun to develop a good sense of self and a healthy need for privacy appropriately bounded by shame.

SUBSTANCE ABUSE AND DISTURBANCES OF THE EMPATHIC WALL

Wurmser (1974, 1978, 1981, 1982) and Krystal (1982) have written much about the early affective environment of the person who will go on to be an abuser of mood-altering substances. Cases like that of Jocelyn make us wonder what becomes of the empathic wall in children raised in a climate of unmodulated parental affect. Although one must postulate constitutional factors that affect ego development, it is likely that, in other families, this wall mechanism can become so overdeveloped that one lives encapsulated from external affect and poorly able to handle one's own. I suspect that such a defensive constellation punishes in later life as much as it protects in childhood. Drugs that are reported to enhance the experience of "feeling," like marijuana, cocaine, and the amphetamines, may work by decreasing the noxious effects of an inappropriately strong empathic wall as well as by interference with the individual's habitual pattern of affect modulation. Other children may grow up with truly inadequate empathic wall mechanisms, more a freeswinging gate than a wall, rendering them oversensitive to the affect around them, and likely to use tranquillizers, barbiturates, and alcohol to dull their senses. In them, "drug use . . . is a pharmacologically induced denial of affect" (Wurmser & Zients, 1982, p. 539).

INTEGRATION WITH OTHER THEORIES

In his microanalysis of the mechanism of denial, Dorpat (1983) has determined the following "four phases of denial reaction: 1) preconscious appraisal of danger or trauma. 2) painful affect. 3) cognitive arrest. and 4) screen behavior" (p. 47). He explains that "cognitive arrest is brought about by unconscious fantasies of destroying or rejecting whatever he considers to be the cause of his psychic pain (or what I have termed the 'painful object')" (p. 47). I believe that it is the normal function of the empathic wall to sense that the pain one is experiencing derives from the object by affective transmission. Dorpat has come quite close to my concept in his suggestion that an affective state deriving from inner conflict has, through denial, been attributed to pain caused by another.

Basch (1982) points out the term *verleugnung* is properly translated as *disavowal,* rather than *denial,* for disavowal implies the vernacular use more central to Freud's meaning—the unconscious version of the self-serving socially acceptable evasions of everyday life, in which there is no hint of psychotic distortion of thought process. He shows that Freud meant to designate disavowal "as the mechanism which defends against traumatic external reality, whereas repression deals with unacceptable instinctual demands" (p. 135). It is his belief that, despite our general assumption that the work of Anna Freud is to be treated as if it were a continuation of that of Freud himself, she deviated from Freud's thinking in assuming:

> . . . that there is a continuum between the use of fantasy by children and the reality-distorting thought disorders of adult psychotics. In doing so she neglects to take into account the continued use of fantasy for all sorts of reasons by many adults functioning on a nonpsychotic level. (p. 138)

"Disavowal," he continues, "prevents the union of affect with percept, without, however, blocking the percept from consciousness" (p. 147).

Finally, Basch states that:

> Conceptual clarity would be served if the term "denial" was used as a collective term for those psychotic or nonpsychotic mechanisms that actually interfere with the perceptual interpretation of sensory signals, while following Freud, using the term "disavowal" only to describe that situation in which the affectively toned meaning that a percept would be expected to have for the self is unconsciously repudiated. (p. 146)

Both senses of verleugnung fit well with the concept that they are preceded by skills learned in the use of the empathic wall and its accompanying gate mechanism. The empathic wall, or gate, conforms to Basch's requirement for a mechanism that "interferes with the perceptual interpretation of sensory signals" as long as one understands that affective resonance is a sensory analog.

The relationship between affective transmission and the repudiation of the "affectively toned meaning of a percept" requires further discussion. Just as affect display can be mimicked (as it is normally in affective resonance and intentionally in the experiment of Ekman *et al.* (1983, cited above), it can be mimed for the purpose of conveying a false communication. The "confidence man," the salesman, and the seducer pull us into a trusting relationship by their use of the verbal tone and facial affect display of affection and caring. The mature person ignores these messages in order to focus better on the verbal, symbolic content of the communication. It is the ability to resist affective transmission that protects us from such sales techniques. Philosopher Alan Watts (personal communication) called this "ig nor' ance," the healthy ability to ignore. Disavowal of an affective percept is initially the function of the empathic wall.

In 1924, the Greco-Russian mystic Gurdjieff addressed the question of the proper attitude with which to begin the study of the self:

> As to self-observation—it is not so simple a thing as it may seem at first sight. Therefore, the teaching puts as the foundation stone the principles of right self-observation. But before passing to the study of these principles, a man must make the decision that he will be absolutely sincere with himself, will not close his eyes to anything, will not turn aside from any results, wherever they may lead him, will not fear any deductions, will not limit himself to any previously erected walls. For a man unaccustomed to thinking in this direction, very much courage is required to accept sincerely the results and conclusions arrived at. (1973, p. 72)

Gurdjieff asks us to live without denial, without isolation, without repression; to live with the soul naked to the light of truth. Yet, as the head turns and the eye blinks to shield the retina from intense light, so the growing ego is protected by a host of mechanisms from overly intense affect. It does indeed take courage and maturity to give up any defense, to stare bravely into the light. The mental mechanisms are not some sort of refuge for the weak. They are a group of protections built into the organism itself, protective systems inherent to the nature of human beings, defenses accumulated through the ages of evolution, recruited even today in the life of an organism struggling for survival.

ACKNOWLEDGMENT

I am deeply indepted to Dr. Léon Wurmser for his constant support and encouragement and for the many theoretical discussions which allowed clarification of my ideas.

REFERENCES

Basch, M. F. (1976). The concept of affect: A re-examination. *Journal of the American Psychoanalytic Association, 24,* 759–777.

Basch, M. F. (1982). The perception of reality and the disavowal of meaning. In *The Annal of Psychoanalysis,* XI (pp. 125–163). New York: International Universities Press.

Basch, M. F. (1983a). Empathic understanding: Review of the concept and some theoretical considerations. *Journal of the American Psychoanalytic Association, 31,* 101–126.

Basch, M. F. (1983b). The concept of "self": An operational definition. In B. Lee & G. Noam (Eds.), *Developmental approaches to the self* (pp. 7–58). New York: Plenum Press.

Beebe, B., & Sloate, P. (1982). Assessment and treatment of difficulties in mother-infant attunement in the first 3 years of life: A case history. *Psychoanalytic Inquiry, 2*(4), 601–623.

Buck, R. (1984). *The communication of emotion.* New York: Guilford.

Demos, E. V. (1982). Affect in early infancy: Physiology or psychology? *Psychoanalytic Inquiry, 3*(4), 533–574.

Dorpat, T. J. (1983). The cognitive arrest hypothesis of denial. *International Journal of Psychoanalysis, 64,* 47.

Ekman, P., Levenson, R. W., & Friesen, W. V. (1983). Autonomic nervous system activity distinguishes among emotions. *Science, 221*(4616), 1208–1210.

Emde, R. N., Gaensbauer, T. J., & Harmon, R. J. (1976). *Emotional expression in infancy: A biobehavioral study* (Psychological Issues, Monograph 37). New York: International Universities Press.

Freud, A. (1946). *The ego and the mechanisms of defense.* New York: International Universities Press.

Freud, S. (1921). Group psychology and the analysis of the ego. In *Standard edition, 18.* London: Hogarth Press.

Galin, D. (1974). Implications for psychiatry of left and right cerebral specialization: A neurophysiological context for unconscious process. *Archives of General Psychiatry, 31,* 572.

Gurdjieff, G. I. (1973). *Views from the real world.* New York: E. P. Dutton.

Kernberg, O. (1967). Borderline personality organization. *Journal of the American Psychoanalytic Association, 15*(3), 641–685.

Kohut, H. (1971). *The analysis of the self.* New York: International University Press.

Krystal, H. (1982). Adolescence and the tendency to develop substance abuse. *Psychoanalytic Inquiry, 2*(4), 481–517.

Lichtenberg, J. (1981). The empathic mode of perception and alternative vantage points for psychoanalytic work. *Psychoanalytic Inquiry, 1*(3), 329–356.

Modell, A. (1978). Affects and the complementarity of biologic and historical meaning. *The annual of psychoanalysis, VI,* 167–180.

Pulver, S. (1971). Can affects be unconscious? *International Journal of Psychoanalysis, 52*(4), 347–354.

Pulver, S. (1974). Unconscious versus potential affects. *The Psychoanalytic Quarterly, XLIII*(1), 77–84.

Rubenfine, D. (1962). Maternal stimulation, psychic structure, and early object relations. *Psychoanalytic Study of the Child, 17,* 265–282.

Sagan, C. (1980). *Cosmos.* New York: Random House.

Scheler, M. (1970). *The nature of sympathy.* Hamden, CT: Archon Books, The Shoe String Press, Inc.

Spitz, R. A. (1965). *The first year of life.* New York: International Universities Press.

Sullivan, H. S. (1954). *The psychiatric interview.* New York: W. W. Norton.

Tomkins, S. S. (1962). *Affect/imagery/consciousness. Volume I: The positive affects.* New York: Springer Publishing Company.

Tomkins, S. S. (1963). *Affect/imagery/consciousness. Volume II: The negative affects.* New York: Springer Publishing Company.

Tomkins, S. S. (1987). Shame. In D. L. Nathanson (Ed.), *The many faces of shame.* New York: Guilford.

Tucker, D. M. (1981). Lateral brain function, emotion, and conceptualization. *Psychological Bulletin, 89,* 19–46.

Tucker, D. M., & Williamson, P. (1984). Assymetrical neural control systems in human self-regulation. *Psychological Review, 91,* 137–152.

Waelder, R. (1951). The structure of paranoid ideas. *International Journal of Psychoanalysis, 32,* 167–177. (Reprinted in *Psychoanalysis: Observation, theory, application. Selected papers of Robert Waelder,* S. A. Guttman (Ed.). New York: International Universities Press, 1976.)

Weisman, A., & Hackett, T. (1961). Predilection to death: Death and dying as a psychiatric problem. *Psychosomatic Medicine, 23,* 232–256.

Wurmser, L. (1974). Psychoanalytic considerations of the etiology of compulsive drug use. *Journal of the American Psychoanalytic Association, 22,* 820–843.

Wurmer, S. (1978). *The hidden dimension.* New York: Aronson.

Wurmser, L. (1981). *The mask of shame.* Baltimore: Johns Hopkins University Press.

Wurmser, L. (1982). The question of specific psychopathology in compulsive drug use. *Annals of the New York Academy of Sciences, 398,* 33–43.

Wurmser, L., & Zients, A. (1982). The return of the denied superego. *Psychoanalytic Inquiry, 2*(4), 539–580.

II

Basic and Applied Notions

The neurological condition called *anosognosia* might remain just another member of the group of curiosities produced by certain discrete brain lesions were it not for its peculiar resemblance to the matter under study herein. In a succinct, matter-of-fact chapter, Shalev describes patients who, as the result of injuries in the inferior parietal lobe of the nondominant hemisphere, demonstrate disorders of the body scheme. When pressed to stare at the paralyzed limb they seem to ignore, some patients will not only deny their "ownership" of that limb but disavow any understanding of how it came to be in their bed. Central to the dialectic of psychoanalytic inquiry is a belief that all people share pretty much the same "equipment" and that all psychopathology can be explained on the basis of varying combinations of such things as drives, defenses, life experiences as integrated into the individual ego, and the societal pressures affecting personality development; this despite Freud's constantly reiterated belief that much we currently hold to be due to intrapsychic phenomena will eventually be traced to the workings of actual biological mechanisms. It is unlikely that the episodes of denial encountered by the psychoanalytic therapist are caused by the discrete lesions that occupy the attention of Shalev, yet it is important that we recognize that a psychological entity may be a manifestation of neurostructural change. In computer language, Shalev describes deficits in function stemming from "hardware" error, whereas the forms of denial or disavowal we study may be understood as "software" problems. An alternative view, not discussed here, might raise the possibility that there is a "denial circuit" that can be accessed by the organism in the manner of a built-in defense. Surely such matters represent the future of psychoanalytic research.

The patient with anosognosia who denies that anything exists to one side of the midline has a world view created (or significantly influenced) by neurological deficit. Sacerdoti and Semi discuss the implications of psychological denial in the formation of the *Weltanschauung* of physically healthy individuals. Whatever we disavow becomes the negative portion of our reality, the unseen that defines the perceived. The authors amplify Freud's belief that adolescence is marked by a shift from a predominantly religious weltanschauung (information accepted on faith) to a scientific world view in which information is accepted only after experiment, study, and personal confirmation. The adolescent is forever being warned that those who do not learn about history are doomed to repeat it, despite the urgent need for such scientific inquiry. Central to this chapter is the authors' injunction to the psychoanalyst: Learn the world of the patient before you presume to alter it—what is denied must first be respected.

The approach taken by Chayes pivots around his trenchant observation that "it would seem as if we are seduced by our own terminology into seeing artificial discontinuities between phenomena which in fact are continuous." Pointing to work by Cohen and Kinston (1984) on the relationship between "primal repression" and repression proper, Chayes suggests the possibility that every defensive operation of the ego starts with denial. Citing work by Le Coultre (1966), he demonstrates that denial may allow the splitting-off of a piece of the infantile ego, which may maintain an independent existence (as seen particularly well in the transference). One is struck by the similarity between this work of Le Coultre, as interpreted by Chayes, and the three "ego states" described by Berne (1964) as "parent," "adult," and "child," and popularized as "transactional analysis." Taking up a theme to be expressed throughout this volume, Chayes emphasizes that denial need not be pathological, for there are many times in the life of an individual when denial allows one to avoid matters that cannot be faced, in order to do what is needed to facilitate the inner growth that will eventually allow the successful handling of what had initially been disavowed. He finds that proper resolution of the conflicts surrounding the separation/individuation phase of development requires such a use of denial. Implicit in this chapter is the view that the mental mechanisms are best understood in the context of developmental theory.

Jappe moves the reader swiftly into the theme of her chapter by describing her own personal experience as a member of the polyglot group of international scholars. Shifting between languages is an experience of "leaping boundaries, of a sense of omnipotence in mastering things but also of the need to forget the pain and bewilderment one felt on perceiving that a word can be so far separated from its meaning that it can be replaced by another and that in the use of a substitute much of the original is surrendered." If the very word *language* derives from the Latin root *lingua,* or tongue, and if we recognize that the language of one's homeland is called the "mother tongue," then the ability to learn many languages (a desirable trait in a European scholar) is in itself a way of becoming split off from the other. Jappe uses case material to develop her premise that empty words, stuffy phrases that convey far less than they promise, are a form of denial, a manifestation of a particular form of relationship to the father. Meaning can be lost when one moves with apparent facility between languages, just as it can be lost when denial strips words of their meaning both in the inner world of the unconscious and in the interpersonal life of the individual. She sees denial as the mechanism central to our attempt to avoid certain perceptions of father; following such defensive operations in childhood, future operations of denial may be tinged with such a relationship to the father.

On the basis of rigorous, carefully replicated research, Shanan demonstrates that the mechanism of denial is neutral with respect to our system of values; he focuses our attention on "what *in* reality has to be denied, and under what conditions." He shows that "denial is a necessary component . . . of adjustment to change," a mechanism that allows change to occur in situations where the inability to disavow the current meaning of a perception might prevent such healthy growth. Rather than accept the idea that aging diminishes the amount of energy available to the individual, Shanan demonstrates that early life is characterized by the accumulation of attachments (with the consequent sequestration of psychic energy into object relatedness), whereas later life is characterized by the work of detachment. Denial assists the redeployment of psychic energy, the adaptation to change. He states that "during the later years and in old age we find a tendency to get engaged in intellectual and transpersonal religious interests in addition to certain (not necessarily pathological) manifestations of living in fantasy." The healthy individual, moving along the axis of time, shifts from intense attachment to a few specific individuals toward a network from which she or he can never be separated. Shanan believes that such conservation of psychic energy can only be accomplished when the healthy use of denial is accompanied by other, mature coping mechanisms. The reader may find refreshing the author's tendency to support his conclusions from large, well-replicated studies, rather than individual case material.

These five chapters may be linked with the three chapters of the next section, on denial as seen in child development, to form thereby a bridge from the purely theoretical matters taken up in the first section, to the essentially clinical focus of the remainder of this volume.

REFERENCES

Berne, E. (1964). *Games people play*. New York: Grove Press.

Cohen, J., & Kinston, W. (1984). Repression theory: A new look at the cornerstone. *International Journal of Psychoanalysis, 65,* 411–422.

Le Coultre, R. (1966). Splijting van het Ik als Centraal Neuroseverschijnsel (Reprinted in *Psychoanalytische Thema's en Varietes*. Deventer: van Loghum Slaterus, 1972).

4

Denial and *Weltanschauung*

Giorgio Sacerdoti and Antonio A. Semi

The problem of a psychoanalytic *Weltanschauung* was faced by Freud, as is well known, in *Die Zukunft einer Illusion* (1927b) where, more than elsewhere, the "vision of reality" corresponds to a conception that is both positive and problematic. More controversially, in *Hemmung, Symptom und Angst,* Freud declared *"Ich bin überhaupt nicht für die Fabrikation von Weltanschauungen"* and, in the *XXXV Vorlesung* (Freud, 1932), he reaffirms that the only psychoanalytic *Weltanschauung* is that of science. However, in all the papers cited, it is stressed that the affects on the basis of religious *Weltanschauung* cannot be disdainfully put aside and that their value for human life must not be underestimated.

Our study started on this polarity between scientific *Weltanschauung* (in Freud's sense) and nonscientific *Weltanschauungen*—ultimately religious, at least in the broad sense. Nevertheless, we were compelled to restrict our investigation to a particular area of psychic life, which seemed to be that which we could approximately call the domain of denial. Within it, the opportunity of distinguishing—as exactly as possible—between what Freud calls *Verneinung* and *Verleugnung*, respectively, becomes imperative.

Those of Freud's writings that are most useful in studying the difference between *Verneinung* and *Verleugnung* are *Die Verneinung* (1925a), *Abriss der Psychoanalyse* (1938), and *Fetischismus* (1927a).

Giorgio Sacerdoti and Antonio A. Semi • Private Practice, Rio de la Crose 149, Giudecca, Venice, Italy.

Negation—for clarity—we shall, from now on, use the German word *Verneinung* as originally intended by Freud—it is described as the modality of thought that allows a repressed representation to be admitted into consciousness in a disguised form. More precisely, *Verneinung* is that form of the analysand's speech that signals to the analyst a repeal of the mechanism of repression. As a consequence of this repeal, a representation can reach the individual's intellectual awareness without being fully accepted (*aber freilich keine Annahme des Verdrängten*) by one who does not feel it as something that is actually his own and affectively meaningful.

Our ability to mobilize the defense of *Verneinung* is central to the possibility of formulating a judgment (*Urteil*) and, second, to the possibility of reality testing (*Realitäts-prüfung*). This latter is necessary not only for a correct perception of the external but also of the internal reality, of the person's psychic reality. Through the *Verneinung*, which operates at the preconscious–conscious level, the person's intellectual life may be enriched by materials indispensable for its functioning.

On the other hand, *Verleugnung* refers to an unconscious defense mechanism of the ego whose purpose seems to be first of all the disavowal of external reality. One example of this process may be seen in the analysis of the fetishistic situation conducted by Freud himself (1927a).

In his paper on fetishism, Freud, with a distinction that we believe still valid, stressed the difference between his own concept of the phenomena and that illustrated by Laforgue (1926). Freud reaffirms that *Verleugnuung* is the word that, in German, appears the most suitable in describing the method by which the fetishist handles the representation of the female genitals.

" 'Scotomization'," writes Freud, "seems to me particularly unsuitable, for it suggests that the perception is entirely wiped out, so that the result is the same as when a visual impression falls on the blind spot in the retina" (Freud, 1927a, pp. 153–164).

This apparently punctilious precision has the purpose of avoiding the mistake of considering the expression "*Verleugnung* disavows external reality" an exhaustive description of the phenomena, whereas it is, in fact, only an ellipsis.

It is therefore worth repeating that *Verleugnung*, to the extent to which it is an unconscious mechanism, addresses representations of external reality that are already present in the ego. The disavowal of external reality is a secondary effect; it comes about only because the representation in the system Pcs-Cs has become unavailable. Therefore those mental operations that are necessary for reality-testing are no longer possible.

In this sense, one can say that *Verleugnung* prevents *Verneinung*. In the typical example, if the representation of "female genitals" is disavowed, it is not possible for the person to say, "It is not true that females have a penis." It is therefore impossible for him or her to examine the latter proposition and acknowledge, through the reality test, that it is indeed "true" for him or her in the sense of being emotionally motivated but false in external reality, that is, unrecognizable in it. The need of the ego to apply the reality test in these cases sometimes produces devastating effects. The *Realitätsprüfung* is applied to the substitute representations, for instance to the fetish, and not to the original representations. This leads to a progressive distortion of both the internal world and the representations of the external world. Freud's paper on fetishism constitutes a sort of shibboleth between his own thoughts and those of Melanie Klein. With Klein, one sees a progressive generalization of the concept of *Verleugnung* and exactly in the sense that Freud attributes to Laforgue. It is not coincidential that Klein (1937) in her paper "*Psychogenese der manisch-depressiven Zustände*" explicitly refers to "scotomization" and, in order to avoid a direct confrontation with Freud, refers her critics to a paper by Helene Deutsch (1933), which confirms the substance of Freud's thought as expressed in *Fetischismus*. In Klein's concept, *Verleugnung* is a archaic defense mechanism whose goal is the entirety of psychic reality rather than a group of specific representations.

Therefore, according to Klein, it is possible for the ego to proceed to begin to disavow a large part of external reality ("zu einer *Verleugnung* eines grossen Teiles des äusseren Realität fortschreiten").

It seems to us that, not only in the previously stated concepts but also in the subsequent development of the Kleinian school, the delicate interweaving of mechanisms that Freud described (in the papers quoted) could not be properly appreciated. In particular, what seems to be lost is the relationship between *Verleugnung* as defense mechanism, on the one hand, and *Bejahung-Verneinung* as a form of thought based on word representations, on the other. Only if one recognizes this relationship and, therefore, clearly distinguishes the two terms, can one see the complicated interplay underlying the phenomenon of disavowal or the avowal of reality; that is true also for the corresponding stages through which an individual analysis will have to proceed again and again.

Regarding denial in the speech of the patient, it seems to us that one must distinguish when denial is implicit or explicit. In the latter case, it is important to have in mind *Verneinung sensu strictiori*, whereas on the contrary, in the case of the implicit form, a number of possibilities are opened. Perhaps we are witnessing the appearance of *Verneinung*, or perhaps we are seeing the impossibility for the patient to have access to this situation; and perhaps, at a deep level, the use of *Verleugnung* instead of *Verdrängung* may be hypothesized.

One may ask whether this range of possibilities may apply (and eventually how far) to the analytic products themselves (this general term is here used on purpose to indicate both the verbal interventions of the analyst during his or her clinical work and psychoanalytic writings).

The circulation of unrecognized negation between analyst and patient (a sort of *Verleugnung* of *Verneinung*) may be both cause and effect of giving preference to nonverbal communication. Bion's paper, "On Arrogance" (1967) seems useful in illustrating what can follow—both in the clinical and in the theoretical fields. This is the case when the analyst misses the opportunity of becoming aware of either his or her own negation or of the patient's negation. Bion concludes his paper as follows:

> In some patients the denial to the patient of a normal employment of projective identification precipitates a disaster through the destruction of an important link. Inherent in this disaster is the establishment of a primitive superego which denies the use of projective identification. (1967, p. 92)

Had Bion taken into account his own and his patient's negations (visible clearly in the case material), the conclusions might be different, that is:

> In some patients the disavowal (*Verleugnung*) of an analytic employment of negation (*Verneinung*) and of other implicit verbal communication precipitates a "disaster" through the destruction of an important link. Inherent in the disaster is the establishment of a primitive superego which uses projective identification in order to avoid an insightful exploitation of *Verneinung*.

We may question the usefulness of centering all our research upon the earliest phases of psychic development and apply it directly in an ever more abstract way to all our concepts and conceptualizations. Such abstraction reaches mystic proportions. It may perhaps be a matter of implicit refusal of the evolving potentialities peculiar to every patient. In this case, we would have to speak of a collusion of the analyst with his or her patient's wish to deny. This would lead to a de facto interminable analysis. Different from this defensive tendency of the analyst in the sense of *Verleugnung* would be a position in which *Verneinung* indicates its tendency to approach the polarity *Bejahung/Verneinung*. Let us return now to the connection—that we declared at the beginning—between *Weltanschauung* and denial.

The term *Weltanschauung* may be understood in two ways: concrete and metaphoric, the latter being the one more commonly used. The concrete meaning, however, has for us psychoanalysts a particular value because it leads back to that period of everyone's life during which visual and auditory representations were formed; these, variously cathected with affects, could be the object of mental operations. In this sense, as Spitz (1958) has shown, the first *Weltanschauung* is a *Mutteranschauung*, from which, through an enlargement of the visual and auditory field, a more complex and rich vision of reality would ensue.

However, it must be pointed out that the word *Anschauung* contains something more than the visual meaning: It is a vision that goes beyond the simple "thing," an affective vision, a conception that has a quality of creativity. The child is creative when, besides exploring space physically, he or she experiences pleasure in communicating his or her discovery of the world and of the language that can describe it. This creativity seems to be strictly connected: to the construction of an ego that is happily aware of existing and functioning and to the two decisions that the function of judgment must take. To refer to Freud once again: (1) whether something perceived (a thing) shall be taken into the ego or not; (2) whether something that is present in the ego as an image can also be rediscovered in perception. In this sense, infantile *Weltanschauung* goes hand in hand with the discovery of the self, of one's potentialities and psychic capacities, of narcissistic and interpersonal gratifications that these potentialities can give. We would say that in this sense the importance of *yes* and *no* (Spitz, 1957) as well as the importance of the discovery of the possibility of lying is basic for the development of the subject as a knowing person.

In this regard, however, mental and verbal processes seem already to be complicated, because verbal negation can have an assertive significance in the child and verbal assertion can also assume a negative significance (concerning one's own autonomy). When a child reacts to the offer of the desired candy, saying, "I don't want it," he or she affirms his or her "ego" by opposing the parents' will; at the same time, he or she negates a wish, allowing its representation to approach his or her conscience.

Now another problem arises immediately for the analyst who is studying how negation evolves. It is the problem of the passage from the purely intellectual admission to consciousness of a representation to its real admission, that is, to awareness of it.

Perhaps—if one notes once again the verbal forms that give expression to this delicate phase—this passage may be called the passage of the "why not?" in the sense that one's attention becomes concentrated—

through a displacement of emphasis in the sentence—on the "not," that is, on the true negation.

Because this passage, however, seems to us difficult and delicate, it is perhaps worthwhile to examine the implications—with reference to *Weltanschauung*—in various situations, in order to try to exemplify the different evolutionary possibilities in negative speech; and this on account of the fact that verbal denial is really a negation or otherwise a form of speech that implies disavowal.

It is perhaps convenient, in view of the preceding, to start from what is probably the watershed of human psychosexual development—adolescence. It is at this age that often, perhaps always, a *Weltanshauung* makes its appearance. The reemergence of instinctual drives of renewed strength makes this *Weltanschauung* into a constellation of defensive structures, yet this may also have an evolutionary meaning insofar as it now actually becomes possible to give new answers to unresolved conflicts.

Thus adolescent *Weltanschauungen* often, implicitly or explicitly, take on negative forms. "No difference at all exists among people" is one of these typical adolescent formulations. It perhaps grants the adolescent not only the post-Oedipal claim of a place of equal dignity with father figures but also the admission to consciousness of a representation of the differences. Such representations allow the individual to handle material that remains highly cathected with feelings and energy derived from the solution of the oedipal complex; a solution that is obviously personal, that is, different for each person.

It is as if the disavowal, through such a *Weltanschauung*, of interpersonal differences would correspond to a search for indifference in order to counterbalance the emotional turmoil connected with the differences. This representation (that each individual is different from the other) is, as we know from clinical practice, very difficult to arrive at in a well-balanced and harmonious way, substantively imbued with neither a sadistic nor a masochistic evaluation of human differences. The sadomasochistic evaluation reveals, in the observation of differences between humans, the wish to maintain the status quo or to reverse it—which amounts to the same thing.

There is in childhood a relative short phase marked on the linguistic side by the play of continuously putting questions or chains of questions to parents (or generally to adults). The interrogation phase of the adolescent is long and—in pathological cases—may have no end. Paradoxically, still worse is the situation in which such a phase of questions has no beginning. For it is only when the individual allows himself or herself to develop this capacity of interrogation or has the possibility of doing so that the phase of growing out of adolescence begins. (This may also never happen or may have a partial development, and, in any case, each solution will be different from the other.)

Intellectualization in adolescence goes hand in hand with the use of *Verneinung.* This may mark a dichotomy, sometimes excessive, concerning the emotional and sexual life of this phase. But it may also be considered a way of enriching the intellect with mental contents otherwise inaccessible, which, in their turn, may be useful—should development continue—in order to tolerate and modulate affects, to cultivate and realize them.

In this sense, using Freud's words, we could say, perhaps, that adolescent *Weltanschauung* is fundamentally a religious vision of the world— based as it is on illusory elements, on *a priori* affirmations, on declared principles that may nevertheless evolve (and actually do evolve in a large number of cases) toward a scientific *Weltanschauung.* The latter would be not so much in the literal sense of the word scientific as in the wider sense of a vision of the world based on an openness to question oneself and reality with the least preconceived ideas; we could say on a willingness to "work through."[1]

Freud himself ironically considered this position (implicitly noting its utopian and therefore illusory character) when, in *Die Zukunft einer Illusion* (1927b), he speaks of "our god λόγος" as "perhaps not a very almighty one." And the development of a capacity for irony is perhaps one of the elements necessary for the formation of an adult *Weltanschauung.* But it is not easy to acquire.

An account of an incident that occurred to an Italian scientist, who was at that time a young man, will be a slight detour to get us back on the subject.

Immediately after World War I, this person was riding the tide in a boat on the Danube. In the same boat there were some orthodox rabbis, with whom he began a philosophic discourse. At a certain moment when the discussion had become relentless, one of the rabbis asked the scientist whether he was a Sephardic or an Ashkenazic Jew. He answered: "But I am not a Jew," and the rabbi said, *"Warum nicht?"* ("why not?").

The incident lends itself to various interpretations. Its effect on the young scientist (who actually had a Jewish ancestor) was one of surprise and hilarity, revealing, we could say in our language, that his affirmation

---

[1]One of us (Sacerdoti & Spacal, 1985) has proposed the distinction between two forms of insight (a word more akin to *Anschauung* than to *Einsicht*), which could be called respectively "dogmatic" and "workable through." Only the first can be "given" to others (as by Bion to the patient of the clinical case cited before).

of not being a Jew was, at least partially, a negation. Concerning the rabbi, we could put the question whether his "Warum nicht?" contained, unconsciously, a *Verleugnung* (in the sense of the unacceptability, for him, of the difference between Jew and non-Jew). In the interaction between the two, we could see the overcoming of the *Verneinung* of the scientist. But, in any case, only in the subsequent account of the scientist is it possible to grasp an ironic, and autoironic element.

Perhaps in the moment of the discussion the protagonists had not yet developed such a capacity. One can maintain, as one of us has documented on another occasion (Sacerdoti, 1987) that a certain amount of latent or unconscious irony had been present in the dialogue between the orthodox rabbi and the scientist.

In latent irony, something is affirmed without knowing (at the conscious level) that the contrary is "true" and therefore that which is verbally affirmed is false (i.e., not emotionally significant). In this sense, unconscious irony could be seen as the negative (in the photographic sense) of *Verneinung:* In the latter, the falseness of a proposition is affirmed without knowing, at the conscious level, that on the contrary, it is true.

It would therefore seem worthwhile for the analyst, during his or her work, to observe the variations of the patient's conscious *Weltanschauung* as it is expressed in a fragmentary way through external events or persons or, even more clearly, through reflections about his or her own value judgments.

Often the patient gives information to the analyst when he or she talks about observations made by others on himself or herself, and often this information allows us to see—through a negation ("I am not saying it, he or she said so and so")—that the patient is changing his or her self-image and that he or she is able to gain an insight of it.

But with the same frequency, the analysand, through his or her own judgments about others or about external events, informs us about the changes that have occurred in his or her *Weltanschauung* about the eventual persistence of adolescent or infantile elements, implying in their turn negations or disavowals.

This matter deals, therefore, with a parameter that is employable—and indeed employed, we believe, by many analysts—but little of this is described and studied. This happens probably because such a study might give rise to the suspicion that the analyst takes on the position of a judge, a personification of the patient's (or perhaps the analyst's own) superego, in contrast with analytic neutrality. This position, as observed by Schafer (1976), might in the end compromise the evolution of analysis itself.

We believe that, on the contrary, attention to the form of the analysand's communication about the variations of his or her own *Weltanschauung* makes it possible to avoid this danger and, instead, to use these messages as a valid indicator of the personal evolution of the patient.

A *Weltanschauung* enriched with ironic elements and based on the capacity of the patient to put interrogations to himself or herself and to others will be the signal that the patient has become capable of developing extensively the second phase of judgment, as described by Freud: to *re*discover in reality (now in symbolic form) what he or she had discovered (also by means of analysis) in himself or herself, *re*cognize his or her own elements in other persons as well as the others' elements in himself or herself.

In conclusion we should like to emphasize the determining characteristic points of our study. In the first place, we have tried to point out the conflict between scientific and religious *Weltanschauungen*. Such a conflict had been noted by Freud, and we have used his terms, his words, while trying to make clear what seems to us to be their meaning when translated into everyday language.

In the second place, we have limited the field of our study to the relationship between *Weltanschauung* and denial, distinguishing the phenomenon of *Verneinung* from the unconscious mechanism of *Verleugnung*. This has led us to propose some hypotheses about the consequences that a misunderstanding between these two very different aspects of psychic life may imply.

If the analyst (through his own *Verleugnung* of the patient *Verneinung*) is so polarized that he or she pays too much attention to the preverbal aspects of the patient's communication, this emphasis may push the patient toward excessive regression, even as it may block the development of the patient's ability (in the psychological sense) to judge.

Such a position of the analyst might have a connection with his or her own *Weltanschauung,* consisting, for example, in his or her belief that in any case all patients have to be considered, at the outside limit, psychotics (and/or children); that is a *Weltanschauung* of the adolescent type.

In valuable psychoanalytic conceptualization as well as in the *Weltanschauung* of patients whose analysis did succeed a sufficient amount of irony and the capacity of self-interrogation ought to be found, without falling into "denial through exaggeration." This, as it concerns psychoanalytic theorization, could consist, on the one hand, in passing from one interrogation to another, never finding anything stable—finally revealing a *Verleugnung* of already acquired theoretical knowledge—or, on the other hand, in the search for the "most archaic experience"—in which a topographical regression is mistaken for a temporal regression (Pasche, 1962). This confusion then becomes the starting point for every sort of (re)constructive affirmation[2] that can also obscure the observation of the changes in the *Weltanschauung* of the analysand. This observation is, in our opinion, of primary interest. With reference to this point, we have indicated the importance of distinguishing two types of *Weltanschauungen:* those that are formulated in negative verbal terms but, for the very fact of using *Verneinung,* may be seen as functioning progressively; and those *Weltanschauungen* that, though formulated in positive (verbal) terms, on account of the underlying use of *Verleugnung,* can only with difficulty undergo progressive developments.

REFERENCES

Bion, W. R. (1967). *Second thoughts*. London: Heinemann.
Deutsch, H. (1933). Zur psychologie der manisch-depressiven Zustände. *International Zeitschrift fur Psychoanalyze, 19*, 358–371.
Freud, S. (1925a). Die Verneinung. *Gesammelte Werke* (Vol. XIV), Frankfurt: Fischer Verlag.
Freud, S. (1925b). Hemmung, Symptom und Angst. *Gesammelte Werke* (Vol. XIV), Frankfurt: Fischer Verlag.
Freud, S. (1927a). Fetischismus. *Gesammelte Werke* (Vol. XIV), Frankfurt: Fischer Verlag.
Freud, S. (1927b). Die Zukunft einer Illusion. *Gesammelte Werke* (Vol. XIV), Frankfurt: Fischer Verlag.
Freud, S. (1932). Neue Folge der Vorlesungen zur Einführung in die Psychoanalyse. *Gesammelte Werke* (Vol. XV), Frankfurt: Fischer Verlag.
Freud, S. (1938). Abriss der Psychoanalyse. *Gesammelte Werke* (Vol. XVII), Frankfurt: Fischer Verlag.
Hoffman, R. S. (1982). Reductio ad absurdum. *International Journal of Psycho-Analysis, 63*, 88–89.
Klein, M. (1937). Zur Psychogenese der manisch-depressiven Zustände. *Int. Ztschr. f. Psa., 16*, 275–305.
Laforgue, R. (1926). Verdrängung und Skomotisation. *International Zeitschrift fur Psychoanalyze, 12*, 54.
Pasche, F. (1962). Régression, perversion, nevrose (Examen critique de la notion de régression). *Revue Francaise de Psychoanalyzé, XXVI*, 161–178.
Sacerdoti, G. (1987). *L'ironia attraverso la Psicoanalisi*. Milano: Raffaello Cortina Editore.
Sacerdoti, G., & Spacal, S. (1985). Insight. *Rivista di Psicoanalisi, XXXI*, 59–74.
Schafer, R. (1976). *A new language for psychoanalysis*. New Haven and London: International Universities Press.
Spitz, R. (1957). *No and yes. On the genesis of human communication*. New York: International Universities Press.
Spitz, R. (1958). *La première année de la vie de l'enfant*. Paris: P.U.F.

[2]One may suspect that, in some of the latter, we find a latent (unconscious) irony, which is sometimes easily perceived by others but which only with difficulty becomes manifest (conscious) in the messenger. This difficulty obviously cannot be overcome through the use of the parody approach that has been attempted by some authors (for instance Hoffman, 1982).

5

Denial in the Use of Language as Related to the Father

GEMMA JAPPE

INTRODUCTION

This chapter is especially dedicated to Hillel Klein: It was he who set up
the train of thought that I shall present. In a moment of refinding, he let
me share—as did Rina Hruoshovski-Moses before—the grief at the en-
forced loss of the German language. Since then, he has helped me to
continue to feel what it is that I too have lost with them, without ever
having had it: the world of our fathers, which was then—and could have
remained—common to us and which, before I was born and during my
early childhood, was corrupted and violated irreparably. At the same
time, I realize most concretely via this very language, how inescapably I
am rooted in the world of the murderers of that time too.

Of course, more terrible things have happened than can be encompassed in the fate of a language; but here and now language is exactly
what reveals our separateness from one another: In order to overcome
this separation, we all find ourselves practicing denial. Neither did we
speak German at the symposium on which this volume is based nor

GEMMA JAPPE • Private Practice, Riesstrasse 21, 53 Bonn 1, Germany.

Hebrew; English was the conference language, the language of two world powers that fought against Nazi Germany.

PERSONAL EXPERIENCES IN THE ACQUISITION AND USE OF A FOREIGN LANGUAGE

Various circumstances during my schooling prevented me from enjoying proper instruction in English at school. My first contact with it was in a kind of children's lesson with exotic games. Later I tried to teach myself by the so-called natural method. During my studies, I practiced on an important and outstanding commentary to Plato's *Timaios,* only available in the English language, and I had, of course, to make up for my meager knowledge of English by turning to the original text for help. I learned to love the language in correspondence with English friends. As secretary of the European Psychoanalytical Federation (E.P.F.), I came across something of which I had never been conscious before: When I had to turn back from the foreign into my native language, my own style suddenly struck me as curiously hollow and strange; I was not sure if I meant what I had written or was caught up in some kind of role play. It was as if to be using English was to be taking part in a game, a venture full of qualms, pleasurable but demanding, as if it were always Sunday and I might take leave of my real, my serious self.

(It was for this reason that I made myself formulate this chapter completely in German and have it translated. My translator is an Englishwoman resident in Germany whose queries have helped me to work out exactly what it is that I want to say.)

Once my attention had been drawn to this phenomenon, I found much to observe in myself and others. For example, every now and then I have occasion to carry out interviews or single therapeutic sessions in Italian. After a certain time, I noticed that none of these initial interviews ever led to a therapy—which I do not of course put down solely to reasons of language—but, more important than that, I was less able to perceive unconscious phenomena, and my abstinence too was impaired. I was under the spell of the sound of this beautiful and much loved language, and unconscious messages did not always reach me the same way as usually. By the same token, I often found it hard to make myself understood when I wanted to offer an interpretation touching on some unpleasant point.

Annemarie Sandler presented a detailed account of a case at the Psycho-Analytical Congress in Madrid in which she told of quite a long phase during which she and her patient both thought each other marvelous, and yet she found the notes she had taken on sessions increasingly boring and unsatisfactory. Possibly this had something to do with the fact that they were both speaking French, the patient's mother tongue and a language Annemarie Sandler knew well. In Israel, in the foreign setting, French may have represented something like an idyllic enclave to the two newcomers.

In a discussion on multilingualism René Diatkine once said of himself, with tongue in cheek, surely, that he was immune to the seductions of foreign languages: *J'ai été toujours fidèle à ma langue* [I have always been faithful to my own language]. At international congresses, there are always complaints about the translation: The professional translators are uninvolved and have little grasp of the subject, whereas colleagues improvising a translation slow the lecture down and in the end distort the meaning. Freud often quoted the play on words *traduttore–traditore* (translator–traitor), and it is really curious that so little analytical thought has been expended on this subject. This "treachery" is a product of denial; the rapid decoding of words spares one the effort of tracking down a meaning hard to grasp.

With little knowledge, many guesses by analogy and stimulated by a week with the sounds of Spanish in my ears, I found I was able to follow in part the contributions of Spanish-speaking colleagues directly. When I could not, I made use of the simultaneous translation and had to realize that it was not so much that words or structures had left me in the lurch but that I had not understood the thoughts. I realized that I could not easily follow the workings of my colleague's mind in reaching a concept and handling it.

CONCEPT INCONGRUITY IN TRANSLATION

When a foreign language is learned, new, unknown words become attached or attributed to well-known things and concepts. A French child is supposed to have said: "That's funny: in French it's called "pain" and it *is* "pain": In German it's called "Brot" but it's still "pain." The arbitrary nature of this process is soon forgotten, but a touch of magic, it seems to me, never quite disappears. Those who, in a foreign country without a command of the language, have experienced how tension can mount (anger on the part of those trying to help, despair on the part of those seeking it) and seen how the sudden appearance of the right word can transform the whole situation at one stroke, will understand what I mean.

This position of helplessness is one to which we never want to be exposed again, and this is why, to my mind, the command of several languages retains a manic touch, born of the pleasure in leaping boundaries, of a sense of omnipotence in mastering things but also of the need to forget the pain and bewilderment one felt on perceiving that a word can be so far separated from its meaning that it can be replaced by another and that in the use of a substitute much of the original is surrendered. The world we dip into in a foreign language is not the world we came from. French bread is really not the same thing as German bread. Even though the psychoanalytical method and Freud's writings have reached many parts of the world, it cannot be denied that Parisian psychoanalysis is different from psychoanalysis in London or in South America or in New York. Work emanating from one school is not easily understood in another because the unspoken traditions of thought cannot be translated with the text. Concepts change their meaning when they are referred to by another word that has its roots in a different history of concepts. This background can gradually, in the sense of a regressive process, overlay the new concept.

Bruno Bettelheim has shown what happened to Freud's language and concepts in the hand of his translator Strachey:

> St. Hieronymous once commented on certain translations of the Bible that they were not so much versions as perversions of the original. The same could be said of the way in which many psycho-analytical concepts have been translated into English. (Bettelheim, 1984, p. 116)

But the perverting of an original does not in itself amount to denial. What in one individual user of the foreign language would be merged appears here in three separate persons: They are, first, the translator in his inevitable and evitable inadequacy, whereby denial may or may not play a part; second, the readers who were ignorant of the original language; third, the psychoanalytical community as a whole, enough of whose members were well able to perceive the distortion. We can see the roots of this collective act of denial. The German language was ostracized in the countries of immigration or under a tabu in the hearts of those who had escaped extermination at the hands of the Germans by the skin of their teeth. At the same time, this denial aided the wish to create a home for psychoanalysis elsewhere and to spread knowledge of it in the New World, if necessary at the price of making it less offensive. This wish also favors an instance of denial still active today, namely that there is an ever-increasing number of contributions to psychoanalysis from countries whose language few of us know, for instance Scandinavia, Finland, Israel.

CONCEPT INCONGRUITY IN LANGUAGE DEVELOPMENT

What we see in translations and the use of them merely repeats in the other direction what has been traced out in the development of language. When I say in the other direction, I refer to the distinction made by Vygotski (see Jappe, 1971) between the original acquisition of language on the one hand, which progresses from all-embracing concepts perceived through the senses, to differentiation and abstraction, and, on the other side, the learning of a language of concepts or of a foreign language in which the learner progresses from a single word to the understanding of the whole system or from the acquisition of a single, clearly defined concept to the matter-of-course use of the whole of it.

At the beginning of language development stands the physical discharge of displeasure in screaming. According to Freud, screaming acquires "the extremely important secondary function of making oneself understood so that man's original helplessness is the true source of all moral motives" (Freud, 1895, p. 318). A mother will satisfy the infant's needs as far as she can; that is to say as far as her wishes and sensitivity will allow. Those signals of need that she does not pick up drop out of the system of communication from which the child's ability to symbolize is to develop. Whether one attributes this dropping out to primary repression or choses to see elements of denial at work depends on whether by denial one understands every nonperception of what was perceptible, or whether one assumes that denial presupposes an already established system of perception—nay, a rudimentary perception of the object of denial. At any rate, symbol formation and the development of meaning are based on the acceptance of a substitute, and a substitute means the partial relinquishing of the object that satisfies the primary needs.

It is seldom that this surrender is carried out in the form of a conscious renunciation; the substitution of words for things can be a manic pleasure. Freud, and Ferenczi after him, saw a relationship between the omnipotence of thoughts and the pride in acquiring language, that is, the ability to use words instead of things. To have a command of words and to play with them helps to mask or deny a person's actual powerlessness against facts and his or her limited ability to act. The price of increasing abstraction is a loss in sensual closeness—a fact that is also denied. This is the cause of permanent recurring misunderstandings between children and adults: As Vygotski has shown (Jappe 1970, p. 117), the two sides may use identical words and mean concepts at an utterly different developmental and abstractional level (functional equivalence).

The affective pathogenic side of this process has been described by Ferenczi as language confusion between children and adults. The child with its pre-genital sexual organization makes the adult a proposal of love to which the adult responds on the level of his sexuality. The child is forced to flee into identification with the aggressor and deny that the attack has taken place because it cannot tolerate the adult's power over it and cannot bear to hate the person it loves; moved by guilt, the adult tries to forget the incident and see that it remains forgotten. Between "normal" concept incongruity—natural in the process of a child's development—and violation of this traumatizing kind one can imagine all the possible quantitative shades and nuances of what we are accustomed to call bringing up and educating. Freud (1905a,b) in his essay on jokes showed what a quantity of inhibition and restriction—unnoticed, and that means denied—is demanded in the normal command of language:

> During the period in which a child is learning how to handle the vocabulary of his mother-tongue, it gives him obvious pleasure to "experiment with it in play" . . . Little by little he is forbidden this enjoyment, till all that remains permitted to him are significant combinations of words. . . . But there is far more potency in the restrictions which must establish themselves in the course of a child's education in logical thinking and in distinguishing between what is true and false in reality; and for this reason the rebellion against the compulsion of logic and reality is deep-going and long-lasting. . . .
>
> Nor, later on, does the University student cease these demonstrations against the compulsion of logic and reality, the dominance of which however he feels growing ever more intolerant and unrestricted. . . . Much later still, indeed, when as a grown man he meets others in scientific congresses and once more feels himself a learner, after the meeting is over there comes the Kneipzeitung (a comic set of minutes, "tavern's newspaper") which distorts the new discoveries into nonsense and offers him a compensation for the fresh addition to his intellectual inhibition." (p. 125 ff.)

SOME METAPSYCHOLOGICAL CONSIDERATIONS

Admittedly it is not always easy here to differentiate between denial and repression. That denial has a part to play in sublimation is a point that Freud (1910a,b) makes in his writing on Leonardo:

> When Leonardo in the prime of his life met again that blissfully charmed smile that had once played on his mother's face when she caressed him, he had long been under the domination of an inhibition that forbade him ever again to desire such signs of tenderness from the lips of a woman. But he had become a painter and so he strove to re-create this smile with his brush. He gave it to all his pictures, to Leda, to Johannes and to Bacchus. It is possible that in these figures Leonardo *denied and overcame* the tragedy of his love-life in the exercise of his art. (p. 189 [emphasis mine])

At this point there is a difficulty that cannot any longer be over-looked: At first it looked as if denial was a reaction occurring in particular situations, as for instance, in the transition from one language to another. Then it became apparent that denial is like a thread running right through the whole development of language and indeed that the growth of language and culture cannot occur without it—and finally, it appeared in the finest of cultural achievements!

A similar difficulty is to be found in Freud's work on negation. The essay begins with some clinical examples and leads to thoughts on what language achieves in the use of the negative form (symbol of negation), then on to the intellectual function of judgment, and finally to the problem of the judgment of what does and does not exist; Freud traces this problem back to the processes of incorporation and expulsion, which (in the final analysis) are derived from the life and death drive.

The symposium of the E.P.F. (Marseille, 1984) on the theme of the death drive made it clear to me that we ought not to think of the death drive as an incomprehensible urge toward annihilation; it can better be understood as an original instinctive reaction of the ego (or of whatever the predecessor of the ego may be) to intolerable disturbances (this explains its close link with narcissism).

It is not hard to see a parallel to denial in this pattern of reaction: Nobody is likely to dispute that denial does away with disturbing perceptions.

Denial as well can occur with greater or lesser intensity; it can be brutal or imperceptible, at various stages of organization, in differing quantities, and it can be permanent or ephemeral. This all tallies with the conception of denial as a derivative of the death drive variously bound or linked with other processes. We are therefore justified in having difficulty finding denial in so many forms. So our problem now is to differentiate between denial and other forms of defense, for all defense serves the purpose of keeping the intolerable away from the ego and can thus also be interpreted as derivatives of the death drive. It has been said, therefore, that denial represents an early form of defense (Anna Freud) or that defense has two phases, an expulsory one and an integrative one, for example, projection (Dorpat, 1983).

We must, therefore, leave the abstract level of metapsychological explanation and return to a description of the phenomena themselves if we want to find something specific to denial.

DENIAL IN TERMS OF OBJECT RELATIONS

In Freud's *Negation,* denial appears literally between the lines. For what divides "lifting of a repression" from the "acceptance of what has been repressed?" Is it not precisely denial that prevents the content (now recognized as thinkable) ("You will think that I want to say something to offend you . . . . The mother . . .) from being accepted. And below the lines we find the footnote:

> The same process is at the root of the familiar superstition that boasting is dangerous. "How nice not to have had one of my headaches for so long." But this is in fact the first announcement of an attack, of whose approach the subject is already sensible, although he is as yet unwilling to believe it. (Freud, 1925, p. 236)

This disbelief, the refusal to believe a thing that may be manifest or that could well be noticed, seems to be peculiar to denial. I am pleased to find that I agree here with H. Sperling, who would like to see the rejection of meaning reserved for the neurotic defence forms of denial. With the concept of belief, we enter the world of object relations, through which we pursue our theme.

Ferenczi has shown, in his study on belief, disbelief, and conviction that belief and disbelief go back to the infant's dependence and counter-dependence on figures of authority. He stresses that adults often put a severe strain on a child's ability to believe, particularly in matters connected with the child's feelings. An example occurs to me here from my own family: My small daughter recently emerged from a shop in a great state of indignation. She had bought herself some sweets, and a woman next to her at the cash desk had admonished her with the words: "They're not good for you, you know?" The little girl had defended herself bravely, "But children like them" and had received a bald "No!" in reply. The woman was morally condemning sweets, but the child thought she was expected to deny the truth of her very real preference for them. Ferenczi's argument on this point culminates in the dictum: "Feeling is believing" (1913/1970, p. 143). By this, he means that we believe in what we can feel, but the possibility remains open that our trust in what feelings and senses tell us might be undermined by the experience of certain forms of dependence.

This idea is supported by Rubinfine's reference to the superego as a dynamic factor in the exercise of denial and to the role of denial in efforts to retain the object, as also to preserve self-esteem against the unkindness of fate. He touches in passing on humor, denial of death, and depersonalization.

At this point I should like to put forward tentatively the idea that denial manifests a particular form of relationship to the father.

CLINICAL EXAMPLE

My patient, I shall refer to him as A., started talking at the beginning of a session in a rather artificially thoughtful way about a feeling of unease. Mentioning Maritta—a young relative who was staying with them—he said he really did think she was awfully nice, he enjoyed seeing her, felt in the mood to do things with her, yes, he'd rather like to give her presents and so on. His feelings toward his wife were rather cooler at the moment, he didn't know why, she didn't move him, he was behaving toward her with considerable reserve, he said. I commented, "You are in love with Maritta." This was met with a lengthy silence. Then the patient said, "If that's being in love, then I must be in love pretty often and with all kinds of women." I confirmed this. The patient felt I was being outrageous, he had meant to sidestep the issue of whether or not he was in love with an offhand, vague generalization and instead he found not only the case of Maritta but many other instances given their full weight. All of a sudden, he was confronted with the question of what he meant to do about being in love.

What interests me particularly in this example is that, protected by denial, he was in a position to enjoy feelings and actions he would otherwise have regarded as forbidden. It was not that he was unconscious of what he was doing and feeling—he was able to describe it in a wealth of words—he simply protested strongly when it came to recognizing what he was doing and giving the thing a name. In this way he succeeded in evading the judgment of his superego. (This would correspond roughly to what Dorpat terms *cognitive arrest* 1983, p. 51). We can also put it this way: The father is cut out and made meaningless in his function and authority.

In fact, in this case, it is a question of an incestuous object: The patient's wife has a brother and Maritta is his wife. A. harbors feelings of intense hostility against this brother, at root jealousy of the close bond between brother and sister. Whereas here the motive of revenge, which may have stimulated love, remained unconscious, in other acts of denial it is closer to being conscious and more obvious. The episode described here forms part of a process of working through that began with a difference of opinion about the payment of the fee by a third party. What is being worked through here is the discovery that the patient has a habit of cheating others and deceiving himself in a way that at first sight seems to be harmless. These actions usually bring him a slight material advantage, but his secret delight is always immense. This delight, which is out of all proportion of the (material) gain, is experienced over the knowledge that an institution or an authority is suffering damage that benefits the patient or is being circumvented or ignored. It is a clear case of attack: The symptomatic actions allow the patient to triumph over the father's power. At the same time, he keeps the triumph a secret even from himself. He never comments on actions like these; he neither condemns nor condones them; they just seem to happen without his admitting his part in them. During the later course of this process of working through, the patient recognized in this unwillingness to judge the characteristic attitude that his parents have always shown toward the Nazi movement. They never, then nor since, confessed allegiance; nor did they disassociate themselves from the movement: They never answered any questions on the subject, and when their son tried to confront them with certain facts and with his knowledge of them, they either remained silent or passed over the question.

To outline the components of identification in the denial, I should like to include a few details about the patient's father and their relation to one another. The father himself never really "had it out" with *his* father, never came to terms with his background. He came from the family of a highly respected missionary, but he did not want to have anything to do with theology. He left home at 17, was conscripted to the national work force and at the outbreak of war to the army, taken prisoner, and on his release after the war was over, he found himself already a husband and father of two children. (My patient was born in 1944, the elder child.) The father set up a business marketing seeds, which not only provided the family income but also gave him the satisfaction of watching his "seed" grow in all the gardens and fields of the area—and in this way, he continued his father's missionary work in the most concrete manner.

My patient seems to have had an intense relationship with his father, longing for him in his absence but also to have suffered cruelty and humiliation at his hands. In puberty and adolescence, his development took a turn unquestionably based on ignoring the father. In his secondary-school days, he began to cheat on a large scale in the pattern described before, behavior that cost him more time and energy than would have been necessary to master his schoolwork in the conventional manner. With his mother's support, he made himself competent in all fields that were a closed book to his father, particularly in music, and finally he decided to study theology in which outwardly he has done very well. So he succeeded in leaving his father far behind him without ever risking rivalry and without any real "showdown." His father's superior physical strength was never challenged, and, in practical matters, the son has remained dependent: Although the father is only a couple of centimeters taller, he is constantly calling attention to the fact that he is a bigger man, and right up and into the time of the analysis, the patient had allowed his father to manage all his finances.

From this it will be clear that the elimination of the father is not the sole component in the process of denial. It may play the major part in single acts of denial, as in the preceding example; but, as an attitude, denial can be seen to have a second, identificatory phase. I follow Dorpat

(1983) in the assumption of a second phase, but I feel that a form of screen behavior peculiar to denial points to the fact that the relationship to the father suffered a particular fate.

The devaluation of the father, presumably the result of disappointment (as the father really *is* a weak figure) or because he was not in a position to fulfill important functions, has the effect of object loss. The lost object relation is replaced on the one hand by fusion with an idealized father imago (in his heart of hearts, the patient believed he was God's favorite, that God himself promoted the patient's fraudulent activities); on the other hand in an identification with the father suspended from his function. Both these relations are feeble because destructiveness has not been digested but left out (in theology the patient does not really feel at home and in his workaday life he feels gauche, a prey to moods and unable to tackle conflicts).

The following dream and what happened when I tried to interpret it will serve to illustrate this fate: The patient is in a cage surrounded by ferocious dogs. The scene is set; it is quite clear that he is to be torn limb from limb. For the moment, he can just manage to ward off the worst by holding out the large glove he is wearing to one of the dogs in such a way that his finger is withdrawn and the dog is chewing around on the empty finger of the glove.

When working with this patient I often find myself in the position of chewing on something that turns out to be an empty sheath. While the patient is talking about fear of castration in his relation to his father, I make a comment on his fear of women. To this he replies that he has no problems at all with women. I contradict him here, reminding him of a series of broken-off relationships and peculiar things in his relations with women and also mention by name the men with whom he has kept up a steady friendship for many years. After a lengthy pause the patient asks me, "How do you come to know all that?" It seems that, in spite of experience to the contrary, he is still holding on to the phantasy that I do not take in or retain anything that he says, as if I were offering him an empty glove finger or an analysis automat (vending machine) for him to chew on and wear himself out. This corresponds to his fear that, once the analysis is over, it will be as if it had never taken place. By reminding him of something I was able—at any rate for a moment—to show him that something in his life was lasting and formed his personal history. The patient was hardly able to let himself enjoy this instance of positive fatherliness. The words with which he meant to express his satisfaction at having discovered something of himself in me became more and more empty and unconvincing. When I pointed out this, he confessed that he was talking in order to be able to look at himself with more distance. It was as if there were someone lying next to him on the couch, making fun of everything and condemning it all. Imagine what his father would say to all this . . . !

In the image of the empty glove and the kennels around him I reocgnize how insufficiently equipped the patient is by means of his hollow father identification; he only protects him provisionally (not lastingly) against his own impulses to bite and archaic drives and wishes that leave him imprisoned in the timeless world of the primary object. Emerging from this session was further material that demonstrated that the empty glove represented the empty words the patient produces to ward off more terrible fears such as the state of depersonalization.

SOME GENERALIZATIONS AND CONCLUSION

I am inclined for this reason, beyond this one case, to adopt the image of the empty glove to describe other instances of empty words, behind which I also suspect a destroyed and patched-up relationship to the father.

This brings to mind what is doubtless a common problem—the trivialization of feelings such as I met often in analysis with the patient, C. Whenever an interpretation touched her too closely, or bewildered her, she answered with "reasonable" everyday maxims of a general psychologizing kind, whose purpose was to make disappear what was disquieting in her feelings. This behavior began to cease when she came to realize how deeply and secretly (apart from overt behavior) her father, whom she had lost in puberty, had submitted himself and adapted to certain standards of the Nazi government and that she herself had a hidden "Jewish" part of her identity that she never acknowledged.

It was the phenomenon of empty language that aroused in me the suspicion that the obvious denial in it had something to do with killing. My clinical work, particularly with patient A., but by no means only with him, has given this conjecture a clearer shape, and so I am inclined to suppose that denial represents identification, or more properly the acting out of fusion with the father, who, whether because of previous defensive actions on the part of the subject or by reason of other conditions, was not able to fulfil his essential function of being a living example in the relationship with the subject's mother and of securing this relationship by the setting of limits and guaranteeing its continuity. Once I had seen this connection, I found further material supporting and confirming it.

Had not Freud interpreted the smile on the faces of Leonardo's figures as denial and as a means of overcoming "the unhappy nature" of the artist's love life, thereby linking it with Leonardo's homosexuality?

Eissler (1980), in his essay on the archaic smile, puts forward the thesis that this smile:

> . . . was the first human document to pronounce life a thing of beauty and pleasure in defiance of the horrors of the human condition. It was a *truly great act of denial* and at the same time an attachment to the world promising pleasure. (1980, p. 245 [emphasis mine])

Eissler sees the source of this achievement in the union of sexual abandonment and complete narcissistic satisfaction in the love of the youth and an older man. This smile "must be the smile of the youth escaping the dangers and horrors of physical intercourse with women and finding sexual satisfaction with a man he loves" (p. 248).

So far we had been talking about the corrupted or damaged father figure but here we are faced with a phenomenon that has its place at the very cradle of occidental civilization as is generally accepted and heavily emphasized by Eissler (1980). The archaic smile was what made it possible for "man to turn his glance to the world around him and let it rest there" (p. 250) and to attain the knowledge of nature, ultimately the basis of modern science. The resulting strengthening of the father principle or even maybe its establishment in the first place (man separated himself from Nature, experienced himself as facing Nature) in no way contradicts the fact that the relationship expressed in the archaic smile had its roots in a situation of helplessness and the experience of inferiority at the hands of supposedly powerful women in a matriarchy and defenselessness against the overpowering forces of Nature. Denial here would take the form of an alliance of the father and the son (or with the young girl, too, in her male aspect: cf. my "Notes on the motif of the choice of caskets") against the mother experienced as ruling over both (cf. Slater, 1968).

The finest products of the human spirit can be traced to this union—including humor. In humor, says Freud, a person treats himself or herself as a child and at the same time plays, from a superior position, the role of the adult toward this child. "It is also true that when the superego introduces a humoristic attitude it is actually fending off reality and serving illusion" (Freud, 1928, p. 166). Freud himself comments not without a touch of surprise that this hardly fits the character of the superego as a "severe master" (p. 388): "Come, look, this is the world that appears so dangerous. Child's play—just fit for a joke" (p. 166).

Even where denial represents the only escape from a reality without hope—of which we shall be hearing a great deal—the alliance is deceptive because it is provisional: Denial produces happiness and rescue for the moment only without in the end being able to ward off the fate that may in fact be made ineluctable by the action of denial itself (as Martin

Wangh never tires of pointing out to us [see Chapter 1]) and often at the price of arousing the revenge of the object that has been excluded and degraded.

The glove in my patient's dream allows him to defend *himself for a while;* the archaic smile immortalizes one moment in time from an era that created Greek tragedy, which deplores precisely this hybris and depicts its inevitable downfall; the hybris of our understanding of Nature, deceptive mastery over its forces, threatens to destroy Nature and the human race with it. Once process affects the next, and, with Nature degraded, our drives become reduced to mechanisms without soul and the father imago becomes an empty shell.

At the end of his book on perversions, M. Khan writes:

> I believe that since the Industrial Revolution and the appearance of scientific technologies in the European cultures man no longer sees himself as made in the image of God or of man but in the image of a machine which is his own invention. (1983, p. 325)

Humans in the image of machines were capable of inventing words like *Endlösung* (the final solution) and *megamorts* and can use them. They are identified with the process of functioning and protected against the horrifying truth of the content of these words.

Of less horrifying proportions but of identical structure is the use of empty words conveying no involvement. For instance, patient A. once tried to get across to me—with all the torture of a confession and more by means of silence and inhibitions than through words—what he and the girl he had first loved had actually done with their bodies. I could feel a tremendous pull on me that conjured up images from my world and almost began to sense his feelings in my own body, when he suddenly put an end to his search for expression with the word *petting.* I was dismissed from the effort to understand and fobbed off with a totally run-of-the-mill expression, with a pornographic catchword.

The beginning of understanding is the attempt to share experience. The word we find together secures the experience of the moment and lends it lasting life and repeatability. Empty words merely create the illusion of our having something in common and form a complicity that excludes emotional reality. With which we have come full circle returning to my opening remarks on the problem of overrapid, pseudounderstanding.

I should not, however, like to close without mentioning a problem that cropped up during my work on this chapter. At first I had intended to collect and analyze examples from everyday life that I thought (following Freud's example) would bring me enlightenment on the process of denial. I thought I had catch phrases in plenty, and I also had in mind things like two articles directly next to each other on the same page of a newspaper, one with the headline "In Their Private Lives People Are Happy Enough," whereas the next begins with the words, "Increasing Numbers of Citizens of the Federal Republic Are Turning to Keeping a Diary to Unburden Themselves of Irritation, Distress, and Worry." But the longer I mulled over the subject the less often I came across such instances, and I no longer noticed empty words. I must have fallen prey to some selective narrowing of perception that I could not seem to alter or affect and I am rather hoping that further discussion will help me to lift that barrier.

REFERENCES

Bettelheim, B. (1984). *Freud und die Seele des Menschen* (dt. v. K. Graf). Düsseldorf: Claassen.

Dorpat, Th. (1983). The cognitive arrest hypothesis of denial. *International Journal of Psychoanalysis, 64*, 47–58.

Eissler, K. (1980). Das archaische Lächeln. In *Zur Psychoanalyse der Objektbeziehungen* (pp. 241–261). Stuttgart-Bad Cannstadt: Frommann-Holzboog.

Ferenczi, S. (1913). Glaube, Unglaube und Überzeugung. In *Schriften zur Psychoanalyse* (Vol. I; pp. 135–147). Frankfurt: S. Fischer. (Originally published 1913)

Ferenczi, S. (1933). Sprachverwirrung zwischen den Erwachsenen und dem Kind. In *Schriften zur Psychoanalyse* (Vol. II; pp. 303–313) Frankfurt: S. Fischer 1972.

Freud, S. (1895). Entwurf einer Psychologie. In *Aus den Anfängen der Psychoanalyse*. Frankfurt: S. Fischer.

Freud, S. (1895). Project for a scientific psychology. In J. Strachey (Ed. and Trans.), *Standard Edition* (Vol. I; pp. 283–343). London: Hogarth Press, 1966.

Freud, S. (1905c). Der Witz und seine Beziehung zum Unbewußten. In A. Freud, E. Bibring, E. Kris, O. Isakower (Eds.), *Sigmund Freud, Gesammelte Werke*. London: Imago, 1940. Frankfurt: S. Fischer, 1960.

Freud, S. (1905). *Jokes and their relation to the unconscious*. In J. Strachey (Ed. and Trans.) *Standard Edition* (Vol. VIII). London: Hogarth, 1960.

Freud, S. (1910). *Eine Kindheitserinnerung des Leonardo da Vinci*. In A. Freud, E. Bibring, E. Kris, O. Isakower (Eds.). *Sigmund Freud, Gesammelte Werke*. London: Imago, 1945. Frankfurt: S. Fischer, 1964.

Freud, S. (1910). Leonardo da Vinci and a Memory of His Childhood. In J. Strachey (Ed. and Trans.) *Standard Edition*. London: Hogarth, 1957.

Freud, S. (1925). Die Verneinung In A. Freud, E. Bibring, E. Kris, O. Isakower (Eds.), *Sigmund Freud, Gesammelte Werke*. London: Imago, 1948. Frankfurt: S. Fischer, 1963.

Freud, S. (1925). Negation. In J. Strachey (Ed. and Trans.) *Standard Edition*. London: Hogarth, 1967.

Freud, S. (1928a). Der Humor. In A. Freud, E. Bibring, E. Kris, O. Isakower (Eds.) *Sigmund Freud, Gesammelte Werke*. London: Imago, 1948. Frankfurt: S. Fischer, 1963, Bd. XIV, 383–396.

Freud, S. (1928b). Humour. In J. Strachey (Ed. and Trans.) *Standard Edition*. London: Hogarth, 1961.

Jappe, G. (1971). *Über Wort und Sprache in der Psychoanalyse.* Frankfurt: S. Fischer.

Jappe, G. (1980). Anmerkungen zum Motiv der Kästchenwahl. In *Zur Psychoanalyse der Objektbeziehung.* Stuttgart-Bad Cannstadt: Frommann-Holzboog.

Khan, M. (1983). *Entfremdung bei perversionen.* (dt. v. W. Klüwer). Frankfurt: Suhrkamp.

Kris Study Group (1969). The mechanism of denial *Monograph III.* B. Fine, H. Wahldhorn, & E. Joseph (Eds.). New York: International Universities Press.

Wangh, M. (1985). Die Herrschaft des Thanatos: Über die Bedeutung der Drohung eines Nuklearen Krieges und der Einfluß dieser Drohung auf die psychoanalytische Theoriebildung. In C. Nedelmann (Ed.): *Zur Psychoanalyse der nuklearen Drohung.* Göttingen: Vandenhoeck u. Ruprecht.

6

Concerning Certain Vicissitudes of Denial in Personality Development

Michael Frederic Chayes

How quaint the ways of paradox,
At common sense she gaily mocks!

Trio: Frederick, Ruth, and the Pirate King
The Pirates of Penzance

What follows is not intended to convey a definitive statement, but rather to give an impression of the development of certain ideas, undergoing change. The lines of argument and tentative conclusions proposed here seem to me to follow naturally by extension from the work of Freud and certain others after him, as well as from my own clinical and introspective experience and understanding. Proceeding from the more general to the more particular, I propose to comment upon our conceptions of defensive operations in general, especially the relationship between denial and repression. In doing this, I will favor a fundamentally unitary concept of the development of defense. Subsequently, I will touch upon certain aspects of the development and vicissitudes of denial in particular, focusing especially on the importance I would attribute to this mode

Michael Frederic Chayes • Private Practice, Burmanstraat 9 hs., 1091 SG Amsterdam, The Netherlands.

of defense for the separation–individuation phase of development and on the roles herein of drive-cathected vision, of "mirroring," of introjection and projection, and of early identification processes. The degree to which pregenital aggression will have been successfully integrated (or not) at the close of this phase will be proposed as the most crucial factor in determining whether denial mechanisms will ultimately have either a chiefly healthy–creative or a mainly pathological–destructive role in the personality organization.

Analysts tend to cherish a bias against the value of denial, doubtless in part because our attention has been primarily focused not on its more benign derivative forms but on its effects in those cases where it produces grossly pathological distortion in the appreciation of, and ability to deal appropriately with, reality. Our orientation toward defenses in general tends to be dualistic: They are inevitable and necessary, whereas at the same time, they are expressive of, or at the root of, more or less pronounced pathology. In fact, of course, *no* mental mechanism—with the possible exception of repression (see later)—is solely and exclusively pathological or solely and exclusively defensive (Wälder, 1930); all depends on its role and functioning within the total personality. The fact that a number of different authors (e.g., Breznitz, 1983; Grunberger, 1975; Winnicott, 1951—to name just three) without apparently having been influenced by one another's work, arrived at the conclusion that denial in the form of illusion (including play) can have, or definitely *does* have, an important beneficial function for both the developing and the adult personality, strongly suggesting that there must be something substantial in favor of this position. It seems clear that denial shows a wide range of variations in its degree of differentiation and elaboration, from the most crude, massive, and primitive to the most subtle, discrete, and refined. Stewart (1970) has presented strong arguments in favor of uncoupling the term for the mechanism from that designating the pathology, that is, to speak not of *neurotic denial* or *psychotic denial*, but rather of *denial in neurosis* and *denial in psychosis*.

Specific defense mechanisms have been enumerated, and attempts to classify them developmentally have been undertaken (cf. Anna Freud, 1936, 1965, 1969, 1970). We can identify them on the basis of their effects in a descriptive, clinical sense, but we know very little about their dynamic mode of functioning, their component mechanisms, and the manner in which these components cooperate (see, e.g., Sandler & Sandler, 1983). One characteristic of both repression and denial is that neither of them operates in isolation: Repression will be assisted, for example, when need be, by projection and denial; denial will regularly be assisted by projection, projective identification, and acting out (see, e.g., Kernberg, 1984).[1]

While preparing the present chapter, it struck me that we lack a fundamentally unitary hypothesis describing the development of defensive processes (cf. also Sjöbäck, 1973), as if we were seeing the branches and fruit of a tree that seems to have no trunk. (I do not intend to dwell here on the neuropsychological and psychophysiological building blocks or prototypes of denial such as have been dealt with by Spitz, 1961.) In addition, I became convinced that justice could not be done to the question of the vicissitudes of the denial mechanism if I were to disregard what seemed to be a basic and unmistakable relationship to repression. From what follows, you will see that my position implies an integration into object relations theory of drive and instinct theory, and ego psychology (cf. Kernberg, 1976, 1980) (favoring object relations theory, which, it is my impression, is and has long been widely misunderstood).

In a noteworthy article by Cohen and Kinston (1984), a coherent and continuous hypothesis of repression is proposed. The authors believe there is a need for an attempt such as theirs because inconsistencies and discontinuities in Freud's ideas concerning repression ("primal" versus ordinary repression; mechanism of action; age at which it becomes established) had rendered the theory of repression alone insufficient when it came to explaining defensive phenomena in narcissistic personality, borderline states, and psychosis, and had led Melanie Klein and others to postulate in such cases the operation of other defensive processes that could not be subsumed under repression. They trace the source of such inconsistencies to Freud's relative disregard of the importance of the role of the environment in early development. In Cohen and Kinston's article, a distinction is established between so-called "primal repression" and what they call "repression proper," the latter denoting a secondary repressive activity aimed against inner percepts or ideas *associatively linked* to the material being maintained under primal repression. The latter material they conceive of more or less in accordance with object relations theory (Fairbairn, 1952; M. Klein, 1946) and Winnicott's conception of the facilitating or mediating environment. One of their conclusions, for which they offer evidence, is that primal repression may occur at *any* time during life, from earliest infancy through adulthood, because it is a result of a failure in the indispensable mediation of, or facilitation by the environment, in meeting a need of the individual so

---

[1]There are grounds for viewing projective identification as a special type of denial, that is, denial by means of action or dramatization.

that the need can be structured as a wish and an aim, with an object.[2] *Note, then, that if it is true that primal repression may occur from earliest infancy, then the onset of the use of denial, if indeed it is the more archaic of the two mechanisms, need not antedate that of repression by more than the merest minimal interval.* As for the other defense mechanisms, which the authors (I think, correctly) consider to be of a different order from that of repression, they resolve the dilemma by calling these "manipulations," which are carried out either with the mediating environment (Winnicott), when trauma and primal repression have occurred early and are massive in nature; *or,* with mental contents, when conflict has been more or less successfully internalized. Unlike Cohen and Kinston, I would not place denial on a par with these other mechanisms, as I am inclined to view denial or repudiation, together with splitting-off, to be the precursor or progenitor of all the other defensive manipulations. (If "denial", very generally speaking, denotes the rejection, falsification or distortion of inner or outer reality, then an element of denial is present in *all* defensive operations.)[3]

In a past paper, Dorpat (1983) concluded that what has been termed *splitting* should in fact be considered to be identical to denial. In preparing his argument, he cites a paragraph in Melanie Klein's 1946 paper, "Notes on Some Schizoid Mechanisms." I was pleasantly struck by the fact that he here referred to exactly the same paragraph that had stuck in my mind as of great significance, though as you will presently see, the meaning that I derive from it differs from that attributed by Dorpat. I shall return presently to question whether in denial the individual also attacks his own thinking processes, a matter which Dorpat finds difficult to accept as put forward by Bion (1959).

Fairbairn (1952), distinctly departing from Freud's structural model (see Kernberg, 1980), envisioned a *splitting off of portions of the ego in libidinal or aggressive relation to internalized object representations* and equated splitting not with denial but with repression itself. Rubens (1984), reviewing Fairbairn's ideas, makes a good case for the conclusion that in fact it is *psychic structure itself* (not structure in the sense of increasing elaboration and differentiation, but in the sense conceived in the struc-

---

[2]Cohen and Kinston also conceive of healthy personality development as meaning development *without repression* (and they offer evidence to show that such a thing may indeed exist). Among other conclusions, they state that pathological development should be viewed as the cause, not a result, of the Oedipus complex.

[3]Certain differences between my own views and those of Kinston that emerged in personal discussion would lead too far afield if enumerated here, but, in my opinion, these do not detract from the essence of the present argument.

tural model) that is equated by Fairbairn with *pathology;* and absence of, or freedom from such structure, with health.

A Dutch analyst, Le Coultre, in a paper published over 20 years ago (Le Coultre, 1966), argues convincingly that splitting of the ego is the central phenomenon in *every* neurosis, illustrating his case with examples ranging from the markedly narcissistically fixated up to and including more simply and purely Oedipal pathology. Whether or not Le Coultre was familiar with the ideas of Fairbairn and Klein is uncertain; in any event he does not refer to them, and his argument follows a different line from theirs. The following summary gives the essence of the steps in his reasoning, more or less as recapitulated by himself:

> The "id" is a mere abstraction, which Freud himself characterized as able only to wish, and no more than that. The very moment the id engages external reality it becomes an ego, and we are no longer justified in referring to it as *id;* at most, as *ego-id.* The ego, in turn, cannot maintain its existence as an ego unless it accepts the drives. What we are accustomed to calling "primary-process thinking" does not, in fact, differ in the essential characteristics of its method of reasoning from so-called "secondary-process thinking," but is merely more childish, magically oriented as to causation, less knowledgeable, less critical and less sophisticated. Moreover, what we call the "reality principle" is nothing more than a more refined, mature and realistic form of the pleasure principle. The conflicts of infantile psychosexual development take place *in the ego,* between opposing tendencies in this ego that is invested with drives and *not* between the ego and the id. In neurotic development, when conflict cannot be resolved in an appropriate fashion, a makeshift primitive way out is chosen, that is, that of splitting off a portion of the infantile ego, which henceforth will not participate in further development. In analytic practice we are dealing with an ego that is split into an adult portion and an infantile portion. The former is typically more controlled and relatively impoverished in respect to drive as compared with the latter. In analysis, which aims to overcome the split and achieve integration of the two portions of the ego, the infantile ego emerges in the transference neurosis in the relationship with the analyst.

As you can see, the ideas of Le Coultre show a high degree of correspondence with those of the object relations theorists and also imply a proposed revision of the tripartite structural model.

To return now to the statement mentioned before, from Klein's 1946 paper, in this article she gives ample credit to Fairbairn (and also to Winnicott), though stressing as well her points of disagreement with him.[4] Speaking of how she conceives of the infant protecting his or her

---

[4]His revision of the theory of psychic structure, which she thinks he ought not to have done; his position that only the "bad," but not the good object or breast is introjected; and what she considers to be his underestimation of the role played by hate and destructiveness in early mental life.

introjected idealized good object from destruction by the bad, frustrating–persecuting introject, she writes:

> The bad object is not only kept apart from the good one but its very existence
> is denied, as is the whole situation of frustration and the bad feelings (pain) to
> which frustration gives rise. This is bound up with denial of psychic reality.
> The denial of psychic reality becomes possible only through strong feelings
> of omnipotence—an essential characteristic of early mentality. Omnipotent
> denial of the existence of the bad object and of the painful situation is in the
> unconscious equal to annihilation by the destructive impulse. *It is, however, not
> only a situation and an object that are denied and annihilated—IT IS AN OBJECT
> RELATION which suffers this fate; and therefore a part of the ego, from which the
> feelings towards the object emanate, is denied and annihilated as well.* (Klein, 1946
> [emphases mine])

Considering the foregoing exposition, I think it not rash to say that
what Klein seems to be giving us here is in fact nothing other than a
description of *primal repression*. For it now seems to me that the establishment of primal repression is effectuated by denial or repudiation, acting
together with a splitting-off operation. It would seem as if we are seduced by our own terminology into seeing artificial discontinuities between phenomena that in fact are continuous.

This, then, would be the first vicissitude of the denial mechanism,
which, once primal repression has been firmly established, is then no
longer recognizable as such. This would also clarify why, when the stability of massive or primal repression is seriously threatened by increased conflictual pressure or anxiety, denial, (once again) recognizable
as such, is seen to be operative in an attempt to restore a stable defensive
equilibrium. The foregoing also helps me to better understand something that has puzzled me from time to time in my clinical work, namely
that there always seemed to have been two quite different kinds of
repression and/or two kinds of target for repression, one discrete (corresponding to "repression proper"), operating in discernible form only
briefly and directed against particular ideas or affects and *not* employing
denial as an ancillary defense; and another (corresponding to "primal
repression"), which seemed to act massively to ward off *entire conflicts*
between an unintegrated infantile portion of the *person* ("ego," as used
by Le Coultre, 1966; cf. Rubens, 1984, on Kernberg, 1980) and primitive internal *object representations,* one or other of the roles being projected onto the analyst in the transference (a state of affairs with which,
of course, we are all familiar at a clinical level). This latter type of
repression paradoxically becomes manifest through the fact of its weakening or lifting, and one regularly can observe that denial is called into
play to buttress the repression as it starts to fail. This also clarifies for me
something else that I regularly experience in my work and that has been

explicity formulated by Margaret Little (1981) and that, as a fact of clinical experience, should be familiar to all analysts; namely that the appearance of (periods of) delusional transference is not limited to frankly psychotic or borderline cases but also occurs in other diagnostic categories such as hysterical characters, perversions, character disorders, psychosomatic conditions, and so forth.

I shall now attempt to touch upon certain concepts that would seem to be of fundamental importance for understanding the ultimate fate of the denial mechanism in the personality.

Let me say that I proceed from an assumption of primary subjective omnipotence (Winnicott, 1951) at the beginning of life, with genuine object relatedness gradually developing in increasing increments and in favorable circumstances being crowned by the establishment of object constancy at about 36 months, the close of the separation–individuation phase. Let us assume, for the sake of seeing where the development of the argument will lead us, that the two fundamental root operations of repression, and of many other defenses, are denial and splitting off, and that denial in turn has two components, an active and a passive one: repudiation or rejection, and withdrawal of attention.

Once the infant has gotten to the point where we can speak of *thinking,* of *mentation,* he or she is also at a point where *mental operations* are no longer mere neurophysiological sequences but *analogous representations, by extension, of body activity* undergoing integration. Thus mental repudiation or rejection would probably be the psychical analogon of ejection, evacuation, or repulsion by either the striped-muscle or the smooth-muscle apparatus, the earliest of which is spitting out (Spitz, 1957, 1961); withdrawal of attention would be modeled on deflecting the gaze or closing the eyes; and splitting off, on biting (see also later text).

At what age can we justifiably conceive of the beginning of mentation? The difficulty about relying solely upon investigations of the type carried out by Mahler *et al.* (1975) in seeking to answer this question is that the observations derived from such work, although of inestimable and indispensable value, depend very much upon manifestations of motility, upon a certain degree of development in the use of language, and of course upon expressions of *affect.* But, there are grounds for supposing that before the use of language develops, thinking, of a symbolic and pictorial kind, has already begun (Castoriadis-Aulaignier, 1976; Klein, 1930; Pines, 1984). Without venturing a guess about at just what age real mentation can be said to appear, it seems not unreasonable to suppose that such processes are already operative in infants under 6 months of age. I do not consider myself a Kleinian, and I am not arguing that the whole of psychosexual development should be "telescoped" into the first 6 months of life, to use Kernberg's (1980) phrase. But I *can* conceive, and I *have* witnessed strongly suggestive clinical evidence that, for example, Oedipal configurations in the sense of early triangular object relations, in which love, jealousy, hate and fear are operative may commence well before genital strivings have become the locus of these configurations; and I *have* seen suggestive evidence, and I *can* conceive of the operation, for example, of what we call phallic strivings and phallic conflict long before the genitals have been invested as the specific locus of these strivings and conflicts (I am not here referring to precocious genitalization that may occur under strain, cf. Greenacre, 1968).[5]

By the time the denial mechanism has become incorporated in the constellation we know as "manic defense," we are now already dealing with a complex, sophisticated, and highly integrated, albeit—in terms of object relations—primitive and magical psychic weapon to parry and to compensate narcissistic injury when the mediating environment does not respond adequately to the child's need. Winnicott (1935) describes manic defense as characterized by a combination of omnipotent manipulation or control and contemptuous devaluation of the object. There is denial of inner reality, particularly of heavy or depressive sensations, and a flight to external reality:

> Conflict is centered in the layer of *mood*. Low is denied by high, death by life, depression by elation [cf. Lewin, 1950]. In the analysis of mood, in the context of this period of development, to feel afraid or depressed means to be small, castrated, weak and contemptible [in the eyes of a ruthless, archaic superego; at this stage of development, one may question whether superego and ego ideal are fully differentiated, one from the other]. The swindler and the imposter escape from [deny] this utterly catastrophic self-valuation by foisting it [projection] upon those whom they deceive: To trust is to be a fool, a "sucker."

---

[5]The value, to me, of Klein's work and the ideas of the Kleinians, lies chiefly in the conception that thought and conflict may begin earlier than has been assumed and that it follows patterns specific to the particular stage of development in which it occurs. I have found Kleinian concepts of early mental conflict to be useful in understanding and interpreting deeply regressive phenomena at a clinical level, without having to embrace the whole of Kleinian metapsychology or having to resort to crudeness of interpretation. Controversy among analysts concerning this area has a long history (cf. Riviere, 1936, and Wälder, 1937), during which the scientific attitude that one would deem desirable unfortunately often seems to have been beclouded by considerations of prestige and personal rivalry (see, e.g., Steiner, 1985). However, interest in earliest mental development persists (see, e.g., the excellent review of recent work by Pines, 1988), and the findings seem to point very much in the direction of the plea I am making here.

For this manipulation and devaluation, we should perhaps assume at least an incipient degree of development in hand–(eye–mouth) coordination and perhaps also of anality. (One must, of course, keep in mind that, in the child or regressed adult in analysis, what we see clinically is *not* identical to the state of affairs that existed in the psyche at the time of very early trauma because further development, however distorted by what has gone before, will have added new defensive operations that are superimposed upon, and have become incorporated with, the original defensive equipment.)

In referring just now to a "psychic weapon," I do not think I use the term ill-advisedly: I would view manic defense as the first highly organized pyschical analogon of the body's physiological response to exceptional stress, when the individual's narcissistic homeostasis is seriously threatened; and as such, as an expression of fundamental vitality. There would seem to be a close relationship between manic defense and the counterphobic attitude; as "fight" in contrast to "flight." Phobic patients have notoriously intense castration anxiety of very early origin and rely heavily on manic defense to counteract this anxiety (J. Bégoin, 1983). It has been observed as well that there exists no other attack that matches the brutality, the viciousness, the mercilessness, and the fury of that by the phobic when he or she feels cornered by the object of his or her phobia (M. Fain, 1983). And my own clinical experience, as far as it goes, confirms this. What I am arguing is for the recognition of denial and manic defense *as reservoirs of the aggression* that must evolve and become integrated into better adapted forms that will remain part of the mature individual's indispensable equipment for advancing his or her legitimate interests in the business of surviving and living.

I would also propose, as a criterion for analyzability that I have not met elsewhere in these terms, that we look in the life history not only for evidence of the individual's potential for containing and tolerating depression but also for evidence of a *capacity to use* (respond to) *trauma creatively,* a resilient turning the tables on misfortune that must draw heavily on a type of denial; in which the primitive mechanism of turning passive into active operates in a constructive fashion, that is, consonant with the vital interests of the individual. (Of course, as analysts, we are aware that the psychic pain that is warded off catches up one way or another with the individual and that there is still a job to be done.)

To turn now to the question of when denial is pathological, and when not, and why, I return to the conclusion that seemed to present itself just now: namely that repression apparently always implies at least some degree of pathology and that (I propose that) primal repression seems to be effectuated by a combination of denial with a splitting-off operation. If this is true, then we can conceive of situations in which denial need not necessarily act in conjunction with splitting; that it need not necessarily lead to repression; and that it need not always be pathological.

Let us begin by examining a feature of that most studied paradigm of denial, fetishism. Freud (1924, 1938), who finally relinquished the belief that the fetishist's appreciation of reality was necessarily worse than the neurotic's, concluded that it was chiefly a question of a difference in the mechanism engaged to deal with the conflict, that is, splitting of the ego instead of repression, that distinguished the two from each other; and that, in fetishism, a consciously held rational belief was manifested side by side with the expression of an unconsciously held, irrational belief that opposed it. He also recognized the use of this mechanism in other areas besides fetishism. Jacobson (1957) considered denial to be characterized by the presence of *both sides of a conflict,* in the form of opposing ideas, *in the ego* (rather than divided between ego and id), where one idea is employed to deny the other. She also pointed out that in fetishism, *one false belief,* that is, that the woman has a penis, is used to deny *a second false belief,* that is, that the woman has been castrated (lost her penis) (see later text).

It was Freud, then, who already acknowledged with his idea of a "third possibility" between neurosis and psychosis, the have-your-cake-and-eat-it-too orientation of the fetishist and of other persons employing the same mechanism. This attitude corresponds to Winnicott's concept of *paradox* characterizing what he called the *third area of experience* (Winnicott, 1951, 1971), which begins with transitional phenomena in the infant some time from 4 months onwards (with individual variations). The transitional object is both "me" and "not-me," and one cannot challenge it by posing the question whether it has been found or created by the infant. In favorable circumstances, this develops into the capacity for the experience of *illusion,* which remains important to the adult to be able to draw upon in bridging the inevitable discrepancy between inner and outer reality (Winnicott, 1951, 1958, 1971). Children's play, of course, which gives them for the first time a degree of autonomy vis-à-vis the mother (Grunberger, 1953), is denial in the form of illusion.

In psychoanalysis, this intermediate area of experience operates as a buffer (Chayes, 1978; Freud, 1914) against catastrophic disillusionment in the unfolding of transference—countertransference phantasy (Green, 1975). This is Winnicott's concept of the use of "potential space," which is also characterized by paradox: that is, through the elaboration of illusion, which fills it, the potential space not only separates, but also connects self with object.

Greenacre (1960, 1968, 1969, 1970), who recognized the early growth-promoting function of the transitional object as opposed to the fetish (which she termed "a focal stopgap for a failure in separation and body ego identity, rendering further development possible, but with a defect") has compared the two phenomena on the basis of their similarities and differences. Both are illusory phenomena. Referring to the bivalence of both the fetish and the transitional object, she uses the term *Janus-faced*. She also applies this term to the quality characterizing the beginning of imitative identification with the mother at the end of the first and beginning of the second year. Greenacre's "Janus-faced" refers, I am certain, to the same bivalent quality to which Winnicott refers as "paradox." Now, going back for a moment to Winnicott, I quote from his original statement, later modified (1951/1975, p. 5):

> In health the transitional object . . . loses meaning . . . because the transitional phenomena have become diffused . . . over the whole cultural field . . . . At this point my subject widens out into that of play, and of artistic creativity and appreciation, and of religious feeling, and of dreaming, and also of fetishism, lying and stealing, the origins and loss of affectionate feeling, drug addiction, the talisman of obsessional rituals, etc.

To this series, we might add wit and humor, ridicule, and the secret (cf. Greenacre, 1958a,b, 1960, 1969a,b); further, the character typologies of the imposter, of the swindler, of other delinquents and of the traitor; and finally, latent or frank psychosis.

Let us examine the pathological end of this series. Whereas normally transference is a ubiquitous phenomenon and our experience of reality is invested by projections from our inner world (cf. Chayes, 1982; Loewald, 1951; Modell, 1969), psychotic persons before the outbreak of the manifest psychosis may compensate by means of a so-called syndrome of hyperrealism, or by the use of a symbiotic partner, as described by Racamier (1980) (cf. Searles, 1965). In the former, the antiprojective barrier is so rigid that the external world seems dead and unreal. When the antiprojective barrier breaks down, external reality becomes flooded with persecutory meaning and the psychosis becomes manifest. In the latter, the symbiotic partner is manipulated so as to respond as a representation of the split-off and projected part of the patient's ego. Abandonment by the symbiotic partner often induces the outbreak of the psychosis.

Jacobson's patient (1957), though perhaps, as she states, not psychotic, nevertheless seemed to me definitely to have a thought disorder, as a consequence of which he experienced affects as though they were discrete *things*. Though Jacobson attributes this to the action of denial, this seems to me to be only partly true: the advanced degree of *fragmen-*

tation in her patient I would attribute in the first place to the effects of repeated *splitting-off* operations. What her patient had to *deny* was not only (as she writes) his deep early *love* for his mother, but, linked to this love, his *archaic guilt* about the magical omnipotent fulfilment of his destructive wishes. The guilt is experienced at age 3 as a narcissistic trauma, and in view of the incomplete separation from the mother at this age, it is possible that the guilt trauma only achieved its pathogenic effect by virtue of the mother's ensuing depression, after her miscarriage. The need that Jacobson's patient had to magically transform the expression on his girlfriend's face through the induction of sexual ecstasy supports this idea.

Searles (1969) describes the analysis of a man with a borderline thought disorder. In the course of analysis, it became understood that the patient had to deny *any* affect in himself because every affective reaction meant to him that he had been successfully *manipulated* by others.

Thinking, I venture to say, must have as its basis *an internalized interaction or dialogue with an introject or internal object representation.* This brings us close to Dorpat's (1983) question whether it is conceivable that an individual would be likely to attack and break up his own thought processes, as suggested by Bion (1959). It is a fact of clinical experience that severely narcissistic patients, when disappointed by the object, cannot combine the two poles of their extreme ambivalence and will magically murder the beloved and loving aspect of the object *and* the part of themselves that loves the object and is loved by it (cf. Klein, 1946), by severing all associative connections with, and denying this part; thus, losing contact with that very part of themselves without which they cannot live (Green, 1979). Dialogue with the loving and beloved aspect of the primary object becomes inaccessible when this part of the ego has been split off, and it seems to me that it would be impossible that this loss, which often must be maintained by repeated splitting operations, would not be disruptive to thinking processes. (Note that this statement implies that thinking processes in such personality structures are not fully autonomous with respect to their introjects.)

Now, how may all this fit into the separation–individuation process, with its differentiation, practising, and critical rapprochement subphases? For the achievement of individuation, one might postulate the cooperation of four general kinds of mental processes (not counting motility and speech): (1) differentiation; (2) introjection/projection and identification; (3) transitional phenomena; and (4) negotiation of, and ultimately tolerance for, ambivalence conflict, leading to object constancy.

Differentiation might be envisioned as taking place in accordance with certain main axes or ordinates, oriented between opposing polarities that are linked with and influence one another and among which one might discern (more can be conceived of):

1. *Corporeal:* One body, fusional $\rightleftharpoons$ two-body, *split*
2. *Energic-affective:* Love (fusional) $\rightleftharpoons$ hate (*splitting,* distancing, evacuating)
3. *Gender:* a. Self: Male $\rightleftharpoons$ Female
         b. Object: Female $\rightleftharpoons$ Male
4. *Narcissistic:* Ideal/complete/perfect $\rightleftharpoons$ damaged/incomplete/imperfect
5. *Mood:* High $\rightleftharpoons$ low

It can be seen here that "splitting" has both a corporeal and an energic-affective component and that denial itself is bivalent: Either polarity may be denied, so that we have both a fusional and a separational type of denial, so to speak. The balance between these two would seem to depend largely upon the environmental response: "good-enough mothering" and "primary maternal preoccupation" (Winnicott, 1956a), which ties in the narcissistic ordinate and the management of ambivalence, where a healthy acceptance of aggression must find its place. The extremes of affect and ambivalence during this period must, I think, make for *instability of valence,* with sometimes rapid switching back and forth between polarities. In the best way, this quality may be preserved in an area of the future personality where it fosters imagination and creativity. (It has been noted that phobic persons are often gifted, creative individuals.) In the worst way, it may issue in permanently paralyzing extreme ambivalence or in untrustworthiness and unreliability. The existence, before the establishment of object constancy, of polarities of such extremes and intensities that they cannot be combined and integrated into a unified whole, implies that in early mental life, once recognition (pain) of a separateness of self from object has begun, a *split* into "good object" and "bad object" must be a *given,* that is, an inescapable intermediate state of affairs universally met with; and that this original *rift* provides the genetic developmental basis, either for fixation at this stage, or/and for later regressive employment of splitting, together with denial, as an extreme defensive measure. (Primal repression and loss of a part of the ego then result.)

Conflicts that are oriented between polarities along axes such as those which I have just indicated, are those that A. O. Kris (1982, cited by Treurniet, 1984) has called "conflicts of ambivalence," in contradistinction to conflicts between or among the three agencies of the psyche according to the tripartite model, which he calls "conflicts of defense." It can easily be argued that the latter so-called conflicts of defense represent merely a special category (class) of ambivalence conflict. However, the point that I should like to stress is that the ubiquity of conflict, rooted in conflict between opposing polarities, and which is one of the essential principles and features of psychoanalytic psychology, derives from or is patterned on the basic physiological—anatomical organization of the nervous system acting on its effector organs: namely the operation in pairs of agonists and antagonists. On both the neurophysiological and the psychical level, well-modulated, evenly matched and finely balanced synergy between agonists and antagonists, or between opposing tendencies, respectively, is a criterion of maturity and good integration. (This approach to the phenomena can be carried through and applied to higher levels of psychic integration, so that, for example, such complex affective states as shame and pride, respectively, can be viewed as the opposing polarities on an ordinate characterized by prominence of exhibitionistic phantasy.)

As regards the establishment of gender identity, Greenacre (1968) has pointed out that concern about castration in the boy and penis envy in the girl are already observable in the second year of life and are colored by anal conflicts at this age; and that *vision* in the sense of excessive exposure to the genitals of the opposite sex and/or the witnessing of wounds or accidents contributes to confusion about gender identity and to castration fears. A family with a dominant mother and a weak or absent father further complicates achievement of a firm gender identity for the boy. Concerning the *fetish*, Greenacre (1969) stresses its "Janus-faced" quality, saying (p. 321) that "the fetish is conspicuously a bisexual symbol and also serves as a bridge which would *both deny and affirm* the sexual difference" (my italics). This is an extremely important point that is too often overlooked, that is, that the fetish also represents for the fetishist his own penis, which he incorporates visually to reassure his fragile sense of maleness in the presence of exposure to the woman's genitals. "To not want to see," literally or figuratively, is characteristic for denial, which is essentially seeing something in order *not* to see something else.

This brings me to the importance of "mirroring" for processes of introjection and identification. It was first Lacan who in 1936 called attention to the 6-month infant's introjection of his own external image seen in the mirror. In this essay, Lacan also reminds us that maturation of the ovary in the female pigeon will only occur *if she sees another pigeon, or her own reflection in a mirror,* before a certain age has passed. Similar phenomena are known in other animal species.

Winnicott (1967/1971) has written of the importance of the mirroring function of mother and family for the developing sense of identity. Pines (1984) has published a long article on mirroring, including the evolution of types of mirroring according to stage of development. He points out the advantages, for differentiation, of mirroring by other people as opposed to mirroring by the glass. He also points out the "Janusian" quality of mirroring, in uniting opposites that are simultaneously identities.[6]

All this strongly suggests that there is reason to believe that *through introjection by vision, we become what we see;* and that this process may be biologically rooted as well.

Once some degree of internal object representation has been established by the process of ongoing introjection, *and once this representation remains present for a certain length of time before being lost,* illusional use of the introject (in the sense of transitional phenomena) can get started, leading to increasing tolerance of the mother's absence. *This is denial as self/object fusion, or incorporation, in the service of establishing autonomy,* and issuing ultimately in stable basic identifications. In a compact and persuasive article, Nicolas Abraham (1978) attempts to show that separation–individuation is achieved *solely* through introjection, in doing which, I think he pushes his case a bit too far. Nevertheless, his ideas, to which I cannot do full justice here, seem extremely valuable. He views the duplicity, or *loss of innocence,* which accompanies the establishment of an introject with the attendant origin of autonomy vis-à-vis the primary object, as the fundamental source of an irrational sense of guilt that is present in *all* cases of neurosis.

Mirroring between persons, of the most primitive, spontaneous kind, that is, before internalized reflectiveness has become established (or before it comes into play), is characterized by the fact that every action elicits a reflected opposing reaction of the same kind from the facing party and particularly so when the context is one of aggression. In this connection I recall to you a second meaning of the word *denial,* which I think I may be justified in doing if indeed the English also denotes an additional or further aspect of the mechanism that is omitted or overlooked when one remains faithful to the German word *Verleugnung: to deny* also means *to refuse (another person's) wish or request.* This, in relation to introjection and identification through mirroring, has bearing on identification with the frustrating object; with the manner in which the frustration is imposed; and on the projections with which the child in-

[6]The identity or equivalence of opposites in the unconscious is manifested in dreams, and in langauge, where the archaic meanings of words are not infrequently the opposite of their current meanings. As the French say: *"Les extrèmes se touchent."*

vests the object; that is *identification with the aggressor* on the basis of mirroring, being *denial as a retaliation for being-denied* (in wish or self). The basis of the *talion law* that rules our unconscious resides, in my opinion, in the role played by mirroring at a time well before separation from the primary object has been effectuated. (Indeed, the superego betrays its earliest origins as situated prior to this time.)

To conclude, I hope to have at least raised some useful questions about the vicissitudes of the denial mechanism and to have shown that it need not always have a pathological significance or function. If, at the close of the separation–individuation phase of development, a reasonable tolerance for ambivalence has not been achieved and basic security and object constancy are not well established, then primal repression of parts of the ego will portend potentially serious trouble: a narcissistic skew in the development of object relations, psychopathy, borderline states, psychosis, and so forth. If denial in the form of illusion can be used creatively and to strengthen autonomy, rather than as a refuge from object relations with which the individual cannot cope and that must be phobically avoided, then denial mechanisms will have found a place in psychic health.

REFERENCES

Abraham, N., & Torok, M. (1978). Le 'Crime' de l'Introjection. In *L'Ecorce et le Noyau* (pp. 123–131). Paris: Aubier-Flammarion.

Bégoin, J. (1983). Intervention at Séminaire de Perfectionnement No. XXV. Paris, January 1983, on "L'après-coup des phobies infantiles."

Bion, W. (1959). Attacks on linking. *International Journal of Psychoanalysis, 40,* 308–315.

Breznitz, S. (Ed.). (1983). *The denial of stress.* New York: International Universities Press.

Castoriadis-Aulaignier, P. (1976). *La violence de l'interpretation.* Paris: Presses Universitaires de France.

Chayes, M. F. (1978). Psychotherapie is Medisch. In *Tijdschrift voor Psychiatrie,* nr.7-8/1978, pp. 427–449.

Chayes, M. F. (1982). *Psychoanalyse en Realiteit.* Paper given at joint meeting of the Dutch and Belgian Psychoanalytic Societies, November 1980; in *Inval,* nr.1/1982, pp. 625–634.

Cohen, J., & Kinston, W. (1984). Repression theory: A new look at the cornerstone. *International Journal of Psychoanalysis, 65,* 411–422.

Coultre, Le, R. (1966). Splijting van het ik als centraal neuroseverschijnsel. In *Psychoanalytische Thema's en Variaties.* Deventer: van Loghum Slaterus.

Dorpat, T. L. (1983). The cognitive arrest hypothesis of denial. *The International Journal of Psychoanalysis, LXIV,* 47–58.

Fain, M. (1983). Intervention at Sémenaire de Perfectionnement No. XXV. Paris, 1983, on "L'après-coup des phobies infantiles."

Fairbairn, W. R. D. (1952). *Psychoanalytic studies of the personality.* London: Routledge & Kegan Paul.

Freud, A. (1936). *The ego and the mechanisms of defence.* London: Hogarth.

Freud, A. (1941). On certain difficulties in the pre-adolescent's relation to his parents. In *Indications for child analysis and other papers,* 1945–1956. London: Hogarth.

Freud, A. (1965). *Normality and pathology in childhood.* New York: International Universities Press.

Freud, A. (1970). The symptomatology of childhood: A preliminary attempt at classification. *The Psychoanalytic Study of the Child, 25,* 19–41.

Freud, S. (1914). Remembering, repeating and working through. *Standard Edition* (Vol. 12). London: Hogarth.

Freud, S. (1924). Neurosis and psychosis. *Standard Edition* (Vol. 19). London: Hogarth.

Freud, S. (1938). Splitting of the ego in the process of defence. *Standard Edition* (Vol. 23). London: Hogarth.

Green, A. (1975). The analyst, symbolisation and absence in the analytic setting, (On changes in analytic practice and analytic experience). *The International Journal of Psychoanalysis, 56,* 1–22.

Green, A. (1979). L'Angoisse et le narcissisme. *Revue Française de Psychanalyse,* Tome XLIII, nr.1, Jan.–Feb. 1979, pp. 45–88.

Greenacre, P. (1958a). The imposter. In *Emotional Growth* (pp. 93–112). New York: International Universities Press.

Greenacre, P. (1958b). The relation of the imposter to the artist. In *Emotional Growth* (pp. 533–554). New York: International Universities Press.

Greenacre, P. (1959). Play in relation to creative imagination. In *Emotional Growth* (pp. 555–574).

Greenacre, P. (1960). Further notes on fetishism. In *Emotional Growth* (pp. 182–198).

Greenacre, P. (1968). Perversions: General considerations regarding their genetic and dynamic background. In *Emotional Growth* (pp. 300–314).

Greenacre, P. (1969a). The fetish and the transitional object. In *Emotional Growth* (pp. 315–334).

Greenacre, P. (1969b). The nature of treason and the character of traitors. In *Emotional Growth* (pp. 365–396).

Greenacre, P. (1970). The transitional object and the fetish: With special reference to the role of illusion. In *Emotional Growth* (pp. 335–352).

Grunberger, B. (1975). *Le Narcissisme.* Paris: Payot.

Jacobson, E. (1957). Denial and repression. *Journal of the American Psychoanalytic Association,* 61–92.

Kernberg, O. F. (1976). *Object relations theory and clinical psychoanalysis.* New York/London: Jason Aronson.

Kernberg, O. F. (1980). *Internal world and external reality.* New York/London: Jason Aronson.

Kernberg, O. F. (1984). *The influence of projective identification on countertransference.* Paper delivered at International Symposium on Projection, Introjection, and Projective Identification, at The Freud Centre, Hebrew University of Jerusalem, May 1984.

Klein, M. (1930). The importance of symbol-formation in the development of the ego. In *Love, guilt and reparation* (pp. 219–232). London: Hogarth Press.

Klein, M. (1946). Notes on some schizoid mechanisms. In *Envy and gratitude* (pp. 25–42). London: Hogarth Press.

Kris, A. O. (1982). *Free association, method and process.* New Haven: Yale.

Lacan, J. (1936/1949). Le stade du miroir, comme formateur de la fonction du je. *Revue Française de Psychanalyse*, 449–455.

Lewin, B. (1950). *The psychoanalysis of elation.* New York: W. W. Norton.

Little, M. (1981). *Tranference neurosis and transference psychosis—Toward basic unity.* New York: Jason Aronson.

Loewald, H. (1951). Ego and reality. *The International Journal of Psychoanalysis*, XXXII, 10–18.

Mahler, M. S., with Pine, F., & Bergman, A. (1975). *The psychological birth of the human infant.* London: Hutchinson.

Modell, A. (1961). Denial and the sense of separateness. *Journal of the American Psychoanalytic Association*, 533–547.

Modell, A. (1969). *Object love and reality.* London: Hogarth Press.

Pines, M. (1984). Reflections on mirroring. *The International Review of Psychoanalysis*, XI, 27–42.

Pines, M. (1988). Mirroring and child development. *Psychoanalytic Inquiry.*

Racamier, P.-C. (1980). *Les Schizophrènes.* Paris: Payot.

Riviere, J. (1936). On the Genesis of Psychical Conflict in Earliest Infancy. *The International Journal of Psychoanalysis*, XVII, 395–422.

Rubens, R. L. (1984). The meaning of structure in Fairbairn. *The International Review of Psychoanalysis*, 11, 429–440.

Sandler, J., & Sandler, A.-M. (1983). The 'second censorship,' the 'three box model,' and some technical implications. *The International Journal of Psychoanalysis*, 64, 413–425.

Searles, H. F. (1965). The effort to drive the other person crazy—An element in the aetiology and psychotherapy of schizophrenia. *Collected papers on schizophrenia and related subjects.* London: Hogarth Press.

Searles, H. F. (1969). A case of borderline thought disorder. *Countertransference and related subjects.* New York: International Universities Press.

Sjöbäck, H. (1973). *The psychoanalytic theory of defensive processes*, thesis. Lund: Gleerup & New York: Wiley.

Spitz, R. (1957). *No and yes: On the beginnings of human communication.* New York: International Universities Press.

Spitz, R. (1961). Some early prototypes of ego defenses. *Journal of the American Psychoanalytic Association*, 626–651.

Steiner, R. (1985). Some thoughts about tradition and change arising from an examination of the British Psychoanalytic Society's controversial discussions (1943–1944). *The International Review of Psychoanalysis*, 12, 27–71.

Stewart, W. A. (1970). The split in the ego and the mechanism of disavowal. *The Psychoanalytic Quarterly*, 1–16.

Stoller, R. J. (1976). *Perversion: The erotic form of hatred.* Sussex: The Harvester Press, Ltd.

Treurniet, N. (1984). Over recente ontwikkelingen van het psychoanalytisch denken. In *Tijdschrift voor Psychotherapie*, jaargang 10, pp. 232–275.

Wälder, R. (1937). The problem of the genesis of psychical conflict in earliest infancy: Remarks on a paper by Joan Riviere. *The International Journal of Psychoanalysis*, XVIII, 406–473.

Wälder, R. (1930). The principle of multiple function. *Internationale Zietschrift für Psychoanalyse.*

Winnicott, D. W. (1958a). *Psychoanalysis and the sense of guilt.* New York: International Universities Press.

Winnicott, D. W. (1958b). *The capacity to be alone.* New York: International Universities Press.

Winnicott, D. W. (1960). *Ego distortion in terms of true and false self.* New York: International Universities Press.

Winnicott, D. W. (1963a). *The development of the capacity for concern.* New York: International Universities Press.

Winnicott, D. W. (1963b). *Psychotherapy of character disorders.* New York: International Universities Press.

Winnicott, D. W. (1965). *The maturational processes and the facilitating environment.* New York: International Universities Press.

Winnicott, D. W. (1971). *Playing and reality.* London: Tavistock.

7

The Place of Denial in Adult Development

Joel Shanan

The purpose of this chapter is to examine the role of denial in the process of psychological development during later adulthood. This analysis shall be undertaken within an assumptional framework that can be considered an extension of the work of Rapaport (1959, 1967) Hartman (1951) and Federn (1952). It is basically ego-analytical, yet emphasizes the notion of energetic transactions between the individual and the societal context in which the process of development takes place (Shanan, 1976, 1982). According to this line of thought, which represents an attempt to integrate ego psychological with system theoretical thinking, the person can be conceived as a multileveled, open system, embedded in and provided with resources from metasystems of essentially social nature, ranging from the partner in a dyad, through family and reference groups to society or culture at large. In this context, the individual is not conceived as only a passive recipient but as intrinsically active in the construction of his or her personal environment. In this vein, psychological development through the life span can be viewed as a continuous and progressive shift in balance between engagement and disengagement of the person on any given level or across different levels of functioning. Thus development as distinct from maturation is conceived

JOEL SHANAN • Department of Psychology, The Hebrew University of Jerusalem, Jerusalem, Israel.

as a complex process of redistribution of psychic or cathectic energy, leading to reorganization of latent structures and overt patterns of behavior. It not only seems logical but necessary to assume that this process of progressive—and at times also regressive—development requires an active giving up of objects to set free energy necessary for establishing novel engagements and consequently for the reorganization of behavior on progressively higher levels of complexity. In the following, it shall be argued that denial plays an important part in this process of coping with developmental change over time.

Although this should hold true for most or all of the life span, the importance of denial in the process of development during the second half of our adult life deserves special consideration. At this stage of life, denial becomes a means of preserving and enhancing integrity in a context in which engagement in new human and (one may venture to say) most other concrete relationships becomes increasingly difficult, if not impossible. Denial can serve adaptive functions as has been recognized by Goldberger (1983), Lazarus (1983), and others far beyond its role as a defense against external threat of mutilation or death. A better understanding of its role in the process of development could deepen our views on life span development and, in particular, of its later stages. It possibly could also broaden our grasp of the construct of denial and its role in adaptation to change. This would require a revision of the more traditional view of denial as a primitive defense, a forerunner in early childhood of what only later is to become an elaborate system of defense mechanisms characteristic of the fully developed adult ego (A. Freud, 1936). Also required is a revision of the more recent position—popular in clinical and medical circles—that stresses, excessively in our opinion, the adaptive value of denial in face of subjectively perceived unalterable threat of death (Eitinger, 1983).

LIFE-SPAN DEVELOPMENT

Although it is true that Freud has to be credited with making the individual the focus of attention as a legitimate entity of scientific inquiry by demonstrating lawfulness and internal consistency in all or most of his or her behavioral manifestations and of his or her development, it is the sociologist Georg Simmel (1950) who is to be credited for his important contribution to the understanding of what constitutes individuality. As a sociologist, he could not but view the individual as part—or, as we would say today, a subsystem—of society as a whole, the metasystem. This part, the individual, is defined by Simmel in terms of freedom, that is, freedom from ties, that, if existent, would make individuality void of meaning. Yet paradoxically he defines freedom, or independence, in terms of dependence, namely as the capacity to choose on whom and or on what to depend. This is not the place to compare Simmel's position on the place of the individual in society with that implied in some of Freud's major writings such as *Totem and Taboo* (Freud, 1938), *Group Psychology and the Analysis of the Ego* (Freud, 1922), or *Civilisation and Its Discontents* (1930). Generally speaking, it seems to me that Freud's ideas on this issue moved over the years—parallel to the changes in his conceptualization of the ego—into the direction of Simmel's position. Simmel's insightful argument leaves no doubt that no human being can be considered as totally independent from others. This, as we know today empirically, is particularly true from a developmental point of view. On the other hand, Simmel had pointed to the fact that no human being can be considered human if one is not ready to grant him or her—in principle—the potentiality of deciding for himself or herself on whom and/or what to depend, that is, to decide where and what his or her place in society should be.

From this vantage point, as well as for a number of other reasons (Shanan, 1976), one can understand human development throughout the life span as a continuous process of becoming psychologically engaged in new, and simultaneously disengaged from, previous social networks. For the first part of the life span, increasing engagement seems to be characteristic for the course of development. During the second part of life, growing disengagement from social commitments and social frameworks is said to be—and indeed is found in empirical research as well as in the clinic—characteristic of psychosocial development. It is interesting to note (and has been possibly overlooked in the past) that Freud put the emphasis on separation rather than on attachment formation in his theories of psychological development. Freud's reluctance to advise psychoanalysis for "older" patients (who today most probably would be considered "young" or "young old") was based on a decrement model of ego development and on the notion of diminishing energy resources. His main scepticism, however, concerned itself with what today we could call rigidity of ego boundaries, self-perception, and ultimately a lowered capacity to enter into new committments or to establish new bonds. Yet, as we know today, from the clinic and from research, there is a great deal of intra- and interindividual variability in the position of the individual on the dependence—independence and consequently on the engagement—disengagement continuum over the life span. In a series of studies, a good deal of evidence has been accumulated in support of a strong relationship between the position of the indi-

vidual in his or her group in terms of engagement and certain aspects of
ego functioning, which we consider central for adaptation, namely the
level of active coping and coping style (Shanan *et al.*, 1976). These studies were carried out in Jerusalem with projective and semiprojective
instruments, such as Murray's TAT and Shanan's sentence completion
technique (Shanan, 1973). They yielded measures of ego functioning in
terms of extent of readiness to cope actively with challenge or stress.
This level of readiness to cope and to some extent coping style were
found to be invariably contingent upon the extent and type of engagement of the individual in social networks. It appeared that people from
late adolescence through later adulthood are ready and able to cope with
age-specific tasks as a function of availability of resources, intellectual,
emotional, and last but not least, material; all of these are contingent, to
varying degrees, upon engagement in social networks. Examples range
from differences found between orphans and children growing up in
normal two-parent families, juvenile delinquents, and normal youth,
through the capacity to adapt to complex tasks, such as prolonged academic studies or certain aspects of service in the armed forces such as
adjustment to seasickness (Gal & Lazarus, 1975) or adjustment to work
after injury (Wolff & Shanan, 1975), adjustment to contact lenses (Mor,
Shanan, & Levinson, 1973), rehabilitation of hemiplegics after CVA
(Adler *et al.*, 1969) as well as adjustment to prolonged and potentially
lethal diseases such as terminal renal failure (Shanan, Kaplan De Nour,
& Garty, 1976). Not in all cases, however, was the readiness to get involved and to cope actively necessarily correlated with a readiness to
perceive reality in all its complexity. Yet on the whole, the more detached a person was, or disengaged from significant social networks, the
greater became the likelihood of his or her coping on a passive level or in
an essentially passive mode.

It seems therefore legitimate to view individuals on a continuum of
having or lacking access—psychological and/or material—to basic gratifications, offered normally by interaction within a social framework to
which the individual or a group of individuals belongs. A state of belonging in which an individual feels gratified psychologically and materially
in terms of the values of his or her group, that is, the group to which he
or she legitimately feels that he or she belongs, we call (social) engagement. Social disengagement, in its extreme form of social stigma, on the
other hand, would be a state in which an individual is led internally or
externally to give up satisfying ties to a person or group of people whom
earlier he or she had percieved as significant others. Thus the term
engagement refers to a perception on the part of the individual of belonging to a significant group, that is, a group offering him or her basic

gratifications and priviledges considered legitimate in a given social context or society. It may be added—and this is important and frequently overlooked in discussions of the relationships between the individual and society—that one of the major priviledges from a psychological point of view consists of the gratifications obtained by helping, serving, or, broadly speaking, gratifying others. The term *disengagement,* on the other hand, refers to the perception of the individual of her- or himself as lacking access to such basic emotional, interpersonal, or material gratifications as a consequence of disruption of communication with a significant group of others, regardless whether the disruption is real, imaginery, voluntary, or forced. It really implies the idea of certain boundary conditions determining the quality and extent of interaction between the person and his or her environment. This definition differs from that of Cumming and Henry (1961) because the latter refers to a process that is initiated autonomously and perceived subjectively as such.

Theoretically, it should become possible to classify states of social interaction both on a perceptual and on a dynamic level, according to the amount and type of engagement actually observed or perceived by the individual. The type and amount of legitimately expected gratification made inaccessible, or the type and number of significant contacts severed, could mark psychological deprivation. Similarly, different periods of psychological development could be classified in this way and could be viewed as parts of a process during which the individual has to cope continuously with the necessity to engage in new and to disengage from earlier affective and social ties. As a necessary condition to achieve this aim, semipermeable boundaries have to be assumed. Attempts to attain "developmental tasks" (Havighurst, 1952) or to resolve "developmental crises" (Erikson, 1950) could then be viewed as transitional situations or phases in which the developing individual has to disengage her- or himself from a given interpersonal, social or—by the same logic—cognitive network, to be able to subsequently engage in new types of social and cognitive interaction. Such transitional states of incomplete or overlapping, double "belonging" engender lack of security, anxiety, and stress characteristic of conflict situations in general and may result in difficulties to develop and maintain a sense of firm identity, self, or ego.

Such an approach to development and to transitional phases of development removes from its conceptual framework the association with drama and psychopathology, as suggested by the use of such terms as *crisis* as used by some authors on the middle and later years, for example, the more or less literary descriptions of Sheehy (1976) or the somewhat better documented ones of Levinson (1979).

The question, of course, arises, by which means or mechanisms can the individual overcome those conflict-charged states of transition from engagement in one network to engagement in a new and different one. It is here where denial may play an important role in general, and in that phase of development that ushers in old age in particular; that is, in the transition from middle to later adulthood. This period of life that stretches today in Western culture over two decades or more is characterized by an increasing likelihood to lose some of one's old friends, one's spouse and, of course, one's parents. There is also, as research demonstrates, a growing susceptibility to illness and physical threat of death. To these experiences of loss and separation, one has to add the less dramatic but nonetheless difficult task of coping with disengagement from the parental role (Gutmann, 1980) when the children are leaving home. This requires a restructuring of the relationships with the departing children as well as with the spouse. On the instrumental level, too, disengagement becomes necessary as one approaches retirement from work. In this latter process, there is not only the threat of losing a major source of satisfaction and self-esteem but also losing the feeling of belonging to an important social network. (Guillemard & Lenoir, 1974), not to speak, of course, of the threat of losing material support in terms of a lowered income following retirement. Finally the aging person is frequently required, if not compelled to disengage him- or herself from values that had guided him or her during all or a great deal of his or her personal development or at least to readapt the hierchy of his or her value system to shifts due to secular change, occuring in his or her environment. One has to adapt to a new style of life, to a "new brave world" around oneself (Shanan, 1982). All this comes with a growing feeling that time is running out and that death has become a real personal possibility, implying the threat of isolation—forever—from contact with other human beings, that is, a "forced" disengagement (Shanan & Weil, 1977) from this world.

DENIAL

Denial, an unfortunate translation of Freud's term *Verleugnung* (meaning to "lie away," to negate), a noun that implies intentionality, that is, activity in the sense Rapaport uses the term, in denying a supposedly existing reality, has been traditionally distinguished from other similar defense mechanisms and in particular from repression by the fact that it serves as defense against threat from the external environment, as opposed to internal, basically instinctual threat. As such, it can be considered conceptually a derivative of the idea of *Reizschutz* (defense against stimulation), an essentially primordial biological mechanism protecting any living system or organism from surplus, that is, noxious stimulation. Denial shares with its hypothetical biological relative the idea of shutting oneself off to protect oneself from dangerous intrusion. It also carries the connotation of an automatically activated mechanism. This being so, it cannot be considered but as an unconscious mechanism, which is not controlled at all or only to some very small extent by the ego. Therein lies most probably also the reason why denial—following Anna Freud (1936)—has been considered a precursor—albeit a very primitive one—of what in subsequent development is to become a defense mechanism of the adult ego. Consequently the use by the adult ego of the defense of denial has been interpreted as due to a state of—at least transient—ego weakness. Depending on the extent to which reality has been "*verleugnet*," disavowed, done away by lying, one has been inclined in clinical circles to view denial as an outcome of deviant or deficient ego development, if not as a sign of severe psychosis.

During the last two decades, denial has come to be considered more and more a potentially adaptive mechanism in situations of extreme, unalterable stress such as experienced by adults in concentration camps or in the face of lethal illness. Common to such situations is the threat to personal integrity and/or one's life, that is, one's psychological and/or physical existence; in Federn's terms to one's "sensate ego," that is, to the boundaries of awareness of one's lasting or recurrent continuity in time space and causality (Federn, 1952). It is not warranted, however, to conclude from this that denial has to be a cognitive "response" to the perception of such threat and is consequently to be analyzed in terms of decision-making or information-processing processes, as some authors in a recent volume on denial of stress (Breznitz, 1983) seem to claim. This purely or nearly purely, cognitive view of denial presupposes a highly rational model of humans. It may be valid for certain types of individuals in certain situations, albeit in situations in which a person is able to give him- or herself a conscious account of what he or she thinks is going on. The position taken here comes closest to that expressed by Goldberger (1983). From the present author's personal experience during World War II in prison and in concentration camp, a decision-making model of denial would hold true probably only for a very small minority of inmates. Not only that, conscious denial did not help them to adapt and to survive. Such attempts at conscious denial would have lead generally to highly unrealistic and nearly always "suicidal" behavior. On the other hand, unconscious denial of the real and deeper meaning of what was expected may have freed energy to view the situation realistically but manageably, within set limits of helplessness. To put it differently, in defining denial, one has ask oneself, "What reality is denied" and why has it to be denied, or more precisely: "What *in* reality has to be denied and under what conditions." The question implies that denial may occur in different forms in different phases of the process of adaptation. In some affinity with Lazarus and Goldberger, one can argue that denial is a necessary component—not necessarily of coping with stress of any kind—but of adjustment to change, in the sense of an internal realignment of energy or interests. It is the type of ego constriction brought about by partial or total withdrawal of involvement or interest from a certain area or object in relation to which the person's aspirations had brought him or her into a state of feeling endangered. Such a state may possibly impoverish a person's capacity for interaction and adaptation temporarily but not necessarily to the point of becoming neurotic or psychotic. In some instances, such a process may function like a regression in the service of the ego (Kris, 1936) and facilitate developmental differentiation. Such differentiation progresses, according to Hartmann (1958), not only through active mastery of demands and tasks by creating new apparatuses—or as we probably would say today, subsystems of the ego—but also, and maybe mainly, by the latter. The new apparatuses perform, on a higher level, functions that had been carried out previously, on a lower level of organization, abstraction, and, one may, assume efficiency. Only extreme phenomena of denial are to be considered as typical—like extreme forms of use of other defenses—for the emergence of deviant development and psychopathology beyond that of everyday life. In the course of normal development, however, denial is necessary, as indicated earlier, for the redeployment of psychic energy in the service of establishing new network connections or structures on an interpersonal, affective, as well as on a cognitive level. Because, as mentioned before, at any stage and at any moment in time the individual disposes only of a given amount of free cathectic energy for investment into new objects and object relations, one has to conclude that a certain amount of such energy has to be withdrawn from previously existing investments in order to be freed for reinvestment into new ones. Denial serves just this purpose, and it serves it in a way by which the denied experiences or the significant parts of such experiences are removed far away from the focus of consciousness to a point from where it is hard to recover them.

Even in the early stages of development, when a steady increase in available energy can be assumed to prevail due to maturational processes, it is hard to believe how all new ties, committments, and investments could be performed, how affective social and cognitive learning could take place without redeployment of available energetic resources.

Even at that early stage, the absence of such redeployment would lead to much more conflict and trauma than usually is observed in the early stages of development. It is therefore not surprising that it is during this period, that is, the pre-Oedipal period, that we find a peak in the use of denial, which, as pointed out by the early authors on the subject, is then considered highly functional from a developmental point of view. This becomes particularly important if one accepts the basic tenet of modern ego psychology, that the ego is not formed only from conflict and that not all of its energy is derived from drive energy but is endowed from birth on (by heredity?) with a given quantity of energy resources of its own.

What is true for the earlier stages of development certainly should hold true for later and in particular stages of late adult development. Even if we do not accept—as in fact we do not—a decrement model during the second part of the life span, one has to concede that in later life *expendable* energy is limited for a number of reasons and the engagement/disengagement balance shifts into the direction of disengagement. On the other hand, those objects and social networks to which the person had been attached, have been over the years, invested more permanently and possibly more intensely than in the earlier stages of development. Consequently, it is safe to assume that as years pass during the second part of life, it becomes more and more difficult to disengage oneself psychologically and factually from such ties.

By now, it should be fairly obvious what shall be the outcome of this argument: denial of earlier attachments or denial of significant aspects of earlier object relations—under which term we subsume relations to inanimate objects and concepts as well—are a necessary, maybe not sufficient, condition for any shift in the engagement/disengagement balance at this stage of life. It is hard to think of this process as entirely controlled by conscious or secondary processes. The more conscious the necessity to disengage oneself from an earlier tie becomes, the more conflict, guilt, and threat to one's integrity is likely to tax the dynamic equilibrium of the person. In such a state of ambivalence, it becomes difficult to arrive at a "free decision" to become independent from previously cherished or valued objects, ideas, beliefs, attitudes, or even habits. Consequently, in order to achieve this with a minimum of energy expenditure, a completely unconscious mechanism has to operate—denial. Denial, in a sense may be regarded as a counterpart to Helmholtz's concept of *unbewusster Schluss*, that is, a psychological mechanism operating at high speed and on a level removed from conscious awareness that can be held responsible for what today in computer language would read "save" and/or "save as." Denial represents an unconscious demand to "delete"—at least from easily available layers of memory or simply—if such a thing is possible (which we don't believe it is)—not to register or to save. This latter process really could be conceptualized as an absence of attempts to assimilate an impression or event as it occurs to you or the avoidance of "engagement" that necessitates energy investment of a basically long-term quality. Another way of looking at it could be in terms of Lewin's (1926) theory, namely to define a particular event by means of an "unbewusster Schluss" as "completed task," which as such can be "forgotten"—albeit without taxing our ego or the system "person" with the necessity to invest effort in remembering, without necessity for an investment, potentially available, even after a considerable lapse of time. This also would imply that the use of denial implies curtailment of time and particularly future perspective. Because the latter is normally shrinking objectively and subjectively during the later part of life, the use of denial becomes if not more adaptive, certainly less maladaptive than during early adulthood or childhood.

This view of denial really implies that what is denied has not necessarily to be a threatening object or event; at least not in the sense of what represents a threat from the external world, labeled as such by an observer. The quality of "external" threat emanates from the consequences for adaptational capacity of maintaining a relationship or staying engaged. Another implication may be that, as in some forms of regression in the service of the ego, denial enables us to disengage gradually from former commitments to safeguard the integrity of our aging ego and self-perception in face of later—presumably stronger—threats of isolation and helplessness. Again, in Lewinian or system theoretical terms, denial leads to a segregation of tension areas, that is, affective and/or cognitive subsystems. Such differentiation may or may not require a shift in boundary conditions, both of internal, between tension systems, and external, that is, in terms of person–environment boundaries. Research findings on old people indeed suggest increasing rigidity of action and goal-directed thinking coupled with an increase in fantasy activity. The latter is found ordinarily to be related to the individual's own past. In younger adults and in children, the same or very similar processes may lead to increased flexibility toward "reality" and fantasy activity directed toward the future, the merely possible and consequently the potentially creative.

In either case, the transformation of internal structure is likely to result in engagement of a new kind—possibly a more energy-saving one than, say, direct interpersonal relationships or work. During the later years and in old age, we find a tendency (Shanan, 1985) to get engaged in intellectual and transpersonal, religious interests in addition to certain (not necessarily pathological) manifestations of living in fantasy. Denial can become, particularly in the later phases of personality development, a perceptual defense, an "unbewusster Kurzschluss" so to speak, which enables the aging person to adjust to the new realities of an increasing social and intellectual isolation during the last phase of life. It is not necessarily death *per se* that has to be denied in the process of normal aging but certain aspects of the ever-changing social context surrounding the aging person. The denial of these aspects may vary, of course, from individual to individual and culture to culture, and within given cultures according to social class and—last but not least—to the personality type to which the aging person belongs, as found in the Jerusalem study of midadulthood and aging (JESMA), a longitudinal study of personality development during the second half of life, determines coping style. The purpose of denial at this stage of life-span development, however, is invariably to maintain for the aging individual a minimum of gratifications, so necessary for the older person for successful adaptation during that period in life.

REFERENCES

Adler, E., Adler, H., Magora, A., Shanan, J., & Tal E. (1969). *Stroke in Israel.* Jerusalem: Polypress.
Breznitz, S. (Ed.). (1983). *The denial of stress.* New York: International University Press.
Cumming, E., & Henry, W. H. (1961). *Growing old.* New York: Basic Books.
Eitinger, L. (1983). Denial in concentration camps: Some personal observations on the positive and negative functions of denial in extreme life situations. In S. Breznitz (Ed.), *The denial of stress* (pp. 199–212). New York: International University Press.
Erikson, H. (1950). *Childhood and society.* New York: Norton.
Federn, P. (1952). *Ego psychology and the psychoses.* New York: Basic Books.
Freud, S. (1938). Totem and taboo. In *The basic writings of S. Freud* (pp. 807–930). New York: Modern Library.
Freud, A. (1936). *The ego and the mechanisms of defense.* New York: International Universities Press.
Freud, S. (1930). *Civilisation and its discontents.* London: Hogarth.
Freud, S. (1948). *Group psychology and the analysis of the ego.* London: Hogarth.
Gal, R., & Lazarus, R. (1975). The role of activity in stress. *Journal of Human Stress, 1*(4), 4–20.
Goldberger, L. (1983). The concept and mechanisms of denial. In S. Breznitz (Ed.), *The denial of stress* (pp. 83–96). New York: International Universities Press.
Guillemard, A. M., & Lenoir, R. (1974). *Retraite et echange social.* Paris: Centre d'etudes des mouvements sociaux.
Gutmann, D. L. (1980). The post parental years. In W. Norman & Th. J. Scaramella (Eds.). *Midlife* (pp. 38–52). New York: Bruner Mazel.
Hartman, H. (1958). *Ego psychology and the problem of adaptation.* New York: International Universities Press.

Havighurst, R. (1952). *Developmental tasks and education*. New York: Longmans, Green and Co.

Kris, E. (1936). The psychology of caricature. *International Journal of Psychoanalysis, 17,* 285–303.

Lazarus, R. S. (1983). The cost and benefits of denial. In S. Breznitz (Ed.), *The denial of stress* (pp. 1–30). New York: International Universities Press.

Levinson, D. J. (1979). *The seasons of a man's life.* New York: Knopf.

Lewin, K. (1926). Vorsdatz, wille und beduerfniss. *Psych. Forschungen,* 733–385.

Mor, E., Shanan, J., & Levinson, A. (1973). Motivation and coping in adjustment to contact lenses. *Journal of Personality Assessment,37,* 136–147.

Rapaport, D. (1959). The structure of psychoanalytic theory. In S. Koch (Ed.), *Psychology: A study of a science* (pp. 55–183). New York: McGraw-Hill.

Rapaport, D. (1967). Some metapsychological considerations concerning activity and passivity. In M. Gill (Ed.), *The collected papers of David Rapaport* (pp. 530–568). New York: Basic Books.

Shanan, J. (1973). Coping behavior in the prediction of complex tasks. *Proceedings of the 17th International Congress of Applied Psychology, 1,* 313–321.

Shanan, J. (1976). Levels and patterns of social engagement and disengagement from adolescence to middle adulthood. In K. Riegel & J. Mecheam (Eds.), *The developing individual in a developing world* (pp. 601–610). The Hague: Mouton.

Shanan, J. (1983). Society in transition and transitional phases of human development. In J. Birren, J. Munnichs, H. Thomae, & J. Marois (Eds.), *Aging: A challenge for science and society* (pp. 112–125). London: Oxford University Press.

Shanan, J. (1983). Consistency and change of personality through the adult years. In M. Bergener & U. Lehr (Eds.), *Aging in the eighties* (pp. 258–271). New York: Springer.

Shanan, J. (1985). *Personality types and culture in later adulthood.* Basel: Karger.

Shanan, J., & Weil, H. (1977). Forced and autonomous detachement. In J. Munnichs, & J. Van den Heuvel (Eds.), *Dependency or independency in old age* (pp. 56–70). The Hague: Martinus Nijhoff.

Shanan, J., Kaplan De Nour, A., & Garty, I. (1976). Effects of prolonged stress on coping style in terminal renal failure patients. *Journal of Human Stress, 2,* 19–27.

Sheehy, G. (1976). *Passages,* New York: Bantam Books.

Simmel, G. (1950). *The sociology of Georg Simmel.* Glencoe, IL: The Free Press.

Wolff, E., & Shanan, J. (1975). Coping behavior and work adjustment. *Bitahon sociali (Social Security)* 9–10, 67–78 (Hebrew).

8

Anosognosia
The Neurological Correlate of Denial of Illness

RUTH S. SHALEV

In the wake of a cerebral lesion, patients may develop a syndrome in which they remain unaware of illness or deny that illness has occurred. Such unawareness or denial is considered to be a true expression of the underlying cerebral lesion and is called anosognosia (Hecaen & Albert, 1978). Neurologically, when speaking of denial of illness, the reference is, for the most part, to denial of hemiplegia, most often a hemiplegia of the left side of the body. The neurobehavioral manifestations of denial are varied and often bizarre. They range from a complete denial and negation of illness, to an indifference or unconcern for the neurological deficit. Some patients will neglect or fail to attend to stimuli emanating from the affected side of the body or even from the extracorporeal space associated with the affected side. Alternatively, a patient may express the opinion that one side of the body is alien to him or her, has disappeared, or actually belongs to a different person (Hecaen & Albert, 1978; Heilman, Valenstein, & Watson, 1984).

The hemiplegic patient with denial will typically refuse to admit the

---

RUTH S. SHALEV • Neuropediatric Diagnostic Unit, Bikur Cholim Hospital, Jerusalem,. Israel.

reality of his paralysis (Hecaen & Albert, 1978). In cases of denial, if the examiner should request the patient lift the paretic arm, the patient will respond inappropriately. Every attempt to show the patient that one side of his or her body is paralyzed is met with indifference or is grossly rebuffed. The patient may accuse the doctor of exaggeration or outright error. In a modified version of this same syndrome, the patient will not deny his or her hemiplegia but will simply react with indifference to his or her inabilities or will find excuses for not being able to fulfill the doctor's request. The term coined for this is *anosodiaphoria* (Hecaen & Albert, 1978).

If the patient demonstrates neglect, he or she will not attend to or will ignore all stimuli presented to the affected side of his or her body. The inattention can occur in one or in many sensory modalities including the tactile, visual, or auditory senses (Heilman *et al.*, 1984). For example, stimuli presented visually to the left visual field or auditory stimuli such as the snapping of fingers (presented to the left ear) will go unnoticed. Patients with neglect might not look to the impaired side on command although able to do so in pursuit of the examiner's fingers. The patient might neglect a sleeve or walk about without a slipper. Food often accumulates in one cheek. Hemispatial neglect is the extension of inattention to the left side of the body—to the space and world around that affected left side (Heilman *et al.*, 1984). The patient might not notice someone speaking or appearing from his or her left side. The patient with hemispatial neglect may fail to eat on one side of his or her plate, will not shave or groom one half of the face or body. If presented with words such as playpen or cowboy, the patient will read them as pen or boy ignoring the left half of the word. If asked to draw a picture of a flower, the result may be just half a flower with the details of the flower on the left side ignored (Hecaen & Albert, 1978; Heilman *et al.*, 1984). Patients with neglect may also fail to recall left hemispatial remote memories, even though the engrams for these memories are not destroyed (Meador *et al.*, 1987).

Alienation is one of the most bizarre of all phenomena in this syndrome. Some patients, although aware that their extremities belong to them, refer to their limbs as though they were separate objects. One patient, when asked to verify visually that her left arm was indeed the direct continuation of her shoulder, replied: "My eyes and my feelings are not in agreement; and I must believe what I feel. I sense by looking that they are as if they are mine, but I feel that they are not and I cannot believe my eyes" (Hecaen & Albert, 1978). Patients who are profoundly affected may even fail to recognize that their extremities are part of their own body. They may complain that someone else's arm or leg is in the bed with them. When confronted with objective evidence, they may still deny that their own limbs belong to them.

The neuropathological correlate of the syndrome of denial of illness is most often seen in lesions of the right hemisphere (Hecaen & Albert, 1978). The area of the right hemisphere that has been implicated most often is the inferior parietal lobule bordering the interparietal sulcus, the supramarginal gyrus, and the angular gyrus. However, lesions within the subcortical white matter disconnecting the parietal cortex from the thalamo-cortical fibres have also been correlated with the hemispatial neglect syndrome (Bogousslavsky et al., 1988). Discrete lesions in the cingulate gyrus and right thalamus have also been implicated in denial of illness (Heilman, Valenstein, & Watson, 1984). Damage to these subcortical areas is consistent with a model of neglect developed by Mesulam (1981) whereby lesions of the cingulate, frontal, and reticular components could interrupt the "integrated network for modulation of directed attention within extrapersonal space." Although the rule is that right-hemisphere lesions cause anosognosia, the syndrome can also result from left-hemisphere lesions. It is likely that the presence of aphasia in left hemisphere damage interferes with the manifestations and diagnosis of anosognosia of the right side of the body.

In humans, the pharmacological basis of neglect is not known. However, experimental studies on an animal model of neglect suggest that disruption of components of the dopamine system may be responsible for neglect induced by subcortical and cortical lesions. Moreover, the use of a dopamine-receptor agonist, apomorphine, had a positive therapeutic effect on the animal model (Corwin et al., 1986).

The early conceptions of anosognosia were predicated on the belief that it was a psychiatric disorder rather than an organic brain dysfunction. The patient was supposedly aware of his or her deficit and could relate to his or her bodily image. The denial was thought to represent a perturbation of the physical personality of the patient or psychopathology of the personality. However, in 1914, Babinski affirmed the notion that anosognosia was not a psychiatric disturbance but the behavioral manifestation of a brain lesion (Hecaen & Albert, 1978). One school of neurological thought, led by Denny-Brown, explained the syndrome of denial by reducing it to a defect of spatial summation following a lesion in the parietal lobe (Heilman, 1979). Other authors suggested that it was the combination of a reduced mental functioning after brain damage, with purposeful defense mechanisms, which produced anosognosia (Hecaen & Albert, 1978).

Weinstein and Cole contended that associated with a decreased level of consciousness and attention was a defense mechanism of forgetting what was psychologically painful to the individual. They referred to anosognosia of the left hemiplegia as aspects not only of the denial of illness but also of other associated unpleasant circumstances. These authors emphasized the idea of motivated drive in which the unpleasant facts of illness are repressed and the catastrophic reaction avoided (Weinstein & Cole, 1963). Their patients would explain away their own presence in the hospital either as a visit to friends or as work there in some capacity. Some expressed the belief that their paralyzed limbs were on the table like false teeth; others said their limbs were lazy, or tired, or sore after injections. Weinstein & Cole believe these perceptions and misperceptions are selected and screened to redefine the patient's situation in terms of his or her new needs, problems, and preexisting social roles. To bolster their argument, these authors note that patients denied not only their hemiplegia but also other disabilities and list ptosis, prosthesis, vomiting, and incontinence of urine as examples. The patients would consistently misname or relocate the hospital. Mount Sinai Hospital was called Mount Cyanide Hospital or Mount Sinai Sanatorium or, if named correctly, would be relocated to another city. Another argument used was that, in spite of their denial of illness, the patients accepted hospital ward routine, medications, and even surgery without question. Moreover, patients who developed anosognosia were identified as having a characteristic premorbid obsessive-compulsive personality. Such patients were reported by their relatives as having always had a strong tendency to deny illness, regarding it as a sign of weakness and failure. Health, industry, and efficiency were ethical values through which the patient maintained a sense of identity. Associated with this was a history of reluctance to go to doctors and a tendency to appear guilty or ashamed when ill or idle. Weinstein & Cole conclude that the neurobehavioral syndrome that appears under conditions of altered brain function when misperceptions or imperceptions exist shows a strong correlation with the habitual methods by which such patients structure their social environment (Weinstein & Cole, 1963).

The concept of denial and neglect developed by Heilman, Valenstein & Watson (1984) and by Mesulam (1981) contrasts sharply with that of Weinstein and Cole. Whereas the latter believe the syndrome to be personality dependent, the former contend that denial and neglect represent a disorder of the attentional-arousal systems. They contend that it is caused by a breakdown in the neuronal networks of the corticolimbic-reticular formation loop. Their reasoning goes as follows: Stimulation of the mesencephalic reticular formation induces cortical arousal and electroencephalographic desynchronization, a physiologic measure of arousal. If the stimulus is unilateral, there will be unilateral electroencephalographic desynchronization. Conversely, a unilateral lesion in the mesencephalic reticular formation would result in a unilateral syndrome of hypoarousal or inattention. Another possible trouble spot in the conjectured loop is the nucleus retucularis thalami. This nucleus enhances thalamic sensory relay to the cortex. However when it is damaged, there is inhibition of the sensory relay system to the cortex. Sensory information which should be arriving at cortical areas is delayed or completely withheld. At the cortical level, polymodal areas such as the inferior parietal lobe can also induce a generalized arousal response. Lesions in the inferior parietal lobe which are clinically correlated with anosognosia are associated with hypoarousal. The patients cannot be aroused to process and judge stimuli coming from the contralateral side of the body. Thus a lesion in this area seems to impair the patient's ability to determine the significance of stimuli, resulting in the neurobehavioral syndrome of anosognosia (Heilman, Valenstein, & Watson, 1984; Heilman, 1979).

Denial of blindness, another (although less common) syndrome of anosognosia, is also known as Anton's syndrome. These patients have bilateral occipital lesions causing blindness but who refuse to recognize and deny their loss of vision. Visual anosognosics act as if they could see, and persist in this behavior despite all evidence to the contrary. They obstinately refuse to learn to accept blindness, even though this incapacity is disorienting, disrupts the pattern of living, and may even be injurious. Occasionally, the anosognosia is manifested by simple indifference to the blindness; the patient failing to complain about his or her disability. Attempts to explain away the visual disorder include invention of excuses related to the environment such as poor lighting, poor glasses, dust in the eye, and so forth (Hecaen & Albert, 1978).

Anosognosia may occur as a paroxysmal event, representing epileptic equivalents, migraine, or transient ischemic attacks. It may also develop following head injury or vascular lesions. Lesions producing this syndrome are located bilaterally in the occipital lobes, destroying both banks of the calcarine fissures and the subjacent white matter (Hecaen & Albert, 1978).

In summary, denial of illness is the behavioral manifestation of a focal neurological deficit. The most common neurological syndrome of denial is that pertaining to a left hemiplegia that results from a focal lesion in the right parietal lobe. These patients will deny, ignore, neglect, or feel alienated from their limbs on the left side of the body and sometimes even to the entire world on their left side. A syndrome of denial concerning blindness from bilateral occipital lesions has also been documented but is far less frequent than the denial of hemiplegia.

REFERENCES

Bogousslavsky, J., Miklossy, J., Regli, F., Deruaz, J.-P., Assal, G., & Delaloge, B. (1988). Subcortical neglect: neuropsychological, SPECT, and neuropathological correlations with anterior choroidal artery territory infarction. *Annals of Neurology, 23*, 448–452.

Corwin, J. V., Kanter, S., Watson, R. T., Heilman, K. M., Valenstein, E., & Hashimoto, A. (1986). Apomorphine has a therapeutic effect on neglect produced by unilateral dorsomedial prefrontal cortex lesions in rats. *Experimental Neurology, 94*, 683–698.

Hecaen, H., & Albert, M. L. (1978). *Human neuropsychology.* New York: Wiley.

Heilman, K. M. (1979). Neglect and related syndromes. In K. M. Heilman & E. Valenstein (Eds.), *Clinical neuropsychology* (pp. 268–307). New York: Oxford University Press.

Heilman, K. M., Valenstein, E., & Watson, R. T. (1984). Neglect and related disorders. *Seminars in Neurology, 4*, 209–219.

Meador, K. J., Loring, D. W., Bowers, D., & Heilman, K. M. (1987). Remote memory and neglect syndrome. *Neurology, 37*, 522–526.

Mesulam, M.-M. (1981). A cortical network for directed attention and unilateral neglect. *Annals of Neurology 10*, 309–325.

Weinstein, E. A., & Cole, M. (1963). Concepts of anosognosia. In L. Halpern (Ed.), *Problems of dynamic neurology* (pp. 254–273). New York: Grune & Stratton.

III

Child Development

In the preceding section, Shanan points out that the act of disavowal prevents the binding of psychic energy to certain perceptions, thus leaving it free to be used for other purposes. The ability, conferred by denial, to redeploy attention and energy does not appear *de novo* in the aging adult; the three chapters that comprise this next section demonstrate how denial may be used by the child, the adolescent, and the parents who must deal with their children.

There is an old joke about two insurance agents competing for the attention of a client. The first claimed that his policy covered one from cradle to grave. Irreverently, the second agent boasted that his policy covered the client from erection to resurrection. In the first chapter of this section, Bar Giora reminds us that before there are children for us to study, there must be adults who engage in sexual intercourse; sexual congress undertaken for the most part in disavowal of its relationship to the process of conception, pregnancy, and child rearing. Save for those few people who practice sexual intimacy with the avowed intent of making a baby, most of us are born into some sort of more-or-less happy denial. And, he suggests, few if any women would be able to survive the ordeal of motherhood without occasional resort to the unawareness afforded by such disavowal. It may not be truly in the interest of either mother or child for the therapist to undo all denial unless the therapeutic milieu can provide remarkable degrees of support. Bar Giora draws heavily on his own experience as a therapist and supervisor to present this intensely humane and empathic chapter.

Denial implies the alteration in fantasy of some portion of external reality in order that the affective response to that altered reality is more

125

acceptable than the affective response to true consensual reality. One can readily visualize a continuum or gradient along which such alterations may be assigned, a continuum where the most mild alterations would be viewed as part of the range of normal, the moderate seen as neurotic, and the most severe and most difficult to maintain, understood by the observer as emblematic of psychosis. Classical psychoanalytic theory requires us to *define* the difference between denial and repression so that in the former what is disavowed will always be some aspect of external reality, whereas in the latter what is removed from awareness is derivative of unconscious conflict related to instinctual wishes. Yet, as many in this book complain, this may be no more than a heuristic device set up to go along with other equally definitional aspects of conventional theory. It is difficult, if not impossible, to state with any confidence that the neurological mechanism for the affect-sparing evasion of external reality differs in any way from the affect-sparing avoidance of internal conflict. As in so many structural aspects of psychoanalytic thought, definitions that create separate realms of cognitive operation are incapable of proof and thus susceptible to confusion, alteration of boundaries, and an astonishing variability of usage in clinical practice.

Eifermann demonstrates the benefit that can accrue from a therapeutic and philosophical attitude free of such precise definition. Her clearly stated intentional avoidance of critical distinction between the fine points that occupy many other scholars allows an understanding of denial in praxis rather than denial in theory. "Rotkäppchen," a story published in 1819 by the brothers Grimm and known variously as "Little Red Cap" or "Little Red Riding Hood," is so well known in our culture that responses or attitudes toward it may be studied in a scientific manner. Whereas many would have been satisfied to evaluate these responses alone, Eifermann makes the trenchant observation that fairy tales are not read in privacy by small children as part of a visual/ intellectual operation but are actually introduced to them as part of an oral tradition. And to complicate further any analysis of fairy tales, Eifermann points out that, in general, these stories are read aloud to children by mother, the person with whom the child is in the most highly charged emotional relationship; a mother who herself has a highly personal emotional relationship to the story in question. Where so much emotion is involved one may expect defenses against emotion to be rampant; Eifermann demonstrates that the telling and retelling of "Little Red Cap" produces a complex and variable system of denials defining that particular mother/child dyad. In reading this chapter, one is drawn to the understanding of the operation of disavowal within a relationship, much as suggested in the earlier chapter of Dorpat, who stated that the mutual acceptance of denial produces family myths. Eifermann's contribution is the obverse of this coin, for each mother's statement of those myths personally important to her shapes the shared myths that then produce the style of denial defining the family.

Infant tended by mother becomes child learning and separating; child becomes adolescent who learns more and separates ever more fiercely. Just as in their earlier chapter, Sacerdoti and Semi called our attention to the world view adopted by the growing adolescent and the implications of that weltanschauung for any understanding of the adult, Erlich leads us into the powerfully emotional world of the adolescent in order that we may understand the importance of denial as a moderating and modulating influence in this tumultuous period of development. One of the potential weaknesses of an edited volume is the repetition created as each author delineates the theoretical/historical background of the matter under discussion. Here this becomes a strength as Erlich adds new perspectives to those already cited.

He states that although most other defenses "affect what happens at the interface of ego and id, the work of denial proceeds primarily at the level of ego and reality." Concentrating on those aspects of reality that pose the most difficulty for the adolescent, Erlich reminds us that what is disavowed may reduce the load of unpleasant affect that discomfits the ego while placing that ego in a precarious relationship to reality. The now classic phenomenologic study by Shapiro (1965) of the impulsive personality made no attempt to define explanatory unconscious mechanisms. Erlich suggests a causal connection between denial and adolescent acting out that may provide a link to Shapiro's earlier observations. Throughout the clinical material by which Erlich illustrates his theoretical perspective runs the theme that the adolescent is likely to disavow those aspects of external reality that produce shame; indeed, it would appear from his clinical work as well as that of Kaufman (1985) and Schneider (1987) that defenses against shame are critical in the development of the adolescent. Where denial replaces critical self-assessment and self-repair, the adolescent is left poorly able to take the role of full-fledged adult. Where denial supports the ability of the adolescent to get on with the task of living and growing while learning enough to make these repairs when strong enough to do so, denial can become a positive tool for growth and development.

REFERENCES

Kaufman, G. (1985). *Shame: The power of caring* (2nd ed. rev.). Boston: Schenkman.
Schneider, C. D. (1987). A mature sense of shame. In D. L. Nathanson (ed.) *The many faces of shame* (pp. 194–213). New York: Guilford.
Shapiro, D. (1965). *Neurotic styles.* New York: Basic Books.

9

The Child as a Challenge to Adult Denial

Rami A. Bar Giora

Prior to his or her birth and even before conception, the child constitutes a challenge to the denial of the adult. Denial of the connection between sexual relations and pregnancy is much more widespread than was previously understood from the data of child and adult analyses. When such denial is present among adults of childbearing age, it can have powerful sequelae, including unwanted pregnancies and unforeseen problems posed by the very existence of the infants issuing from them. This denial of the connection between intercourse and pregnancy has its own strong roots in childhood, for even Oedipal fantasies rarely involve thoughts of procreation; hedonistic interests of equal strength also abet adult denial. In situations of physical intimacy and excitement, it is easier not to consider the connection between the pleasure of the moment and long-term parental responsibilities, or at the very least, the connection between the sexual act and pregnancy.

The anticipation of the newborn thus presents a serious challenge to the tendency toward denial already existing prior to conception. This anticipation can either strengthen denial or cause the opposite—shake the denial and bring about a reorganization of perceptions and behavior. This is my main hypothesis, and I shall attempt to show how the

Rami A. Bar Giora • ILAN Child Guidance Clinic, P.O. Box 8125, Jerusalem 9108, Israel.

child possesses special power to challenge the denial and other similar defensive systems of the adult, although of course she or he is not the only force in life that challenges denial.

The decision to enter into pregnancy burdens the wide range of flexibility in mental life, for some frustration is inevitable whatever decision is taken. An internal negotiation for or against pregnancy, or whether to become pregnant now or later, cannot be compromised— one cannot decide to become only slightly pregnant.

Once pregnancy has begun, the forces opposing the pregnancy can take many forms, according to their intensity and the personality organization of the people involved. Thus we can see denial of pregnancy *ad absurdum*, with total disregard for the conditions necessary for the development of a normal pregnancy, such as proper diet, rest, medical follow-up, abstinence from, or restriction of, smoking and alcohol. One can observe attempts to cover up the pregnancy with clothing, an overemphasis on "keeping busy" and other ways of suppressing the pregnancy from consciousness. All of these phenomena contain some elements of denial of pregnancy. At times, this resistance is displaced from the fetus to other areas of the body or other bodily functions. They, rather than the fetus, then become the object of discomfort, complaint, and anger. Overzealous medical attention to these complaints will only magnify the challenge to denial of the fetus. After all, it is easier to focus on one's aching stomach or painful back, than to blame the infant that lies between them. Most pregnancies, whether wanted, unwanted, or partially unwanted, conclude in birth, and thus denial is pushed into the corner by the undeniable reality of the growing fetus. The baby is to the denial of pregnancy as the noonday sun to one who claims with closed eyes that it is midnight.

The choice of method of delivery is in itself an excellent example of different types of denial. For example, the method of Leboyer supports denial of the aggression inherent in the expulsion of the fetus from the uterine paradise. Alternatively, anesthesia may assist in the denial of the pain and fear associated with delivery.

After birth a new chapter begins, which also may arouse the need for denial. We shall suggest a general outline in which the infant serves as a crystallization point of adult aversion and hostility, against which denial is mobilized.

The birth event is a milestone between two periods in the journey of parenthood. The first period is the pregnancy, which causes escalating physical, physiological, and psychological changes. These changes bring fatigue and disturb the homeostasis to which the mother is accustomed and thus threaten her sense of well-being. The second period on the way to parenthood begins after the birth. The beginning of this period has been rightly termed the time of "pregnancy outside of the womb." It also limits the mother's mobility and causes increasing fatigue as a result of the accumulating burdens of feeding, daily care, and the discrepancy between the sleep–wake cycles of mother and infant. On top of these burdens, one often sees the emergence of psychological difficulties side by side with the joy of parenthood. These psychological difficulties were described by Paul Dewald (1980, p. 48) as follows:

> Becoming a parent represents another important maturational crisis in the life of the adult, requiring a variety of new forms of adaptation and experiences and at times involving a considerable reorganization in regard to previous patterns and levels of function. Not only are there marital, social, economic and personal lifestyle changes required, but the role of being a parent has multiple associations intrapsychically in the individual's relationship to his or her own childhood and parents.
>
> For example, the infant and young child's helplessness may activate fears of aggression in the parent; the necessity of providing for the child's needs may activate feelings of envy in parents whose own needs were not satisfactorily fulfilled in childhood; parents may reverse passive experiences from their own childhood to active ones and repeat toward their own children what they experienced from their parents; parents may unconsciously identify with their child and vicariously enjoy giving it satisfactions which the parent did not receive as a child; parents may perceive the child as a threat and experience various competitive feelings toward the child; the sibling position, sex, appearance, and innate talents of the child may have specific associational meanings for the parent in relationship to his/her own childhood experiences; etc. These are only a sample of the types of conflict which may be activated in the parent by the birth of a child.

After Dewald's concise formulation, let us see how Winnicott (1947, p. 201) describes the phenomenon of maternal distress:

> The mother, however, hates her infant from the word go. . . . We know about a mother's love and we appreciate its reality and power. Let me give some of the reasons why a mother hates her baby, ... The baby is a danger to her body in pregnancy and at birth. The baby is an interference with her private life, a challenge to preoccupation. . . . The baby hurts her nipples. . . . He is ruthless, treats her as scum, an unpaid servant; a slave. She has to love him, excretions and all, at any rate at the beginning. . . . she must not be anxious when holding him. At first he does not know at all what she does or what she sacrifices for him. Especially he cannot allow for her hate. He is suspicious, refuses her good food, and makes her doubt herself, but eats well with his aunt. After an awful morning with him she goes out, and he smiles at a stranger, who says: "Isn't he sweet?" If she fails him at the start she knows he will pay her out for ever.

Winnicott (1947, p. 202) continues to develop this idea and writes:

A mother has to be able to tolerate hating her baby without doing anything about it. She cannot express it to him. If, for fear of what she may do, she cannot hate appropriately when hurt by her child she must fall back on masochism. . . . The most remarkable thing about a mother is her ability to be hurt so much by her baby and to hate so much without paying the child out, and her ability to wait for rewards that may or may not come at a later date. Perhaps she is helped by some of the nursery rhymes she sings, which her baby enjoys but fortunately does not understand?

> "Rockabye Baby, on the tree top,
> When the wind blows the cradle will rock,
> When the bough breaks the cradle will fall,
> Down will come baby, cradle and all."

This is not a sentimental rhyme. Sentimentality is useless for parents, as it contains a denial of hate, and sentimentality in a mother is no good at all from the infant's point of view.

It seems to me doubtful whether a human child as he develops is capable of tolerating the full extent of his own hate in a sentimental environment. He needs hate to hate.

Every parent experiences this struggle with hostile feelings; some cope successfully, although at the price of occasional failures, whereas others are defeated and drawn into a vicious cycle of disappointment, despair, and anger against the child who is seen as the cause of the parent's suffering. Such defeats are seen in the battered-child syndrome, in full or partial abandonment, cruelty, or other forms of neglect.

Leon Shelef, in his book *Generations Apart: Adult Hostility to Youth* (1981), and Lloyd de Mause, in *The History of Childhood* (1974), examined different approaches to child rearing, according to current and historical texts and demonstrated that parental cruelty toward children, which today would lead to criminal liability, was commonplace in previous centuries. Hatred of the child was accepted and frequently added its part to the other devastating enemies of childhood, such as plagues, infectious diseases, hunger, exposure to cold, and other noxious influences.

The nature of the parent did not change as quickly as did the social and judicial concepts relating to defense and protection of the child. Whereas the social acceptability of parental expressions of hostility have radically changed, the hostility itself remains unchanged. Freud (1915, p. 137) writes:

> If the object is a source of unpleasurable feelings, there is an urge which endeavours to increase the distance between the object and the ego, and to repeat in relation to the object the original attempt at flight from the external world with its emission of stimuli. We feel the "repulsion" of the object, and hate it. This hate can afterwards be intensified to the point of an aggressive inclination against the object—an intention to destroy it.

The reader may well ask whether, if all these things are true, a parent must have a tremendous amount of love, tolerance for pain and disappointment and the ability to minimize difficulties and to maximize enjoyment of the positive sides of the child in order to achieve a positive balance. If not, how can any of us survive childhood at all? David Gutman (1980, p. 501) writes:

> It could be said that the evolutionary rationale of narcissism has less to do with the preservation of the self than with the preservation of the parent-child bond that is vital to species as well as individual survival.

So, narcissistic love and adoration of the child may help to counterbalance hatred.

Winnicott (1956, p. 300) asked himself what solution could be offered for the possible crisis of motherhood and the difficult demands that arise after birth. He coined the phrase *primary maternal preoccupation,* that is to say, a heightened devotion and responsiveness, an intensive mobilization of empathy and concern for the baby, a kind of adaptive monomania. This preoccupation is like a psychological "baby bonus" that fortifies the mother at the critical moment as a countermeasure against fatigue, exhaustion, and the tendency to blame it all on the newborn. This tendency causes her to perceive the newborn as bad, and, as a result of the aversion and hostility toward the baby, the parent perceives himself or herself as bad. Thus the need for denial.

Freud (1921, p. 101) writes:

> The evidence of psychoanalysis shows that almost every intimate emotional relation between two people which lasts for some time—marriage, friendship, the relation between parents and children—contains a sediment of feeling of aversion and hostility which only escapes perception as a result of repression.

What justifies repression also justifies denial (see Chapter 6).

As we follow the various methods of the parent's struggle with his or her hostility toward the child, hostility that (as we have seen) has so many sources, one can discern a number of common strategies:

1. Reversal—as in overprotection and reaction formation of varied form.
2. Projection onto another—such as the parent of the parent or his spouse or onto another person like the child's nurse.
3. Attempts to escape by withdrawal or distancing from the child.
4. Adopting a program of premature socialization by strict education and discipline, rationalized by the ideals of order, cleanliness, proper behavior, and the like.
5. Counterbalancing hostility by splitting, that is grandiose glorifi-

cation of the child. Freud (1914, p. 91) saw in this the reenact-
ment of childhood narcissism in the parent.

In all of these patterns of defense, hostility is experienced as a
negative quality that must be denied. Thus denial is essential in order to
preserve the parent's self-esteem. Of course there are extreme cases in
which hostility predominates and either becomes egosyntonic or leads to
complete breakdown. Generally, the hostility comes in manageable
doses—most parents manage to deal with hostility in some adequate
manner, based on a healthy coping personality. The child himself or
herself helps the parent deny his or her hostility if he or she creates only
the "average expected difficulties," which do not overtax the parent and
are balanced by positive emotions that the child evokes in his parents.

Difficulties that overtax the parent's coping abilities may cause so
serious a challenge to denial that the parent can no longer enlist the most
comfortable and generalized defense strategy—putting things off—
"mañana"—for one cannot put off crying, hunger, or developmental
deviance. So often one encounters parents for whom the central experience is not the fact of their hostility toward the child, but their guilt- and
shame-based anger over the fact that the child has "forced them to be
bad."

A mother reports during counseling: "I felt terrible that I let the
baby cry without going to him as they had instructed me in the well-baby
clinic. Then I felt terrible when I picked him up angrily and he wouldn't
calm down. Either way, I would be a bad mother, and I hated myself."

Another father in the course of psychotherapy said: "When I have
to dress him Saturday morning, his wildness drives me crazy. I hate to
force him to get dressed, because I feel like I'm pulling his arms out of
their sockets, and I hate to force him to take medicine when he doesn't
want it. I hate to be a bad father, and I get terribly angry at him when he
forces me to be the 'bad guy.'"

This mother and father, like many others, were quick to cling to the
dynamic lines suggested or approved by their therapists, such as an
invitation to recall childhood experiences of their own or to view their
anger toward the child as being displaced from their husband or wife
and the like. Both for parents and for beginning therapists, it is much
more difficult to confront directly the anger toward the child and the
threat that children evoke against the denial of parental hostility.

This hostility is associated with the feeling "I am a bad parent" that
becomes translated into "I am bad"—one of the most sensitive areas of
self-esteem. As the child grows and attains the ability to communicate
verbally, he or she often may come to play a role similar to that of the

famous boy in Hans Christian Anderson's story, who cried out "but the king is wearing no clothes!" The image of the innocent child, still uncorrupted by lies, distortions, or manipulations, is very popular in folktales, parables, and jokes. The child is often portrayed as a compass showing the way to truth, however unpleasant that truth may be. Thus the expression "the child is the true natural philosopher." In the context of parenthood, this smile of surprise and pleasure can easily change to shock and embarrassment when the child attacks denials to which the parent has grown accustomed.

"But Mother, you said that chocolate makes holes in your teeth and toothaches," says a 4-year-old little girl to her mother, who cannot reply immediately, because her mouth is stuffed with chocolate. When she can finally swallow it, she screams: "Get out of the room, you little brat, you can't talk that way to your mother."

Another boy, 3 years old, tearfully says to his father who has reprimanded him for saying "son of a bitch" at the table: "But Daddy, you used to laugh, at first, when I said it."

An 11-year-old in family therapy says to his mother: "Even when you give me good advice you're angry at me, even when you call me darling." The mother, not supported by her husband, who sits nodding his head as if to say "that's exactly right," says she is going to leave the room. Her actions are not understood, and she is perceived as the "bad guy." She indeed walks out, but in subsequent treatment sessions the very perceptive comment of her son stimulated a very important discussion for the mother and the family. Most children, even though they have heard Anderson's beautiful story, eventually join the club of denial users. Karl Menninger (1942, p. 31) referred to this when he wrote in *Love against Hate* about the crimes unwittingly committed by mothers against children: "The greatest crime of all, perhaps is the inculcation of a dishonest, hypocritical philosophy of life." A dramatic example of the child's joining with denial is the "denial by two," or "denial by three," which we can see in families where incest or sexual abuse has continued for years.

The adolescent years often bring frontal clashes between the systems of denial of the parents and the behavior or verbal provocations of their children. For example, the traditional areas of conflict—such as double standards in the code of sexual behavior or pretenses of good citizenship side by side with criminality of varying degrees. All these areas may stand out as points of controversy between parents and adolescents. Usually the claim is that "you parents demand of us what you don't carry out yourselves" or "you pretend to be what you aren't."

Often such arguments between the adolescent and his or her parents are displaced onto society in general, the school system, the government, and so forth. Sometimes they pass beyond the verbal level into "acting out." For example, a 14-year-old girl, brought back by the police after spending a few nights in another city, passing from bed to bed and discotheque to discotheque, was referred for psychological evaluation. Her mother, a woman embittered by a difficult life, yet showing traces of physical beauty despite the passage of many years, cried out and beat her breast in anguish: "You see, I told her not to do it, that's exactly what I told her, so many times I told her." At my request, the mother spelled out exactly what she had told her adolescent daughter:

> You'll be walking down the street and be thinking to yourself what a shitty life this is and everything, and be in a lousy mood, and then, all of a sudden, a shiny American car will pull up with a sharp-looking guy inside. He'll ask— "Where are you going, babe, I'll get you there. Come on in and have a good time. We'll go to a movie." That's exactly what you have to be careful of.

The daughter's behavior for a brief interlude was directed by exactly what her mother so much denied and thus presented a most serious challenge to the mother's denial.

Another interesting area related to denial is the encounter between the child in psychotherapy and the novice therapist, as he or she takes his or her first professional steps. Among these young therapists one can easily discern two attitudes: those that either created the need in the first place for working with children or later strengthened the desire to do so.

One attitude might be termed *the altruistic* in the sense of Anna Freud. Its essence is the denial of feelings of rejection and distress from the therapist's own childhood and reinforcement of reversal by overidentification with the child in therapy. The child is then showered with love and affection just as the young therapist would have wished to receive.

The second attitude might be called "the overly benevolent." Its essence is a tendency to overpermissiveness toward the child, accompanied by an accusing attitude toward the child's parents and teachers and covert competition with them.

The therapist who adopts the second attitude possesses excellent rationalization. Common sense tells him that "love conquers all" and that proper affection will overcome distress and misfortune; thus the theory of the modification of bad internal objects by positive corrective experience.

This tendency toward overpermissiveness, overcriticism of parents, and competition with them is often tied to denial of the therapist's aversion and intolerance of the child's behavior that closely resembles the parental anger. Such a beginning therapist will typically enjoy the initial "honeymoon" period that may occur in the first stages of treatment and be unaware of their tendency to encourage the child in continuing this phase of positive transference, just as they may be overwhelmed later by expressions of negative transference. Deep down inside, they are hurt at expressions of resistance such as lateness or missed appointments. They may have partial blind spots for situations that are painful for the child, such as cancellation of therapy sessions, vacation by the therapist, or the appearance of the therapist in the company of other children or colleagues. These therapists may have a tendency to be overly responsive to the child's requests, to readily change the hour of therapy, and so forth. They must feel they are "being good," are providers of comfort, and certainly are not "pain causers." Underlying this attitude is denial of the child's suffering and the adult's hostility toward him—a "denial of bad by doing good" as it were.

One young therapist perceived the wild play of a child in his treatment as reflecting infantile rage of a deprived child. Without being aware of it, he directed the child to sandbox play by removing all balls, darts, metal objects, and wood-working tools—anything with which the child might hurt himself—and thus reinforced his own image of the child as displaying regressive play in the treatment situation. He would often restrain the child physically and described how the child would transform during a fight against such restraint and suddenly melt into the arms of the therapist.

During a discussion about another case, this same therapist heard about aspects of homosexual passive wishes in children that may find expression in surrendering themselves into the arms of the adult. Immediately there was a radical change in his therapeutic approach because he was shocked by the thought that he was arousing something negative or perverse in the child in his treatment.

This same therapist, in diagnostic situations, would help children being examined in subtle ways, almost breaking the formal rules of the test. On the Rorschach, he would feel completely in tune with the answers of the child, only to discover later that in fact he was not so sure of their location and meaning as he had been with the child at his side.

On another occasion, he agreed to a request to accompany a child in treatment to his house from the clinic because of a bully who was lying in wait for him and would beat him up on the way home. It turned out that the child's complaint was indeed correct. The therapist followed the child at a short distance and caught the bully red-handed. When he described the event in supervision he was agitated as never before: "Children can be so irritating and violent, the only thing that would stop that bully from picking on smaller children is a good slap in the face."

He continued and said, "He was really afraid to go home, I couldn't just say to him, 'You have to work things out by yourself.'" When he was asked whether he did not think that perhaps the child's parents could help him come and go from the clinic, he replied: "To tell the truth, if he had parents who cared about him he wouldn't be in treatment to begin with." In his anger at this question, he saw his supervisor as an unempathic parent, too rigid, and as inhibiting the spontaneity and affection of the therapist who correctly perceived the child. This novice therapist was honest and learned a lesson from his young patient, who was an expert at provoking children and adults stronger than himself. The double challenge he had experienced from the child and his supervision brought him to a deeper understanding. He denied an inner world of conflicts and anxiety through helping the weak and correcting the bad in order to maintain "good feelings." This experience was well used in his own personal therapy. He summed it up at the end of the year: "What I brought up in therapy from my work was much more significant than that which I brought from my daily life." In my opinion, this type of "denial by the opposite" is an adult continuation of what Anna Freud called "denial by word and action."

Another young child therapist, who in the army had always been a devoted and successful field officer, made a personal discovery one day, during the course of a treatment session with a young boy, which would have been impossible to make under the burden of army duty.

His young patient, using a toy jeep, was proceeding to kill cows and farmers, overturning everything standing in the way of his super war vehicle; and the young therapist found himself quite rudely interrupting the child's play. This act was extremely uncharacteristic of him because, as a rule, he behaved with great gentleness and consideration. He later stated that he had taken a giant leap forward in self-understanding at that moment.

However, one also meets different beginning therapists who, under the stress of similar confrontations and challenges use what we may call "denial by the opposite" but which they would prefer to call "turning to the different." By this I mean those who shifted to behavior, simplistic family and supportive therapies, thus saving themselves the pain of uncovering and reintegration. Methods of helping parents by therapy, counseling, or parent groups may be divided alike between those who bypass denial by adapting a manipulative approach and those who encourage with deeper psychic reality.

I have presented some ideas and vignettes illustrating the power of the child to challenge adult denial that can be found in parenthood and in child therapy. Thus, the adult may find himself or herself at a

crossroad: either to use this challenge constructively for therapeutic re-
education and reintegration of his or her personality or to misuse it by
means of forcing his or her defenses on the child.

REFERENCES

de Mause, L. (Ed.). (1974). *The history of childhood*. New York: Harper Torchbooks.

Dewald, P. A. (1980). Adult phases of life cycle. In S. I. Greenspan & G. H. Pollock (Eds.), *The course of life: Psychoanalytic contributions toward understanding personality development* (Vol. 3, pp. 35–54). Bethesda: National Institute of Mental Health.

Freud, S. (1914). On narcissism. In *Standard edition* (Vol. 14). London: Hogarth.

Freud, S. (1915). Instincts and their vicissitudes. In *Standard edition* (Vol. 14). London: Hogarth.

Freud, S. (1921). Group psychology and the analysis of the ego. In *Standard edition* (Vol. 18). London: Hogarth.

Gutman, D. L. (1980). Psychoanalysis and aging: A developmental view. In S. I. Greenspan & G. H. Pollock (Eds.), *The course of life: Psychoanalytic contributions toward understanding personality development* (Vol. 3, pp. 489–518). Bethesda: National Institute of Mental Health.

Meninger, K. (1942). *Love against hate*. New York: Harcourt Brace and Co. N.Y.

Shelef, L. (1981). *Generations apart: Adult hostility to youth*. New York: McGraw Hill.

Winnicott, D. W. (1947). Hate in the countertransference. In *D. W. Winnicott collected papers* (1958), through Pediatrics to Psycho-Analysis. New York: Basic.

Winnicott, D. W. (1956). Primary maternal preoccupation. In *D. W. Winicott collected papers* (1958). New York: Basic.

10

Adolescent Denial
Some Psychoanalytic Reflections on Strength and Weakness

H. Shmuel Erlich

The question of the chronological classification of the mechanisms of defense is an old one. Anna Freud, in her classic monograph (1946), has already touched on it and reached the conclusion that it should probably best be left alone. "Instead," she wrote, we should "study in detail the situations which call forth the defensive reactions" (p. 57). This chapter is correspondingly not going to advance the untenable position that there is in any way an association between the developmental crisis of adolescence and the emergence of the mechanism of denial.

Both clinical and developmental experience make it abundantly clear that denial appears in relatively early childhood. Once it appears, it becomes a constant, if only potential, feature of intrapsychic functioning throughout life. We may assert that *some* capacity for the differentiation of self from external reality is a prerequisite for its emergence and a condition for its occurrence. This assertion would still hold true even during later developmental stages when the correlation between quality and level of self-differentiation and the usage of denial tends to become, at least on the surface, more problematic and complex. Nevertheless, it is

H. Shmuel Erlich • Department of Psychology, The Hebrew University of Jerusalem, Jerusalem, Israel.

still true, and this is the position I take in this presentation, that a rudimentary capacity for differentiating self from external reality is to be seen as the *sine qua non* for the development, if not the recourse, to the mechanism of denial.

Following Anna Freud's suggestion, we have actually learned a great deal about the nature of specific defenses by studying the vicissitudes of the situations that called them forth. Why under certain circumstances one prefers a particular defense mechanism to others may shed light on the defense itself. It seems to me that the same process could fruitfully be undertaken in the reverse: We may gain a good deal of understanding about a particular situation or phenomenon by studying it through the prism of the defense mechanism employed to handle it. Such a study must rely, of course, on some previous knowledge of the defense in question.

I propose to look at the developmental crisis of adolescence through the operation of denial, or disavowal. In doing so, I do not mean for a moment to suggest that adolescence is exclusively under the sway of denial as a defense mechanism, that this is the only or even main defense during the period, or that they are somehow uniquely associated with one another, so that adolescence (more than other developmental periods) can be characterized by denial. I do not think that such assertions can be proven, nor that they are particularly reasonable. But I do believe that a special fit can be shown to exist between some of the tasks and conflicts faced by the ego of the adolescent and the method of handling and resolving conflictual tasks afforded by denial. Furthermore, I believe that an understanding of this fit can greatly enhance and contribute to our understanding of both adolescence and the operation of denial.

Although most clinicians would agree that, compared to other age groups, adolescents are no less, and probably even more so, disposed to deny, very little seems to have been written on the specific use, or meaning of the utilization of, denial in this period. As early as 1957, Jacobson pointed to a linkage between denial and action, seen in analysis as the tendency toward acting out: To the extent that acting out serves to avoid the emotional response to memory, it is a form of denial. In a later and much celebrated work, Jacobson (1964) seems to have set the stage for what has been the predominant theme in the adolescent literature, namely the association of denial in adolescence with the adolescent's need to counteract the emotions associated with the experience of his limitations: the internal life of the adolescent is dominated by the struggle between the upheaval produced by a seductive, libidinal id seeking to shake off the iron grip of a sadistic superego. This struggle is denied as externally he or she flaunts his or her independence of thought and action. The adolescent may make a great show of his acceptance, or rejection, or rebellion against various philosophies, views and patterns of action. In reality, however, "for a long time he may not be able to achieve more than a pretense of independence, maintained with the aid of such denial and isolation mechanisms" (1964, p. 184).

Echoing this theme, that the adolescent resorts to denial as a way of combating his helplessness and limitations, Blos (1963), writes of the predilection of some adolescents to take refuge in the "magic of action and gesture" and sees in this action a manifestation of the adolescent's "need to deny his helplessness through action, to affirm by exaggeration his independence from the archaic omnipotent mother, to counteract the regressive pull to passivity by denying his dependence on reality itself" (1979, p. 259). If the adolescent's efforts to resolve the conflicts presented by the incest taboo and bisexuality should flounder, he "protects himself by a stubborn denial of any self-limitation, that grave affront to narcissism" (p. 480).

In a similar vein, Blos sees in the obedient son, who is ready to submit to the omnipotent, idealized good father and to trust in him, an attitude that is not based on anything realistic, and therefore something akin to denial (1979, p. 386). In all these descriptions, denial is associated exclusively with the smallness, weakness, dependence, and vulnerability of the adolescent vis-à-vis the parental figures, or of the adolescent ego faced with limitations to its narcissistic aspirations and in its dealings with unresolved negative Oedipal issues.

Let us turn at this point from this brief review of the salient features of the treatment of adolescent denial in the literature to an equally brief examination of the mechanism of denial in and of itself. Freud referred to disavowal in a few telling contexts: In connection with castration anxiety (1923), particularly as it stems from the recognition of the anatomical differences between the sexes (1925) and in relation to fetishism (1927b); in discussing religion (1927a) and the pains of living; in studying the commonalities and differences of neurosis and psychosis (1924); and finally, in describing the mechanism of the splitting of the ego (1924, 1936, 1940). Two central characteristics emerge very clearly from Freud's treatment of the subject: (1) the relationship between denial and reality and (2) the intimate tie between denial and splitting of the ego. I would like to underscore and develop these two aspects, because I see them as intrinsically and significantly related both to adolescence and to adolescent denial.

Denial is always in some focal relation to an aspect of *external reality*. Stated differently, when we speak of denial or of disavowal, we are referring to that special psychological way by which something that is "really real," so to speak, something that is really there and to which we bear a real relationship, is rendered psychologically nonexistent, that is, is nullified by the ego. This is clearly different from those other defenses that primarily or exclusively affect internal reality and by which the ego strives to make shifts and alterations only in our inner, psychic reality. Whereas the latter affect what happens at the interface of ego and id, the work of denial proceeds primarily at the level of ego and reality. The most immediate implication of the recourse to denial is therefore the fact that it places the ego in an extremely hazardous, or at least in a highly complex position in regard to reality.

Because reality testing is a *sine qua non,* essential aspect of the ego, the denial of a facet of external reality immediately places a tremendous burden on the continued integrity of the ego and threatens its ability to maintain adequate function. Clearly, such crass handling of reality cannot go unnoticed or uncompensated. Sooner or later, with a greater or lesser degree of psychiatric righteousness, the culprit ego will have to face the music. But we are still left with the question: Why does the ego resort to a defense that endangers its very existence, and how does it manage to survive such a potential self-destruction?

An easy solution to this problem may have been found if we could have relegated denial to the period of earliest childhood, when reality testing is still rough and poorly established. Or, if we could make the assertion that denial operates only in adults undergoing severe regressions, for example, psychosis, and thus once again to regard denial as characterizing only those states in which ego pathology is both rampant and severe. Perhaps quantitative factors are indeed at work, alongside qualitative ones. Indeed, we speak at times of "blatant denial," referring to those instances where the aspect of reality denied is so preponderant that to deny it would have required a much greater expenditure of psychic energy, or suspension of good reality testing, then merely to ignore some relatively minor or unimportant aspect of reality. This is clearly not the case, however, and indeed would be a misleading way of applying the concept.

In answering our question, two points present themselves. In the first place, far from being involved in repudiating minor or inconsequent aspects of reality, denial is typically called upon precisely when very painful, highly charged, and conflicted issues are at stake. If this is not the case, the ego is far more likely to call upon defenses of lower costs to itself, for example, displacement, avoidance, negation, or repression. We are probably correct in asserting that the ego is forced to call upon denial when faced with a piece of reality highly regarded by it but also extremely threatening and at the same time almost unavoidable by any other means.

Second, we must remember that *we may properly speak of denial only when and where it coexists with otherwise good reality testing*, as Anna Freud has already established (1946). If this condition were not observed, we would have to restrict ourselves to speak of denial only where regression is an accompanying process or defense. It is, of course, true that we frequently meet with denial in psychotic and otherwise regressed patients. But it is equally true, as I am certain everyone has encountered, that we also find denial in nonpsychotic persons, even if such encounters may be accompanied by feelings of incredulity or dismay. Indeed, what is called "psychotic insight" is usually achieved only when the ego is no longer capable of denial. We may perhaps even hazard making a risky statement in this connection, that to the extent that we do find denial in psychotics, this may be testimony to the fact that some good, more adequate reality testing may still be preserved. The higher incidence of denial in psychotically regressed populations may indeed not reflect lowered reality testing *per se* but rather another facet of denial, namely the tendency toward splitting of the ego; a tendency prevalent in such populations and that may facilitate recourse to denial.

Thus we approach the second characteristic of disavowal, which complements and sheds light on the first. If denial requires that good reality testing continues to prevail in the rest of the ego, whereas a highly charged aspect of reality is being denied, the implication can be only one: That the ego has undergone a psychological process we have come to regard as ubiquitous, namely, it has split or divided itself into different parts. Thus some portion of the ego experiences reality in a manner that can be described as being in adequate, realistic contact with it, whereas other portions behave and respond in a highly distorted way, as if whatever is regarded or sensed as frightening or obnoxious does not really exist at all.

How is all of this related to adolescence and to adolescent denial? Before we answer this question more directly, let us take a second look at one of Freud's last papers in which he establishes the role of this splitting of the ego in the operation of denial. I refer to Freud's paper, "A Disturbance of Memory on the Acropolis" (1936). In it, the octogenerian Freud tells the 70-year-old Romain Rolland the story of an incident that took place in 1904, when Freud was 48. On a holiday trip to the Mediterranean seaboard with his younger brother, they both had difficulty accepting the advice of a friend in Trieste not to proceed to the island of Corfu, as they had planned, but instead that they take the boat to Athens. Despite their gloomy mood and indecision, they followed this suggestion. When finally standing on the Acropolis, Freud had the surprising thought: "So all this really *does* exist, just as we learnt at school!" Freud's introspective account goes on to introduce the notion of the splitting of the ego:

> The person who gave expression to this remark was divided . . . from another person who took cognizance of [it]; and both were astonished, though not by the same thing. The first behaved as though he were obliged, *under the impact of an unequivocal observation,* to believe in something *the reality of which had hitherto seemed doubtful.* . . . The second person, on the other hand, was justifiably astonished, because he had been unaware that the real existence of Athens, the Acropolis, and the landscape around it had ever been the object of doubt. What *he had been expecting was rather some expression of delight or admiration.* (p. 241 [emphasis mine])

Freud's continued analysis of this fragment of experience centers around the feeling that to be given the actual opportunity to see Athens aroused strong feelings of incredulity, regret and even depression—it was too good to be true! The fulfillment of this long-standing wish actually gave rise to a subjective experience of derealization, which is akin to depersonalization. It asserts that what is perceived is unreal and aims to defend the ego by disavowing a piece of reality. But the denial is not merely of something in the here and now but of something made meaningful through its intimate significance within one's past. It is in this connection that Freud's account becomes more eloquent but also immediately and openly pertinent to adolescence:

> It is not true that in my school days I ever doubted the real existence of Athens. I only doubted whether *I should ever see Athens.* It seemed to me beyond the realms of possibility that I should travel so far—that I should "go such a long way." This was linked up with the limitations and poverty of our conditions of life in my youth. My longing to travel was no doubt also the expression of a wish to escape from that pressure, like the force which drives so many adolescent children to run away from home. . . . When first one catches sight of the sea, crosses the ocean and experiences as realities cities and lands which for so long had been distant, unattainable things of desire— one feels oneself like a hero who has performed deeds of improbable greatness. (Freud, 1936, p. 247 [emphasis mine])

What is then stirred up, however, by the joy of the fulfillment of such long-standing childhood dreams is the sense of guilt:

> It must be that a sense of guilt was attached to the satisfaction in having gone such a long way: there was something about it that was wrong, that from the earliest times had been forbidden. It was something to do with a child's criticism of his father, with the undervaluation which took the place of the overvaluation of earlier childhood. It seems as though the essence of success was to have got further than one's father, and as though to excel one's father was still something forbidden. (p. 247)

Freud's personal account is not merely revealing—it strikes the chords that I believe are the real issues around which adolescent denial can most cogently be understood and met. For to view adolescent denial as being couched primarily in weakness and vulnerability is to distort our understanding of what happens at this crucial developmental crossroads. It is true that a good deal of adolescent experience involves issues of vulnerability and hence of weakness—certainly internal, and so to some extent also, on external weakness. And yet such emphasis seems to miss the picture in some crucial way. The adolescent arrives at this stage of development slightly out of breath, so to speak: He has been panting and postponing for so long, in fact, for all of his life. He has deferred burning wishes and aspirations for genital fulfillment, Oedipal strivings, competition for supremacy and primacy, for strength and wisdom, for power, accuracy, and control through knowledge—for so long, that, for all he knows, these needs, wishes, fantasies, and aspirations may indeed be only the myths invented by his elders in order to subjugate and control him. His experience as a child in the world of adults, whom he looks up to and wishes to emulate, has been governed by a highly specific, constantly repeated, implicit injunction, underlying all his encounters with frustration, delay of gratification, and postponement of self-indulgent fulfillment. That injunction, clearly etched in his memory, says— "Not now, later, when you grow up." And now he suddenly finds himself standing in disbelief, with a mixture of joy and incredulity, on top of his Acropolis—he has finally arrived, or so it seems.

It seems to be of small wonder that the overwhelming sense of adolescents should be one of derealization and depersonalization whenever they are faced with the new evidence of their senses—with the reality of their being as big, frequently as powerful, and to their mind certainly as smart, as their elders. It is reality that tells them, in no uncertain terms, that the time has come to call in their debts, to collect the long-deferred promises. Reality also tells them that, should they only begin to allow their wishes some expression, they could not really be stopped. The sense of power and strength, the intoxicating nearness of the spoils of victory, are almost overwhelming.

What are the obstacles to the adolescent's realization of his potential? A great deal has been written and said on this subject, so I will only briefly allude to the main themes. The most serious obstacles stem from the fact that those early aspirations are intimately tied to the same libidinally invested, infantile figures. The reawakened threats of incest, on the one hand, and the tremendous pulls to passivity and dependency on the other, require renewed and redoubled efforts at separation–individuation (Blos, 1967) as well as a shoring up of the old Oedipal renunciations (A. Freud, 1958).

It very quickly becomes painfully obvious to the adolescent that his having arrived at his Acropolis, at the attainment of adultlike physical stature, sexual prowess, and the capacity for truly abstract logical and cognitive manipulations are not quite what he had hoped for and imagined all through childhood. It is as though an eager guest has arrived too early at a party that has not quite started yet and finds himself detained in the foyer by his embarassed hosts—"for just a little while longer." His forced detention may prove very valuable to him. It actually enables him to proceed with the internal work of modifying and remodeling psychic structure and object relations that are his real ticket to adulthood. Thus, he can gradually develop the capacity to escape the regressive pulls of passive-maternal and negative-Oedipal strivings. He may remodel his superego along milder, more reality-appropriate lines. His renunciation of the Oedipal longings opens the door to extrafamilial relationships in which fuller expression of drives and wishes will eventually be possible and even welcome. Through homoerotic, narcissistically invested first-love relationships, he can integrate his narcissistic aspirations and strengthen sufficiently his sense of self so as to allow for his subsequent embarkation on heterosexual love relationships. Finally, out of these new capacities both for object relations and vis-à-vis his own self, a new sense of identity is shaped and consolidated so as to be serviceable for times to come.

We can see and appreciate the importance of the adolescent delay before reaching full adulthood. But to the *adolescent,* the experience is one in which he must constantly engage in massive denial. He must deny his *strength,* the reality of much of his attainments, so as not to face prematurely the full consequences of what and where he really is. In other words, he must deny the reality of having arrived at the party, or at the Acropolis, so as to be able to go on delaying and postponing. But he must equally vehemently deny his weakness, his second-best or "not-quite-making-it-yet" status. For to fully accept and experience those portions of his reality that are weak and childlike immediately threatens him with unbearable, if covertly desired, headlong surrender to his longings for childish passivity, with total capitulation to those forces he strains to escape.

It is precisely this sense of the admixture of strengths and weaknesses that arouses in the adolescent incredulity and joy on the one hand, and tremendous fears and guilt over regressive wishes on the other. He typically handles this dilemma by splitting his ego, by experiencing and presenting himself as strong, potent, sexual, and capable on the one hand, while also showing himself to be weak, small, vulnerable, asexual, and incapable. This split in his ego enables one part of his self to deny the *real* existence of the other, and yet for *all* of him to go on and accept the continued but necessary delay a little bit longer. Subjectively, the experienced split in the ego gives rise to states in which he either feels himself to be unreal, as in depersonalization, or experiences his external reality as unreal, as in derealization.

Depending of course on a variety of other factors that govern the overall state of ego strength, it is here, in this conflict between his strength and weakness, that we may look for the source of many of these adolescent experiences of a slightly dissociative nature.

I would like to stress that these dissociative experiences are by and large at a subclinical level. They are another one of these sources of confusion that make the diagnosis and treatment of adolescent phenomena such a difficult task. We must also recognize that, much as they are a feature of the adolescent's subjective experience, these ego splits and the denials that are grafted onto and made possible by them, are not at all easily verbalized or shared by the adolescent. This, of course, is a source of much consternation to the adults interacting with him, as they can never be certain of which frame of mind they will find him in, and their response to his denial often ranges from rage to exhaustion.

IMPLICATIONS FOR TREATMENT AND CLINICAL ILLUSTRATION

In the hands of the clinician dealing with and treating adolescents, awareness of these subjective states, of the predilection to splitting, and the constant conflict between weakness and strength, regressive surrender, and dangerous triumph, forms a powerful tool. Once he or she understands these conflicts and the developmental impasses from which they derive, he or she can approach the adolescent much more easily. For as much as the adolescent finds it difficult, if not actually impossible and unthinkable, to verbalize these notions for the adult, he is extremely appreciative and relieved when the adult, or the therapist, takes the lead in verbalizing these conflicts for him. The relief is usually very dramatic and the need to deny will usually subside quite strikingly. Our failure to verbalize and interpret these needs may contribute to a deepening split in the ego, fostering the adolescent's move in the direction of an "as-if" personality, or to a deeper consolidation of a "false self." Such issues must be approached early and forthrightly in adolescent treatment.

A brief clinical vignette follows in order to demonstrate some of the issues raised here.

Tamar, an 18-year-old girl, came to see me in the midst of real turmoil and crisis in her life. She had spent the last year and a half forming a group of youngsters who, like herself, were interested in doing their compulsory army service in the special format available to Israeli youth, combining regular army training and service with life and work on a kibbutz. As this group which she put together was not sponsored by one of the political or apolitical youth movements, concerted and sustained efforts on her part were required. Her success was obviously no mean achievement, and a real tribute to her initiative and leadership. Just before they began their official period at the kibbutz, she had spent time abroad, again feeling socially very successful. She arrived from that experience to the kibbutz feeling like "a new person." Her exuberance continued for several days, until the following incident took place. The counselor attached to their group (several years older and much admired by all the girls) showed some interest in her. He invited her to his room, and when she was there, he took hold of her hand. She became very flustered, asked, "What's this supposed to mean?" and when he spelled out more clearly his interest in and attraction to her, she bolted and ran out. Over the next few days she became increasingly restless, tearful and agitated.

She felt terribly ashamed in the presence of the rest of the group, as if they knew what had happened to her, and was unable to work with or join them on social gatherings. Even entering the dining hall became unbearably painful. Several days later, she left the kibbutz and the group, and withdrew from the program in a way that clearly burned her bridges behind her. She moved back to her home in town and shortly thereafter came to see me.

Tamar is a big, vibrant, active, and lively girl. She is also a strikingly sensitive, attractive, thoughtful, and verbal person. The dramatic quality of the events and the emotional upheaval that accompanied them were indicative of an impulsiveness and even a measure of self-directed inner violence and aggression, which soon emerged more openly in depressive affect, a tendency to escape the world and hide under her bedcovers, and even some suicidal ideation. Despite these indications of how seriously upset and buffeted she was, Tamar was and still is very far from being psychotic, schizophrenic, or of borderline pathology. She has maintained a firm grip on her object relations throughout, continues to be socially active, to work, and to manifest no deficiencies whatsoever in her overall ego functioning. Her central and repeated question is a puzzlement—How could this have happened to her, of all people?

Space does not permit much elaboration. Let me therefore summarize the answer that began to take shape as we attempted to understand and deal with her puzzlement. Tamar had lost her father early in her childhood, yet she denied any feelings attached to him or the loss itself. Her proneness to denial was further prominently demonstrated in her revelation of a shameful childhood secret: For about 3 years, while in the early school grades, she would masturbate quite openly in class. She remained impervious to all requests by her mother and teachers to stop her habit, professing not to understand what they wanted of her, and simultaneously not having any conscious appreciation of the sexual pleasure she was deriving from it. At the same time, however, she was so embarrassed and ashamed that she actually gauged her progress in life by the gradual distancing and disappearance of all those who were privy to her secret and shame. Thus moving on to high school was an important step in that direction; her trip abroad was another. Finally, her beginning a new life on the kibbutz meant that she was literally on new social and emotional grounds, thoroughly untainted by her past.

Her encounter with sexuality, in the form of the advances made by the counselor, was doubly significant and meaningful. She was suddenly, without warning or adequate preparation, thrust into a sexualized situation, with strong Oedipal overtones, in which she was frightened by the upsurge of her own barely repressed wishes. But this is only one part of the story, the more conventionally acknowledged part. She had also made valiant efforts to overcome, master, and deny these feelings and wishes so closely linked with her ego passivity and weakness. She saw them as part and parcel of her shame as a small girl, of what she was then unable to contain and hide. Now, she felt, she was finally big, strong, powerful, and successful—"a new person." As this "strong person," she would no longer have to fear those embarassing and dangerous impulses, nor would she have to experience her passivity and helplessness before them. She had *repressed* her sexual wishes and Oedipal longings for her father. But she now *denied* the *meaning* of the subtler forms of the man's attention, or of the situation she would find herself in if she went to his room. Feeling herself strong and invincible, she could give no way to those feelings and wishes that meant she was simultaneously also small, desirous, potentially weak, and passive. Quite obviously, then, her sudden confrontation with the same wishes immediately broke down the denial and brought the "weak" and the "strong" persons in her, as it were, to a head-on, impossible conflict.

An important component of working through the dynamics of this conflict centered on her proneness to such denial. This took the form of becoming acquainted with her subjective experience of mild derealization. She would not, even though she could, distinguish clearly and carefully between reality and fantasy, between dreamlike inner states and the actualities of the situations she would find herself in. Once the diffusion of this boundary was pointed out and described, the different subjective experiences became almost immediately familiar to her. The enhancement of her observing ego allowed her to describe them with some distance, and gradually she exercised control over them.

This tendency to ego splitting, with the attendant lowering of reality testing and self-esteem, and heightening of her proclivity to denial, though well circumscribed, was clearly reflected in many later instances. The usual pattern was one in which she would allow herself to enter situations that could not even be described as compromising, of which she had been given ample notice by the man involved, yet she would deny the clear warnings and inuendo, leading to some real unpleasantness and misunderstanding. She would later laughingly comment about the "unreal" nature of these events, saying that these were things that would ordinarily happen only in movies. She was actually quite taken aback when her little sister presented her with a poem in which she had clearly described her as confusing light and darkness, dreams and reality.

SUMMARY

I have reviewed the particular fit between denial and adolescent development and experience. Denial, in my view, involves some aspect of reality and is made possible by a split in the ego. In the adolescent, the real attainment of adultlike possibilities creates an enormous conflict between the need and wish to exercise these new capacities, the guilt and shame aroused by them, and the fear of equally potent regressive childhood pulls. The adolescent, caught between his real strengths and weaknesses, tends to split his subjective experience accordingly, denying through action or gesture whatever is more disturbing at the moment. This is a necessary step for further integration of ego identity and personality. Yet it is also a source of difficulty for the adult and therapist dealing with him. Early verbalization and forthright interpretation of this dual difficulty is a real relief for the adolescent and is generally accepted by him with gratitude.

REFERENCES

Blos, P. (1963). The concept of acting out in relation to the adolescent process. *Journal of the American Academy of Child Psychiatry 2*, 118–136. Reprinted in Blos, P. (1979) *The adolescent passage*. New York: International Universities Press.

Blos, P. (1967). The second individuation process of adolescence. *Psychoanalytic Study of the Child, 22*, 162–186. New York: International Universities Press.

Blos, P. (1979). *The adolescent passage*. New York: International Universities Press.

Freud, A. (1946). *The ego and the mechanisms of defense*. New York: International Universities Press.

Freud, A. (1958). Adolescence. *Psychoanalytic Study of the Child, 13*, 225–278. New York: International Universities Press.

Freud, S. (1923). The infantile genital organization: An interpolation into the theory of sexuality. In *Standard edition* (Vol. 19, pp. 141–145). London: Hogarth.

Freud, S. (1924). Neurosis and psychosis. In *Standard edition* (Vol. 19, pp. 149–153). London: Hogarth.

Freud, S. (1925). Some psychical consequences of the anatomical distinction between the sexes. In *Standard edition* (Vol. 19, pp. 248–258). London: Hogarth.

Freud, S. (1927a). The future of an illusion. In *Standard edition* (Vol. 21, pp. 5–56). London: Hogarth.

Freud, S. (1927b). Fetishism. In *Standard edition* (Vol. 21, pp. 152–157). London: Hogarth.

Freud, S. (1936). A disturbance of memory on the Acropolis. In *Standard edition* (Vol. 22, pp. 239–248). London: Hogarth.

Freud, S. (1940). Splitting of the ego in the process of defense. In *Standard edition* (Vol. 23, pp. 275–278). London: Hogarth.

Jacobson, E. (1957). Denial and repression. *Journal of the American Psychoanalytic Association, 5,* 61–92.

Jacobson, E. (1964). *The self and the object world.* New York: International Universities Press.

11

Varieties of Denial
The Case of a Fairy Tale

RIVKA R. EIFERMANN

Fairy tales have traditionally been examined by psychologists and psychoanalysts primarily from the viewpoint of the child: what the child projects into the tale; with whom he or she identifies; what symbolic representations are unconsciously perceived in the tale; and how he or she is affected by being exposed to it (e.g., Bettelheim, 1976). Thus far, however, little attention has been paid to the fact that a story comes alive only as an *interactive process* between storyteller[1] and receiver—*both of whom* have needs, wishes, fantasies, *and* defenses that draw them together, with the story as their common focus.

It is the centrality of this aspect of storytelling to which I will draw attention herein. I shall base my discussion on the Grimms' tale *Little Red Riding Hood*, entitled *Rotkäppchen* in the original, and perhaps better translated as *Little Red Cap*. Using only specific aspects of the story, my analysis of this tale will demonstrate how one defense mechanism, namely denial, becomes operative in both mother *and* child during the course of their collaborative undertaking. Much can be learned from specific attention to this dyad, particularly that of mother and daughter.

Despite its happy ending, *Little Red Riding Hood,* both as told by the

---

[1]By "storyteller" I mean the person telling or reading the story to another, or its writer.

RIVKA R. EIFERMANN • Department of Psychology, The Hebrew University of Jerusalem, Jerusalem, Israel.

155

Grimm brothers and in its numerous variations (Zipes, 1984), as well as various of its watered-down versions, has cruel and frightening aspects. Nevertheless, the tale has retained its popularity, as evidenced by the incessant flow of new editions and versions that appear. Mothers often introduce it to their children, and the children then request repeatedly, endlessly, that it be read to them. I propose to illustrate how both teller and receiver of the tale provide one another with a setting in which denial is reciprocally exercised in ways that are mutually relevant. (The denial is in act and in fantasy, of reality as well as of feelings.)

I do not mean to imply that the aspects on which I focus are necessarily those most central to the tale. Nor do I wish to maintain that denial is the defense mechanism, let alone the aspect of the mother's or the child's personality that is the most prominent in the reciprocal undertaking on which I shall dwell. What I intend to demonstrate is that there is a narrative (Schafer, 1983; Spence, 1982) that draws together these particular aspects of the situation, and that, through this narrative, new light is thrown on the process involved in listening to and telling this tale—and others.

Before I proceed, I shall present an outline of the original *Rotkäppchen,* for the benefit of readers who may be unfamiliar with the tale:

> Once upon a time there was a little girl who was loved by everyone. Her grandmother gave her a little red cap, which she always wore, and she was therefore called "Little Red Cap" (Little Red Riding Hood). One day her mother sent Little Red Riding Hood to bring some cake and wine to her grandmother, who was ill, instructing her to walk nicely and quietly and not to run off the path, and to be polite as she enters grandmother's home.
>
> Grandmother lived in a forest, and, upon entering it, Little Red Riding Hood met a wolf. Not knowing that he was a wicked wolf, Little Red Riding Hood patiently answered his questions as to her destination, and saying, "you surely must know it," told him how to identify her grandmother's cottage. The crafty wolf then tempted Little Red Riding Hood to look around, to enjoy the pretty flowers and singing birds, and the little girl, who then "opened her eyes," decided to pick a fresh nosegay for her grandmother. She ran from the path, deeper and deeper into the forest fancying, as she picked a flower, that the prettier ones were to be found there.
>
> Meanwhile, the wolf ran straight to grandmother's cottage and, pretending to be Little Red Riding Hood, entered, went straight to grandmother's bed, and devoured her. He then put on grandmother's clothes and laid himself down in her bed.
>
> When Little Red Riding Hood had picked so many flowers that she could hold no more, she remembered her grandmother and resumed her journey. The cottage door was open—she felt peculiar upon entering, and said "Good Morning" but received no reply. In bed lay her grandmother, looking very strange. With bewilderment, Little Red Riding Hood exclaimed ". . . what—big ears," "big eyes," "large hands," her grandmother had, to which the wolf replied soothingly; but his response to ". . . what a terribly big mouth you have (grandmother)" was to jump from bed and swallow her.

Having appeased his appetite, the wolf fell into a deep sleep and snored. A huntsman who was passing by was surprised by the snores coming from the old woman's cottage. He entered the room, took a pair of scissors, and after a few snips at the wolf's stomach, Little Red Riding Hood, frightened but unharmed, jumped out, followed by a weak but alive grandmother.

Little Red Riding Hood then fetched heavy stones with which they filled the wolf's body, and when he awoke and wanted to run away, he fell down at once, and died. The huntsman took the wolf's skin and left, and Little Red Riding Hood and grandmother happily ate and drank what the little girl had brought. Grandmother revived, and Little Red Riding Hood thought to herself, "As long as I live, I will never again leave the path, to run into the forest, when my mother has forbidden me to do so."

My narrative relies on: (1) general features of the situation—of the tale and of mother and child in interaction; (2) parts of a student report, written for one of my university seminars, in which the student in question recalled *Little Red Riding Hood* and a childhood preoccupation that accompanied the telling of the tale; (3) sections of a pair of tape recordings from each of two mothers, first the mother reading the tale to her daughter, and then the child retelling it; and (4) a specific revision of the tale, written by a mother–writer, with the purpose of making it less cruel and frightening. Thus, the data on which I base my construction does not contain specific, personal associations of the kind that are necessary for an individual analysis in depth of either the object relations involved in each case, or of specific fantasies (conscious or unconscious) that the tale evokes. Additionally, in my references to *Little Red Riding Hood,* I do not examine symbolic representations of the kind that a classic and long-surviving tale such as this invites, and that, indeed, have been applied to it and similar tales (e.g., Bettelheim, 1976; Burton, 1978; Cath & Cath, 1978; Diamant, 1977; A. Freud, 1967). As my analysis is confined to the overall significance of the tale rather than its meaning to any one individual,[2] the more detailed and idiosyncratic meanings of the data obtained from the people quoted in what follows is beyond the scope of this chapter. This level of analysis has implications throughout for my usage of the term *denial.* It also means that the narrative I construct is in the nature of a general description and will vary both in emphasis and personal meaning when applied to individual cases. I shall return later to these and related issues.

Let us begin with the act of mother reading the tale to her child. By carrying it through to its happy end, mother may be providing her child with a readymade fantasy through which, as Anna Freud (1936) put it, the child can deny the reality of her smallness and dependence: Whereas the tale at first emphasizes Little Red Riding Hood's vulnerability and

[2]In later articles (Eifermann, 1987a,b) I qualify this statement.

helplessness, eventually and by contrast, it is she who turns to be the most resourceful and physically strongest figure in the tale. In *Little Red Riding Hood,* the fact that the girl is little is even part of her name, and her particular vulnerability due to her youth and size is made harshly explicit in the story through the thought expressed by the voluptuous wolf, "What a tender young creature! What a nice plump mouthful!" Yet, as the story unfolds, the advantages of being "little" rather than a grandmother are clearly described: When saved by the huntsman, "the little girl *sprang* out of the wolf's stomach," while grandmother emerged *"hardly able to breathe"* (my italics). Then, the child takes over altogether: "Little Red Riding Hood . . . quickly fetches great stones with which they filled the wolf's stomach." Thus, not only is Little Riding Hood physically faster and more agile than her grandmother, she now proves—*in denial* of what is realistically feasible—to have more presence of mind, to be more practical, and to act faster than even the huntsman. Moreover, she is not only the leader in this whole operation but its main executor. And, as if all this were not enough, she turns also out to be strong enough to carry "great stones" and to do so "quickly." In fact, we are told that the stones were so heavy that when the wolf woke up and wanted to run away "he fell down at once, and died." It is interesting to note, in this connection, that it is in the early English translation of the story (1884) that the German *Rotkäppchen* is accurately rendered as *"Little* Red Cap." From that point in the story when, through denial of her smallness and consequent physical weakness and dependence, she becomes master of the situation in the tale, "Little" is dropped from her name, and she is henceforth known as "Red Cap." Such a use of denial in the process of a story I call "denial in fantasy."

However, before such a denial in fantasy can take place, mother leads her child through a tale of adventures that scare not only Little Red Riding Hood but also the little listener to the tale. Before going into how mother may be dealing with her part in this cooperative undertaking, I shall present, from data collected in one of my graduate seminars in the Department of Psychology at the Hebrew University (Eifermann, 1985), illustrations of how the child copes, through denial, with the anxiety-provoking aspects of the tale. The first instance is that of a student who, many years after her childhood encounters with the tale of *Little Red Riding Hood,* and with the image of the wolf in Grandmother's bed, still responded to these events with denial reminiscent of the fictional protagonist, Little Red Riding Hood herself.

According to the original Grimms' Tale (1819), when Little Red Riding Hood drew the curtains of her grandmother's bed, she was facing a grandmother who was "looking very strange": "Oh, grandmother," she exclaimed, "what big ears you have!" And hearing the gentle reply: "The better to hear you with," she persists with "Oh, grandmother, what big eyes you have!" Again, the reply—"The better to see you with"—only leads to a further anxious enquiry, "Oh, grandmother, what large hands you have," which calls forth: "The better to seize [*packen*] you with." The child, at this point horrified, insistently and, it seems desperately, still demands reassurance, "But, grandmother, what a *terribly* [*entsetzlich*] big mouth [*Maul*] you have!" (my italics). (*Maul*, the German word used here for mouth, is only applied with reference to *animals*.) "The better to devour you with," comes the reply. And, the tale continues, the wolf had scarcely said this, than, with one bound he was out of bed and swallowed poor Little Red Riding Hood.

In the large variety of drawings of "grandmother" in bed that I have examined, it is the wolf that lies there, quite unmistakably. And children who look at these drawings unhesitantly recognize him for what he is. Thus, it is Little Red Riding Hood's *denial* of the "reality" in front of her (once we combine picture with tale) that drives her to seek help and reassurance from the very source of her terror—and this is what leads to her (temporary) doom. It seems that the same mechanism was still partially alive in our student, as she recalled the tale of Little Red Riding Hood. In an assignment in which all students were asked to reconstruct the tale of Little Red Riding Hood as they recalled it and to add some associations to it, this student commented: "As a child I always thought, 'How could Little Red Riding Hood be so stupid that she did not recognize that it was the wolf!'" And yet, in her reconstruction of the tale, this same student, having quoted Little Red Riding Hood's questions to Grandmother, remarked, "One could add another question, 'Grandmother, why is your belly so very swollen.'" It is as if, to this day, she retains her anger toward Little Red Riding Hood for her desperate and catastrophic need to deny, yet, at the same time, the child within her carries Little Red Riding Hood's denial even a step further: Although *her* Little Red Riding Hood explicitly knows about the swollen belly already filled up with Grandmother (and hidden with a blanket in all pictures!), she *still* persists in turning to "grandmother" for reassurance. It is as if she (the student and her Little Red Riding Hood) is saying: The more evidence there is for horror, the greater the need to deny it. Thus the student seems to reveal the frightened child within her through these traces of her original identification not only with Little Red Riding Hood's anxiety but also with her manner of attempting to cope with it.

My second example comes from transcribed recordings of a mother reading the story to her little girl, and the girl's reactions during the reading.[3] I have selected the section of the reading in which Little Red Riding Hood first encounters the wolf. The child who hears the story, and not for the first time, clearly needs to fend off the anxiety this encounter triggers in her: She already knows that the wolf "is lying." Her denial of the threat, by turning the situation into a game, is particularly striking:

As her mother reads, ". . . and there behind the tree, there was hiding ———," the child intervenes with a fearful scream "Oh the wolf!" And then, as her mother repeats (in a sinister voice) "the wolf," the child again screams. But, just a little later, when her mother quotes the wolf telling Little Red Riding Hood in a sweet voice, ". . . don't be afraid, I'm a friendly wolf," the child, now in the role of an observer who knows better, inserts, "He is lying." But she soon steps back into the role of Little Red Riding Hood, responding to each of the wolf's guesses about what is in her basket with great enthusiasm and complete involvement: "Would you like me to guess? Well, in your basket you have . . . perhaps eggs?" "No!" she cries out. And when her mother continues quoting from the story, "Little Red Riding Hood did not reply . . . 'Perhaps cheese?'", the child laughs. To the next question, "Perhaps cake?", she responds with a great joyous "Yes!" Denial takes over, and the pleasure of the immediate guessing game supercedes that which she had just explicitly recognized about the wolf, namely that he is not trustworthy.

I shall now turn to mother[4] and to how she deals with her part in the cooperative undertaking. There is no doubt that, among many other things, often protective and loving, that she does in the act of reading the story, mother also exposes her child (who is a willing partner) to a tale of cruelty and fright. I do not mean to imply that that is all there is to the story or, indeed, to the exposure. Our interest here is, however, in how mother deals with this particular aspect of it. We have recordings (collected as part of the research project already quoted), of two mothers who read variations of the tale to their children.[5] It is very evident, in both the readings and in the verbal exchange between mother and child, that, among many other things, each mother insists and expands upon the more anxiety-provoking aspects of the tale. Retrospective interviews indicated that neither mother was quite aware of doing this.

One mother, as she was reading *Little Red Riding Hood* to her 4½-

---

[3]These recordings were obtained as part of our ongoing research project on object relations in the storytelling situation.

[4]In three later papers (Eifermann, 1987a,b,c), I present partial self-analyses regarding my own internalized mother, as unconsciously presented here.

[5]I would like to thank each mother and child for their generous permission to study and publish their recordings.

year-old girl, stopped her flow of reading (she was herself reading the particular version for the first time), and inserted a question. The following exchange transpired:

MOTHER: Just a minute, what has happened to Little Red Riding Hood. I haven't understood. Did he swallow Little Red Riding Hood or did he not swallow Little Red Riding Hood?

GIRL: [In a protesting voice, simultaneous with Mother's repeated question] No, no, he didn't swallow.

MOTHER: Oh, he didn't swallow Little Red Riding Hood.

GIRL: Because she ran so fast.

MOTHER: Little Red Riding Hood ran fast. When *I* was a little girl I was told that he *did* swallow Little Red Riding Hood . . . and you were told that he *did not* swallow Little Red Riding Hood?

The mother, who cannot quite follow this version of the tale, dwells on the scary topic rather insistently—has the wolf actually *swallowed* or has he not *swallowed* Little Red Riding Hood? The child's repeated protest does not deter mother, nor does she take the girl's explanation, "because she ran so fast," as a possible invitation to leave it at that. She shares her more gruesome childhood tale with her, again repeating, "did *swallow* Little Red Riding Hood," "did not *swallow*."

Another exchange runs as follows:

MOTHER: The brave huntsman entered the house . . . he caught the wolf, opened her [a slip of the tongue] stomach [Mother laughs briefly], took out grandmother who was in perfect condition and only somewhat frightened.

GIRL: Why?

MOTHER: Why was she frightened? . . . Well, really, think that *you* were in the stomach of the wolf . . . would you not be frightened?

Mother, who seems to understand her little girl's question to mean "Why was she frightened," in an effort to explain, puts the gruesome situation in as concrete and direct terms as possible. The exchange continues:

MOTHER: No? What would you be?

GIRL: A little glad, actually . . . !

From the exchanges between our second mother–daughter pair, I have chosen a section in which it is the 6½-year-old child who tells a version of the tale to her mother. We can see how the mother draws the child back to a gruesome part of the tale that the child overlooked.

GIRL: . . . and the house was not terribly far, but at the edge of the forest, with windows, in the shape of a heart, terribly beautiful, and . . . ehm, in front there were four trees and . . . a lawn.

MOTHER: Yes.

GIRL: And a garden . . . and . . . he swallowed grandmother and Little Red Riding Hood, but the guard, there was a guard who walked [heard] there, when, eh, the wolf was snoring and thought it was grandmother. Then, he went in, ehm, to see how grandmother was, and saw that it was the wolf and caught him, and put him in the zoo, and [quickly] took out grandmother and Little Red Riding Hood, who ate what Little Red Riding Hood had brought.

MOTHER: Where did he take them out of?

GIRL: He took them out of the stomach of the wolf.

MOTHER: So in the story the wolf swallowed them [her]?

GIRL: Yes.

The child dwells and elaborates on the pretty and romantic aspects of the tale: the beautiful house, the garden. Mother asks about a gruesome detail that her child skipped in her telling and returns yet again to another that is frightening. Without claiming that it is representative, it seems that this data indicates that, for whatever conscious and unconscious reasons, mothers will sometimes expose their children to more gruesomeness than the tale, or the child, invites. Thus, it is also possible that mothers' often-expressed concern about the possible harmful effects of the gruesome tale on the child may contain an element of denial that there may be such a tendency toward the children in themselves.

Before expanding on one such case, of a mother who revised and published *Little Red Riding Hood*, I would like to add a few words concerning the nature of my illustrations. I want in this way to make explicit what, in my opinion, only too often remains implicit when legitimate conclusions, drawn on the basis of limited data, are taken out of context: I have already said that my intention here is to focus on a specific aspect of the mothers' behavior, but that any personal statement about them is beyond the scope of this paper. In saying this, I mean neither to be apologetic nor "protective" toward the mothers I have quoted (and shall quote in what follows). I mean, rather, to differentiate clearly between different levels of analysis, the aims of which do not overlap. The data I present are entirely sufficient for my purpose: I believe that I have demonstrated that mothers will at times expose their children to more cruelty and fright than is either invited by the child or determined by the script; and I shall further demonstrate that denial may at times be operative in the process of such exposure. Yet it is quite outside the aim of this presentation, and indeed its possibilities, to draw any more detailed conclusions about any specific mother or mother/daughter dyad. For, without viewing the data in a context that enables careful analysis of background, emotions, and motives, its more specific meanings remain unknown. Thus, for example, the quotations I have presented do not evoke the general affective atmosphere in which the exchanges have taken place. More specifically, when the first mother tells her child, ". . . when *I* was a little girl I was told . . . ," she may be predominantly expressing her need to share her tough childhood experience with her child, or to compare herself favorably with her mother, or to expose her child to cruelty in a more protective way than she experienced her own exposure. The possibilities are many and varied, and so are the motives underlying them, as well as their implications for the mother/daughter relationship. Similarly, when the second mother asks her child about the more gruesome parts of the tale, which the girl has skipped, mother may, for example, be unconsciously helping her child, under her protective guidance, to make explicit what she knows the child knows but dares not say. Yet gruesomeness and cruelty are then made explicit by the mother (even though it may be a minor by-product and regardless of the fact that the predominant personal motives for the act remain unknown), and denial may then be involved.

Dvora Omer, an Israeli writer in her own right, has revised and published (1979) a collection of the Grimms' tales in Hebrew. She introduces her collection with the following words (translated from Hebrew):

> [This is] a personal and true story of a writer who is also a mother (of three) and an educator (by profession). . . . I have tried to remain as true to the original as my motherly conscience would allow. I exclude most cruel descriptions and emphasize positive motives. . . . I also emphasize the distance of the world of fairy tales from reality—in the characters, in time and in name—so as to enable the children to cope more easily with contents that may be frightening.

In what follows, I shall demonstrate that Dvora Omer is not successful in her attempt. While she excludes some of the frightening details and the cruelty from the tale, she introduces and elaborates on other such features, ending up with a story no less gruesome than the original. Further, Omer's (unsuccessful) attempt reveals denial of some of her own unwanted feelings.

One of the revised scenes is that in which the huntsman ". . . took a pair of scissors, and began to cut open the stomach of the sleeping wolf. When he made two snips, he saw the little red cap shining, and then he made two more snips, and the little girl sprang out." In her attempt to reduce the curelty inherent in the story and the fright it might produce in a child, Omer writes instead: "He took a big knife from the kitchen and opened the wolf's stomach. And the gobbler was so tired that he never noticed that the huntsman took grandmother and Little Red Riding Hood out of his stomach." (Some further reduction in anxiety might have been afforded by reversing the order of these sentences, saying first that the tired wolf would not realize what was happening, making it quite explicit that the wolf did not feel anything when he was being cut open, rather than when grandmother and Little Red Riding Hood were taken out of his stomach.) In any case, any horror about the wolf's agonies that her first sentence might evoke, or fright that it provoke (the child might imagine that the wolf is about to wake up in agony and attack the huntsman!), is immediately alleviated. And yet, this more humane attitude toward the wolf is, surprisingly, not extended either to Little Red Riding Hood or to her grandmother. Quite the contrary, their agonies are dwelt upon and elaborated so that they exceed the original. The Grimm brothers describe the events after the wolf had swallowed up Little Red Riding Hood as follows: "When the wolf had appeased his appetite, he lay down again in bed, fell asleep and began to snore very loudly. A huntsman was just passing the house . . ." Thus, the brief, scary description is immediately relieved through the happy coincidence of a rescuer appearing on the scene right away. But Omer chooses, instead, to dwell on the horror and agony of it all:

> Since his stomach was full, it was no wonder that the wolf felt tired. After the delicious and voluptuous meal, he returned to grandmother's bed and fell into a heavy sleep, making loud long snores.
> And thus, an hour passed, 2 hours passed. Grandmother and Little Red Riding Hood were caught in the dark, narrow stomach of the wolf. While the wolf lay in the soft and comfortable bed of the old woman, sleeping deeply and snoring loudly. Then a huntsman passed near grandmother's house. . . .

The slow passage of a long, agonizing time is thus described in detail, and in quite realistic terms—contrary to our reviser's declared intention "to emphasize the distance of the world of fairy tales from reality." In Omer's effort to achieve this distance, she uses such devices as the repeated reminder to the child that "this is just a story." Thus, she replaces the classical opening of the Grimms' tale, "Once upon a time there was a little girl" with "Close to the *betwitched* forest, *where many stories and fairy tales are woven,* there lived a dear little girl" (my italics). In the same spirit, she replaces "Little Red Riding Hood did not know what a wicked creature he [the wolf] was" with "Little Red Riding Hood did not know that the wolves in stories and fairy tales are bad, usually very [bad]."

Omer finds it difficult, in terms of her conscience as a mother, to expose (her) children to the excessive cruelty and threat which she finds in the original Grimms' tale. In this she denies some other, contrary aspects of her feelings, which nevertheless find direct expression in her revision of the tale. (At the risk of repeating myself, I would like nevertheless to add that this is not a personal analysis of the writer, which I would in any case consider inappropriate. I do not have access to the personal constellation necessary for any statement regarding Omer's general motives, predominant defenses, or indeed any aspects of her as a person.) This version, which is very popular, enables many a mother to go along with her denial. The fact that her child is, for her own reasons, a willing accomplice in such (indirect) aggressiveness helps maintain the interaction.

I have tried to illustrate how mother and child cooperate in telling and receiving the tale of Little Red Riding Hood, with its anxiety-raising, cruel, and frightening aspects. I have said that mother and child provide one another with a setting in which denial is reciprocally exercised in ways that are mutually relevant. Mother, as agent, scares the child, but at the same time gives him or her the opportunity to deny both smallness and anxiety. The child, reciprocally, provides mother with a setting in which she can tell such a tale, while denying some of the feelings she expresses through it toward her child. I should add that the whole situation of mutuality and togetherness, even closeness, in which the telling of the tale usually takes place, brings to the fore complementary aspects of this same situation: namely the child's feelings of security and well-being in having mother close to her and mother's feelings of closeness and protectiveness toward her little girl (Winnicott, e.g., 1971, deals extensively with these issues). These factors of course *also* keep the interaction going, yet at the same time they contribute to an atmosphere in which denial of other feelings (on which we have focused in our illustration), is facilitated.

I would now like to make brief reference to certain theoretical positions implied in my presentation, in particular my use of the term *denial*. I have not, in my construction, gone into any detail about the kinds of "denial" to which I refer, nor have I discussed any of the theoretical issues associated with the concept. Yet I would argue that my varying uses of the concept could be more or less understood in context and, moreover, that no more was required for the purposes of the present analysis. For example, I would be surprised if anyone, at any point within the present context, understood me to refer to denial as a psychotic *mechanism* (e.g., Freud, 1924; Klein, 1946) or to deal with *subject matter* that belongs to psychosis, in Stewart's (1970) sense. Yet, within a narrower range of application, I *have* used "denial" in a variety of senses. I will even go so far as to say that my use of it in a not too specific manner has enabled me to remain with the mainstream of the issue under discussion, although "at the cost of oversimplification," as is so often said. Furthermore, it has enabled me to remain with a general idea, without committing myself prematurely to a specific stance, or in a manner more precise than that permitted by the material at my disposal.

Let us, for example, examine more closely my treatment of Little Red Riding Hood's encounter with the wolf in her grandmother's bed. Even leaving aside the questions that might be raised concerning analysis of a fictional character (Oedipus is, of course, the most prominent case of this kind used by psychoanalysis), many other issues may yet be raised. For example, I have said that when she persists in questioning "grandmother" about her strange appearance, Little Red Riding Hood is denying the (external) reality before her. One might, therefore, ask whether the little girl was, simply, so stupid—as our critical student suggests—as to be unable to put two and two together, and thereby indeed be unable to "recognize" that it was the wolf. This cannot be inferred, however, from the Grimms' tale. For, despite the absence of any warning from her mother (in the original tale as told by the Grimm brothers) against talking to any stranger, let alone to greedy wolves, and despite her ignorance about wolves ("Little Red Riding Hood did not know what a wicked creature he was, and was not at all afraid of him"), she is alert and suspicious, and her rising anxiety can be clearly sensed in the description of her entrance into her grandmother's cottage:

> She was surprised to find the cottage door standing open, and when she went into the room, she had such a strange feeling that she said to herself, "Oh dear! how uneasy I feel today, and at other times I like being with grandmother so much." She called out, "Good morning," but received no answer; so she went to the bed and drew back the curtains. There lay her grandmother with her cap pulled far over her face, and looking very strange.

So what was it that was going on at this point? Was the little girl unconsciously denying the actual (extrapsychic) *perception* (viewed by Linn, 1953, and Roshco, 1967, as an early defense, therefore later associated with severe disturbances)? And, if Little Red Riding Hood's denial *was* at the perceptual level, was it *complete* or incomplete (Sperling, 1958)? In other words, did she adhere to a perception of a very strange grandmother, or did she have glimpses of the wolf? Or, would her denial be altogether more appropriately described in Trunnell and Holt's terms (1973) as "a failure to fully appreciate the *significance or implications* of what is perceived"? (italics in the original throughout). Yet such a view of the occurrence carries within it "the paradox of denial" (Spence, 1983), namely that "because it functions in a partial manner, denial allows *some* information to register" (my italics). In the case of

Little Red Riding Hood, does the information register bit by bit, as the increase in anxiety, reflected in the wording of her questions, suggests? Perhaps we are back with our student, who, as a child, considered Little Red Riding Hood "so stupid?" Not stupid, perhaps, but at the level of cognitive development of the preoperational child, when she or he is as yet incapable of simultaneously comprehending a number of relevant dimensions (Piaget, 1928)? Perhaps her increasing anxiety, yet adherence to "grandmother" to the last of her questions, reflects partial comprehension, due to the level of her cognitive development? There is no way these or similar issues regarding specific mechanism(s) at work can possibly be settled in the "case" of Little Red Riding Hood. Where real, live people are concerned, further data can be obtained, depending, of course, on pragmatic circumstances; but, in the case of fictional characters, this is impossible.[6] Nevertheless, I think that my analysis of the fictional character, as well as the more extensive analysis of mother and of daughter in interaction around her tale, has value for opening up a new avenue of thought. Indeed, had I tried to make more sense of it than possible, I would have found myself so entangled with the unresolved specifics of the "denials" to which I have referred, that my general line of thought would have been entirely lost.

I thus express the position that, although precise delineations of the range and meaning of a concept are sometimes necessary, a demand for precision will be counterproductive at other times. I am not arguing against periodic reexaminations of psychoanalytic concepts. Such efforts help us gain better understanding of and command over the meanings of concepts, and within a necessary historical perspective (e.g., Sjoback, 1973, Trunnell & Holt, 1974, Chayes, Chapter 6 this volume; Wangh, Chapter 1 this volume). But once a basic mastery of the problematic issues surrounding the concept is gained, and its major connotations are known, we nevertheless continue to use it in different ways and with different depths of meaning, depending on our theoretical orientation and also on the extent of our exclusive commitment to one specific position. For example, many will shift back and forth between their use of the dynamic concept of "The Ucs" of the topographical model and the descriptive concept of the structural model, despite the theoretical disharmonies involved in such shifts (Sandler, 1984). Similarly many of us will shift in our use of "denial" from one sense to another. The range of its usage and the discursive circumstances under which greater or more limited restrictions are imposed on its usage are dependent on theoretical orientation and exclusivity of commitment and, perhaps even

[6]I would like to thank Ruth Nevo for clarifying this point with me.

more so, on personal view. One author's use will always remain another's misuse. One thinker may argue, "I'd rather be precisely wrong than vaguely right" (Patrick Suppes, personal communication), whereas another will claim, "The cost of precision will be offset, I believe, by the gain in evocativeness and significance" (Schafer, 1983, p. 34).

There is a related issue to which I would now like to turn briefly. Although my presentation expresses a position on the usage of concepts, I am not concerned with theoretical issues associated with the concept of denial. To take but one brief example, I say, following A. Freud (1936), that the child denies the *reality* of her smallness and dependence and thus reduces the consequent anxieties that this evokes. Anna Freud has been queried about her use of the term *objective anxiety* (based on "objective [external] facts") in this context (Sandler with A. Freud, 1985) and has argued (with reference to the specific case discussed) that the child "thought it was real, so for him it was real anxiety, namely objective anxiety, whether it was so in fact or not." Carmi (1984) emphasizes that such an extension of the concept of "reality" imposes great strains on Anna Freud's own theoretical premises, according to which excessive use of denial is inconsistent with (external) reality testing. My analysis enables me to accept A. Freud's earlier, straightforward statement that the external reality of the child's smallness and dependence produces anxieties that can be fended off or decreased by denial in fantasy. Although I am aware that I have thereby circumvented the weighty theoretical issues that remain unresolved when the concept is applied more widely, I do so because these issues are not of direct concern to me here and, moreover, because I believe that in the present context I have made, with the aid of this concept, heuristically productive observations, notwithstanding the unresolved theoretical issues.

Let me complete my presentation with one additional remark. In my illustrative analysis, or in other words, in the narrative constructed herein, I have emphasized the collaborative enterprise of mother and child around aspects of *Little Red Riding Hood* and the opportunities for reciprocally exercised denial that this enterprise offers. Of course, aspects of the same data can be, have been, and will yet be viewed from quite different angles. As a matter of fact, in my preceding reference to Piaget, I have already implied one such possible alternative emphasis with regard to Little Red Riding Hood's behavior. Our data is always multidetermined and more or less limited. As in the process of our work with our patients, so also in reexamining the present data: Aspects of it can be retold differently without having the various constructions necessarily be mutually exclusive.

ACKNOWLEDGMENTS

The data quoted in this paper were collected with the aid of a grant from the Sturman Center for Human Development, the Hebrew University of Jerusalem. I would like to thank Kariel Pardo for his fruitful comments on an earlier version of this paper.

REFERENCES

Bettelheim, B. (1976). *The uses of enchantment.* New York: Alfred A. Knopf.

Burton, A. (1978). 'Beauty and the Beast.' A critique of the psychoanalytic approaches to the fairy tale. *Psychocultural Review, 24,* 241–258.

Carmi, M. (1984). A critical discussion of the concept of denial (disavowal) in psychoanalytic literature. Unpublished master's thesis, The Hebrew University, Jerusalem.

Cath, S., & Cath, C. (1978). On the other side of Oz. Psychoanalytic studies of fairy tales. *Psychoanalytic Study of the Child, 33,* 621–639.

Diamant, L. (1977). Clinical contribution to dwarf symbolism. *Psychoanalytic Review, 64,* 611–620.

Eifermann, R. R. (1985). Teaching psychoanalysis to non-analytic students through work on their own dreams. *Psychoanalysis in Europe, 22,* 38–45.

Eifermann, R. R. (1987a). Fairy tales—A royal road to the child within the adult. *Scandinavian Psychoanalytical Review, 10,* 51–77. Also in Stork, J. (Ed.), *Das Märchen—ein Märchen? Psychoanalytische Betrachtungen zu Wesen, Deutung und Wirkung der Märchen* (Märchen—eine Via Regia zum Kind im Erwachsenen). Stuttgard-Bad Cannstatt: Frommann-Holzboog, 83–116.

Eifermann, R. R. (1987b). Interactions between textual analysis and related self analysis. In S. Rimmon-Kenan (Ed.), *Discourse in psychoanalysis and literature* (pp. 37–56). London: Methuen.

Eifermann, R. R. (1987c). "Germany" and "The Germans": Acting out fantasies and their discovery in self-analysis. *International Review of Psycho-Analysis, 14,* 245–262. "Deutschland" und "die Deutschen"—Agieren von Phantasien und deren Entdeckung in der Selbstanalyse. *Jahrbuch der Psychoanalyse, 20,* 38–55.

Freud, A. (1936). *The ego and the mechanisms of defense.* London: Hogarth Press.

Freud, A. (1967). About losing and being lost. *Psychoanalytic Study of the Child, 22,* 9–19.

Freud, S. (1924). The loss of reality in neuroses and psychoses. In *The standard edition of the complete psychological works of Sigmund Freud,* Vol. 19. London: Hogarth.

Grimm, J., & W. (1819). *Kinder- und Hausmärchen.* München: Winkler Verlag (1949).

Grimm, J., & W. (1884). *Grimms' household tales.* (Margaret Hunt Ed. and Trans.). London: George Bell & Sons.

Huss, R. (1975). Grimms' The table, The ass and the stick: A drama of the phallic stage. *Psychoanalytic Review, 62,* 165–175.

Klein, M. (1946). Notes on some schizoid mechanisms. In *Envy and gratitude, and other works 1946–1963.* London: Hogarth Press and the Institute of Psycho-Analysis.

Linn, L. (1953). The role of perception in the mechanism of denial. *Journal of the American Psychoanalytic Association, 1,* 690–705.

Omer, D. (1978). *Fairy tales of the magical palace.* A Selection of the Brothers Grimm Tales, translated and revised. Tel Aviv: Joseph Schreberk. (In Hebrew.)

Piaget, J. (1928). *Judgement and reasoning in the child*. London: Routledge & Kegan Paul.

Roscho, M. (1967). Perception, denial, and derealization. *Journal of the American Psychoanalytic Association, 15,* 243–260.

Sandler, J. (1984). Reflections on some relations between psychoanalytic concepts and psychoanalytic practice. *International Journal of Psychoanalysis, 64,* 35–45.

Sandler, J., with Freud, A. (1985). *The analysis of defense: The ego and the mechanisms of defense revisited.* New York: International Universities Press.

Schafer, R. (1983). *The analytic attitude.* London: Hogarth Press.

Sjoback, H. (1973). *The psychoanalytic theory of defensive processes.* Lund: CWK Gleerup.

Spence, D. P. (1982). *Narrative truth and historical truth.* New York: Norton.

Spence, D. P. (1983). The paradox of denial. In S. Breznitz (Ed.), *Denial and stress* (pp. 103–123). New York: International Universities Press.

Sperling, S. (1958). On denial and the essential nature of defence. *International Journal of Psychoanalysis, 39,* 25–38.

Stewart, W. (1970). The split in the ego and disavowal. *Psychoanalytic Quarterly, 39,* 1–16.

Trunnell, E., & Holt, W. (1974). The concept of denial or disavowal. *Journal of the American Psychoanalytic Association, 22,* 769–785.

Winnicott, D. W. (1971). *Playing and reality.* London: Tavistock Publications.

Zipes, J. (1984). *The trials and tribulations of Little Red Riding Hood.* London: Heinemann.

IV

Clinical Implications

Wurmser opens this section devoted to the clinical manifestations of denial by reviewing the terms defined so far in this volume. He asks that we restrict the use of the term *denial/disavowal* to situations in which some portion of external reality has been excluded from conscious awareness; denial means "not knowing." *Repression,* in the strictest sense, refers only to drive-related material and thus must be defined as "not wishing." Pointing out that in isolation the individual has kept apart cognitions or ideoaffective complexes that if joined might cause unwanted emotions or degrees of emotion, Wurmser defines isolation as "not linking." It would be useful to add to this list the mechanism of dissociation, in which the individual has already been flooded with emotion of an intensity higher than optimal, due perhaps to the failure of any or all of the other mechanisms named previously; in dissociation we acknowledge the existence of the affect but remove from it our identity. Thus dissociation involves "not identifying." Wurmser has devoted many years of painstaking work to the psychoanalytic investigation and treatment of patients with chemical dependency and substance abuse, pointing out that the pharmacopoeia is a chemical modulator of affect. This chapter contains two sections—a series of clinical cases illustrating how denial operates in severe psychopathology and a model by which to explain impulsive action.

Drawing from broad experience with the group of patients labeled "borderline," Stone elucidates a biopsychosocial understanding of the interaction between environment and neurophysiological capacity. Chosing several examples in which the manifest psychopathology is altered in terms of intrinsic and/or extrinsic contributions, he shows the

ubiquity of denial as a mechanism that facilitates the more widely her-
alded characteristic defenses of this group, such as projective identification and splitting. In his discussion, these assertions are placed in metapsychological context contrasting their varying congruence with the
schemata of Lichtenberg, Kohut, Masterson, and others. Although the
synthesis may not have reached its final form, this chapter may stand as
an example of the search for continuity between biological substrates
and psychological structures.

Many readers will find Friedman's chapter both informative and
disturbing, the balance between these emotional reactions weighted by
our own need to deny his carefully assembled evidence. In a series of
prior publications describing years of painstaking psychoanalytic investigation of homosexual men, Friedman has concluded, in direct opposition to conventional psychoanalytic wisdom, that some people may be
considered both homosexual and psychologically healthy. Using Freud's
well-known criteria that psychological health implies happiness in both
work and love, Friedman has described a series of men who have been
homosexual from earliest life, have never experienced heterosexual fantasies, have never experienced the fear of women and of heterosexual
sexuality usually assumed as the basis of homosexuality, and who have a
lifelong history of successful, loving interpersonal relationships as well as
success in a chosen field of work. There is a growing body of psychobiological research suggesting that at least some portion of gender identity is influenced by hormonal factors operating during intrauterine life;
one statement of this theory might be that notwithstanding the chro-
mosomal pattern otherwise defining gender, some "switch" in the brain
is immutably turned in the direction of maleness or femaleness by this
intrauterine hormonal environment. Such theories are attractive not
merely because they offer some understanding of the fact that homosexuality has been found in all eras and in every possible culture but that
they explain how a sexual orientation counter to the continuance of the
species can be a natural phenomenon.

Friedman presents data from a large and growing cohort of homosexual men whose earliest sexual fantasies were homosexual. Because
such fantasies are clearly skew to those of his peers, the growing boy
learns to hide them in a number of ways. To the extent that denial is
used to hide from these fantasies (what Wurmser calls denial as "not
knowing"), this boy tends to create false or pseudomasculine scenarios in
an attempt to feel "normal." Friedman presents compelling evidence
suggesting that middle-aged men who leave home, marriage, and family
to take up an openly homosexual life are those who had in this manner
denied their early homosexual identity. Psychological health for a boy

with primary homosexual identity would seem to imply open acceptance by himself and by his milieu of such an identity. The function of denial here is to allow the boy to adjust to the unreal expectations of his environment. In contrast to the role of denial in the adolescents described by Chayes (where denial protects the individual from the emotional avalanche associated with conflicts for which he is temporarily unprepared and with which he will deal when more mature), the pseudomasculine compromises offered by denial produce an intrinsically unstable product, one that cannot resolve the tensions involved.

Musaph discusses the perimenopause as a biological given handled by women with varying degrees of denial. Part and parcel of the international movement awakening both men and women to the nature of societal understanding of femininity and feminine role assignment has been the awakening in some women of a wish to remain youthful and "fully" feminine forever, despite the clear injunction of most leaders of this movement that female health must involve realistic acceptance of female biology. Other examples of denial cited by Musaph include the tendency of physicians to deny the presence of illnesses in their own families.

Many of those who heard the work of Baider and Edelstein presented at the symposium in Jerusalem on which this volume is based were moved to tears by their description of seven patients who devised highly creative fantasies disguising the facts and implications surrounding serious and frequently fatal malignant illnesses. The theoretical matter of the chapter is clear—here fantasy reaching delusional intensity was used to bolster massive denial of illness. Baider and Edelstein worked with these patients by accepting the fantasized or delusional material as if it were normal, thus entering the personal system of the patient and forming relationships of extraordinary power that allowed maximum therapeutic efficacy. Several discussants suggested that such action on the part of the therapists paralleled the loving relationship of mother and child engaged in fables and fairy tales; it seemed as if therapist and patient were making use of a channel of opportunity available to everybody but generally disavowed as irrational or unrealistic. This chapter illustrates one of the major premises of the volume itself—the mechanism of denial is not immutably pathological but may be used in the service of psychological health. The act of forcing a dying patient to renounce a psychologically healing fantasy, when we can offer nothing to heal the physical illness, may be an example of denial on the part of the therapist.

Weisman also asks, "What is wrong with denying? Does it help to deny, and does it take away hope?" He points out that undue pessimism is as much a product of denial as undue optimism, and that "hope is a product of self-esteem." Describing his lifetime study of patients with cancer, Weisman offers a balanced survey of the importance of denial in both healthy and dysfunctional adaptations to severe illness. Central to his approach is a careful evaluation of the patient's personality and style of coping, for the premorbid adjustment will influence the development of psychopathology during terminal illness. Weisman describes patients whose calm is based not on denial but on clear understanding, as well as patients in whom any specific element of their clinical condition may be disavowed in order to produce such calm. He differentiates between cognitive denial, in which a person disavows some element of external reality, and existensial denial, in which some aspect of the person is disavowed by his or her milieu.

So much of what one discovers depends on what one sees. Dieter Ohlmeier was asked by his cardiologist colleagues to apply psycho-analytic methods of investigation to the problems presented by a group of young men with a history of recent myocardial infarction. As he states, "*Work,* usually in the sense of feeling chronically overworked, offers a form of protection as well as an opportunity to attain a form of rational control over their human environment" (p. 262). Incapacity to work produces severe anxiety in these men for whom identification with the superior replaces any working through of the relationship with fa-ther. "The superior, finally, is no longer perceived in the form of a living person; in his place one finds an 'organization' with all its 'suprain-dividual' mechanisms and regulations." Observed both in structured group therapy and (in one case) formal psychoanalytic treatment, these men exhibited denial as a protection against self-awareness at nearly all levels studied.

Each of these chapters suggests a different use for denial; indeed, one might suspect that each author describes a different mental mecha-nism. But taken as a unit, these several chapters demonstrate what is the major point of this book: The mechanism of denial represents a first line of defense for an individual confronted with an unacceptable percep-tion. Where confrontation with reality might allow percept to trigger affect, disavowal of the perception maintains the organism relatively free of unwanted or unacceptable affect. What we have traditionally seen as a mechanism only impeding the development of the mature personality may now be understood as a mechanism protecting the per-sonality itself from disintegration, whereas other, perhaps reparative mechanisms may be brought into operation. Where denial favors dys-function, it must be undone; where denial protects, it must engender respect.

12

Blinding the Eye of the Mind
Denial, Impulsive Action, and Split Identity

Léon Wurmser

INTRODUCTION

Falstaff (*Henry IV*, pt. II, a. I, sc. II) responds to the Chief Justice's exclamation: "You hear not what I say to you," by claiming: "Very well, my lord, very well. Rather, an't pleases you, it is the *disease of not listening*, the *malady of not marking*, that I am troubled withal." Eventually the Justice gives in: "But since all is well, keep it so. Wake not a sleeping wolf." Whereupon Falstaff gives that quintessential answer that could be the motto for all his followers unto this day: "To wake a wolf is as bad as to smell a fox."

There is no question that this "malady of not marking" refers to what we have come to call denial. But what is denial?

Reading the discussion about denial and its relation to the other defenses, especially repression and isolation, one may be reminded a little of the confusion of tongues at Babel, and it may be therefore appropriate to begin with one of the Midrashim about the Tower of

---

Léon Wurmser • Private Practice, 904 Crestwick Road, Towson, Maryland 21204.

Babel: "And let us make a name [as monument]: The School of Rabbi Ishmael taught: Shem, a name, means nought else but an idol":

וְנַעֲשֶׂה–לָנוּ שֵׁם. תְּנֵי ר' יִשְׁמָעֵאל אֵין שֵׁם אֶלָּא ע"ז.

And so asks Juliet: "What's in a name?"

We all who work with words know, however, how much indeed depends on clarity and explicitness, but also how it is often not possible in the realm of inner reality to define clearly what we mean; the borders are unsharp, the concepts of what is experienced overlap and flow into each other. Yet, still, they can retain an identifiable core.

Not only are names important as part of a more differentiated understanding, but names dictate action and determine our treatment approach in ways that are often damaging. Let me then try quickly, without sinking too deeply into the terminological controversy, where I see the usefulness of the terms that occupy us in this volume. We can only accept terms if they can be clearly related to observations that can be shared between patient and therapist, not merely propounded at panel discussions and round-table seminars of analysts.

Freud says, in "Repression" (1915): ". . . the essence of *repression* lies simply in turning something away, and keeping it at distance from the conscious." In that it applies to all defense, for us today, this is too broad. The specification relevant for us comes in his description of primal repression, *Urverdrängung*: ". . . *dass der psychischen (Vorstellungs-) Repräsentanz des Triebes die Übernahme ins Bewusste versagt wird*" (*Gesammelte Werke* XIV, p. 250), "[. . . which consists in the psychical (ideational) representative of the instinct being denied entrance into the conscious" (Freud, 1915, p. 248)]. Repression means therefore primarily *not desiring—a block against wishing.* By tradition, another act of No or blocking has also been assigned to repressing: *not remembering.*

"*Verleugnung*"—denial or *disavowal*—is described as "*Einerseits verleugnen sie die Tatsache ihrer Wahrnehmung . . . die Verleugnung der Wahrnehmungen.*" (*Gesammelte Werke* XVII, p. 134) ["he disavows his own sense perceptions . . . disavowing the fact of their perception." (Freud, 1940, pp. 202–203)]. Equally Anna Freud (1936) says: ". . . to get rid of unwelcome facts by denying them." Thus denial means *not perceiving—a block against,* a disavowal and disclaimer of *what has been seen or heard or sensed* (cf. also Waelder 1951, p. 221).

Isolation is described by Anna Freud (1936) as removing "the instinctual impulses from their context, while retaining them in consciousness . . . he severs the links between his associations and isolates ideas from affects . . ." (p. 35). So isolation means *not connecting*—keeping inner experiences apart.

"Freud pointed out in 'The Unconscious' (1915) that defense is always directed against affect," writes Basch (1983, p. 146). Fenichel states, "Thus in the last analysis any defense is a defense against *affects*. 'I do not want to feel any painful sensation' is the first and final motive of defense" (1945, p. 161). This would imply that these defenses are not directed against impulse, memory, perception, and thought as such, but against the affects linked with them. Would this then mean it is the affects that are detached and eliminated from wish and memory in repression, from perception in denial, and from thought in isolation? Would then, in all of them, the No mean: "I do not want to feel"?

DENIAL AND SPLIT IDENTITY

Trunnell and Holt maintain that one should distinguish denial in the *vernacular* sense, the phenomenological assertion of an untruth, "literally seeing but refusing to acknowledge what one sees," the result of all successful defenses; versus denial in the *scientific* sense, "the defensive failure to appreciate fully the implications of that perception" (1974, pp. 782–783).

I believe that the question of its vernacular use—in distinction from its psychoanalytic meaning—can be solved rather simply. The vernacular refers to its (pre-) conscious use, whereas denial in the technical sense is, as defense mechanism, dynamically unconscious. I prefer to use a different term for such conscious version of the defense, though; and it seems to me that the term negation, *Verneinung*, used by Freud in 1925, is suitable for that purpose. Such a conscious saying No to perceived reality accompanies, as Trunnell and Holt indicate, all successful defense.

Distinguishing more sharply Basch wrote (1983):

> . . . that conceptual clarity would be served if the term '*denial*' was used as *collective* term for those psychotic or nonpsychotic mechanisms that actually interfere with the *perceptual interpretation* of sensory signals, while, following Freud, using the term '*disavowal*' only to describe that situation in which the *affectively toned meaning* that a percept would be expected to have for the self is unconsciously repudiated. (p. 146)

> Disavowal—Verleugnung—involves the separation of personal meaning from some perceived aspect of external reality judged to be potentially anxiety provoking. . . . Disavowal prevents the union of affect with percept, without, however, blocking the percept from consciousness." (pp. 146–147)

Defense in general consists in "treat[ing] an experience as if it did not, after all, matter to the self and, therefore, is not submitted for review by consciousness" (pp. 148–149). The move "from primarily factual into personally meaningful experience" (p. 151) is blocked in disavowal. It is not the perceptual reality but its meaning that is blocked by "*Verleugnung*," disavowal (p. 127): "*Verleugnung is a repudiation of the meaning of reality, not of reality per se . . .* [it is] a self deception in the face of accurate perception" (p. 134). "Disavowal is designated as the mechanism which defends against traumatic external reality, whereas repression deals with unacceptable instinctual demands" (p. 135). (This in reference to Freud's "Outline" of 1940.) Such repudiation of the meaning of perception is supported by a protective fantasy (p. 136).

In short, then, "disavowal . . . is not a distortion of perception *per se*, but only a defense against that percept's personal significance . . . Perceptual defense encompasses more than disavowal," (p. 145) namely psychotic denial, negative hallucination, hysterical blindness, withdrawal, and the like, collectively encompassed by the term *denial*.

Dorpat (1979) refers to denial as refusal "to accept the meaning and implications of his perceptions" (p. 107) and as "the unconscious repudiation of some or all of the total available *meanings* of an event to allay anxiety or other unpleasurable condition. . . . Denial is the reality repudiating aspect of what defenses do" (1983a, p. 223). Dorpat extends our understanding of denial with his important addition that "the *cognitive arrest* in denial reactions prevents the subject from fully and accurately symbolizing in words whatever it is that he has defensively negated" (p. 229). He sees its essence in this cognitive arrest:

> The dynamic defensive function of denial is carried out by the active *exclusion* of information *from focal attention*, i.e., explicit conscious awareness. . . . In denial, the subject shifts his focal attention from disturbing stimuli emanating either from himself or from the environment to less disturbing stimuli, fantasies or ideas." (1983b, p. 48)

Denial, then is the collective term used for all forms of defense directed against perception. Percepts may refer to the outside world, or they may refer to the self and the inner world; hence denial may affect self- or object-representation. Such defense may remove from focal attention specific cognitive meaning (or significance) and affective tones that could arouse anxiety or pain. That subtype would be called *disavowal*. In addition to disavowal, there are much broader sweeps of perceptual blockage that remove facts (not only affectively toned meanings) from representations. This is denial in the broader sense, as in massive—delusional—distortions of perceptions or those perceptions found in altered states of consciousness, especially those induced by intense rage or panic. All defense mechanisms, including all forms of denial, are unconscious. The conscious correlates of these mechanisms include lying or hiding certain painful truth from oneself; or negation, which stands similarly in a specific relation to disavowal.

To this point we have discussed denial as a mechanism used by the ego to alter perception and meaning. Let me now focus on the "denial of affects". Dorpat (1983b) describes in his case vignettes how one patient attempts "to deny both her anxiety over the impending break in the analysis and her anger toward the analyst" and how the other spoke in a confused and confusing way "to avoid awareness of [her] painful envy" (pp. 50–51). Thus the implication is that perception of affect is warded off by this mechanism as well.

But what is the *perception* of affect? Is this *different from feeling the affect*? Before continuing we have to ponder this curious gap: that there appears to be *no separate* defense with the aim of *not feeling*.

Along with the general neglect of affects in psychoanalytic theory, the general tendency to disregard affect as a part of inner reality sui generis and the traditional view of affect merely as a derivative of "Trieb," there exists no clear theoretical conception of one defense mechanism specifically directed against feeling some affects. Because however, analysts have dealt more with feelings than with anything else, such a gap could not remain open, and so all three terms have been used to label the observation that patients *defend* against certain affects, that they cannot *feel* certain feelings—they *repress, deny,* and *isolate* feelings; hence the difficulty in differentiating these three defense mechanisms vis-à-vis affects.

The revolution in theory made necessary by modern infant research forces us to develop new terms that describe the methods by which the ego handles what many believe to be "innate" affects. Basch (1976) suggests that we reserve the term *feeling* for our awareness of these innate affects; thus I suggest that the experience of *not-feeling* is best described

TABLE 1. Survey of Defenses

Unconscious	Meaning of defense	(Pre-) conscious
Repression	Not desiring/wishing; not remembering	Renouncing
Denial	Not perceiving	Lying, hiding the truth
Disavowal	Repudiating the meaning of perception	Negation (denial in vernacular sense)
Affect blocking	Not feeling	Suppression
Isolation	Not connecting	Concentration

by Fenichel's (1945) term *affect blocking*. I have tried to summarize this group of related definitions in Table 1.

Yet I have still avoided the question of whether there is a real difference between avoiding awareness of an affect and the blocking of the feeling itself. Would the former—the avoidance of awareness—be affected by the defense of denial as here defined, whereas the latter—the blocking of the feeling itself—would refer to the direct experiencing of the affect? The first would pertain to the self-representation, the other to direct self-experience. Can one block the former, while clearly feeling the latter?

Wherever there is denial, there is also some registration of what has been so blocked. I agree with Dorpat when he correlates this with the distinction between "focal awareness" (Schachtel, 1959) and the "tacit knowing of subsidiaries" (Polanyi, 1964). This intriguing doubleness of knowing and not knowing had been called by Freud the "splitting of the ego." But that does not fully answer the question about the role of affect in denial. Let me approach this from a different direction.

Basch (1983) suggests that both the registration of affects (as part of the self-representation) and the affectively toned meaning of a percept are eliminated by denial/disavowal. Yet what is the meaning of "meaning" in this context? It surely is not the logical and semantic sense of that important word. Rather it would be circumscribed as *"value to oneself,"* and we should not be surprised if that inner valuing authority—the superego—has its mighty hand in it when we deal with disavowal and denial on a massive scale, as in depersonalization.

Perhaps we can go one step farther. Does the affective tone or meaning of perception belong to the same type of experience as affects like anxiety, sadness, anger, shame, guilt—quite independent from the intensity of the latter? Clinical experience seems to indicate that the disturbances of these two groups are at least distinguishable though often concomitant. The depersonalized person says it paradoxically: He *registers* emotions he has but does not quite *feel* them. Federn (1952) adduced the metaphor of ego boundaries and their cathexis to explain the difference, but I am not sure whether we need this. Basch explains it by the distinction of episodic versus semantic memory, of left and right-brain processes. Perhaps it is, however, not necessary to go beyond psychological understanding and resort to explanation by physiology.

Does not perhaps the difference lie simply in the sanction given by the superego to parts or all of perception? I think of a kind of validation from "above"—the seal of inner approval: "This is of *value* for me and can be accepted." And its opposite: "I cannot accept such value and must disavow it, deprive it of meaning."

This may pertain to anything we perceive—without or within. We may feel any affect—let us say joy or anger—with or without such validation from above. In the latter case, we register it, we do not even necessarily block it, we "feel" it and yet "don't" feel it.

It is like in an insolent institution: An individual is registered but treated as a nonperson if he loses the approbation of those above. He walks around; he is being seen, but nobody greets him, he is ignored, his existence is disavowed.

Thus *disavowal* (or denial in the narrow sense) *works at the behest of the superego:* To that purpose it *withdraws validation and valuation from certain percepts* or certain *processes of perceiving.* That is all that it can do. Neither are the affects or impulses blocked by it, nor is the cognitive part of perception necessarily impaired—except, as Dorpat states, it may be removed from focal attention, so that even the *facts,* not only their meanings, are omitted from percepts—denial in the broad sense.

Whenever there is extensive disavowal we find a curious *oscillation* between two part identities. The *avowal* of one *part identity* necessarily means the *disavowal* of the other—hence the tremendous importance of the narrowing down or falsifying of perception by denial.

More generally I find these concepts of the *denial of one's identity,* the assumption of a *part identity,* the *conflict* between such part identities, and all this under the sway of opposite parts of the superego, of tremendous importance, yet not much commented upon in our literature. In fact, something of this appears to play a role in all the patients I get to know well in treatment. Living such a part identity—an *"adopted or imposed identity,"* as one of may patients called it—arouses an uneasiness that one is not in touch with one's feelings. Such a "pseudoidentity" (or "false self," in Winnicott's phrasing, "persona" in Jung's) is particularly pronounced as the surface manifestation of severe shame conflicts; but the entire duality of such part identities, that splits much of life asunder, can often be understood as massive conflicts between the shame part of the superego and its guilt part.

The duality of denial and countervailing fantasy has impressed me less than this *duality of two alternate part identities*—part personalities of great complexity and in sharp conflict with each other that use denial as their main weapon against the other and the underlying *conflict between opposing superego parts* (intrasystemic superego conflict; "superego split").

To pursue the issue of that double identity and double denial in depersonalization still further: Whereas there may be *some* affect blocking, the claim of "I don't feel anything; nothing touches me" can be understood not so much as an absence of emotions than as having the meaning: "Some, or most, or all of my perceptions have lost their personal significance, i.e., their affective tone, for me; I have to disavow such meaning because looking, hearing, and touching would arouse too much anxiety or could be too painful—I have been or will be punished for it by loss and abandonment, or by mutilation, or, and that especially so, by humiliation." Why? "Mostly because of that part of me—that part identity—that must be disclaimed and disowned." In fact the question arises whether there are any *large*-scale attempts at repression without at least some attempts at blocking the meaning aspects of perceptions, that is, denial "mobilized against the leakages of repression" (Wangh).

Why would that have to be so though? I suggest, for three reasons: (1) the process of perceiving may itself have become so charged with unacceptable wishes—with impulses for merger or power (as in psychotic shame, in psychotic denial, but also in severe general inhibitions in cases of quite regressive neurosis); (2) the percepts may have assumed such a threatening quality (e.g., during and after severe trauma, like in Holocaust survivors); and (3) the perceiving self has to be disclaimed as "foul, gross, and disgusting" as one of my patients kept calling herself. The deeply ashamed person is particularly prone to such chronic depersonalization.

What holds true for depersonalization is applicable to altered states of consciousness more generally, as the following example of a young physician shows who manifested a characteristic sequence leading up to an act of at times severely damaging *pseudostupidity*:

It would begin with a sense of helpless rage. To understand that feeling, it is necessary to know that his parents had pushed him and his younger brothers, in the most one-sided, blind, irrational way from early childhood on, into becoming doctors, saying: "You don't need to have these games or play with such toys, because you will be a doctor: you don't need to learn this—why should you be interested in literature, or learn to write composition, or be concerned about finances, if you want to be a doctor?" They imposed a one-sided view of him and of his brothers that had a nearly delusional quality and caused disastrous consequences.

The sequence at issue would begin with intense, but helpless rage, followed by guilt and shame, and end in a specific act of pseudostupidity [such as snorkling without appropriate gear and almost drowning, failing to hospitalize a patient with ventricular fibrillation, entrusting his check deposits to an employee who had already shown her lack of truthfulness, signing up for an insurance policy without reading the form] that would be followed by a state of pervasive sadness and crying without clear source.

Beneath this pattern lies one of greater dynamic significance:

> I feel in a constant trap of anger and guilt. I am stuck in it. Whenever I showed disagreement at home, my mother would start crying and yelling: "After all I did for you, you no-good louse, this is the thanks I get. You are good for nothing." And the father would scream: "You are killing your mother. You will say the Kaddish. You are very religious, aren't you?"

Then he tries to undo or wipe out the angry thoughts. He goes blank or severs by isolation the blind affect of anger/anxiety/sadness from empty ideas without affect. Such images include cutting off his wife's legs during intercourse or moving his index finger up and down during a lecture or a show, "having the crazy thought to shoot the person" and of course undoing it right away. Or what is being spoken appears just confusing, an empty noise without meaning. What is most important, however (and I quote his recounting of playing chess, of boxing or tickling matches, or of actual fights with brothers or father):

> I would not see the catastrophe coming. And suddenly I would be totally overwhelmed. With chess I could not see, I could not foresee his plans, and suddenly I was beaten. I would ruminate and obsess, plan and plan, in order not to be overwhelmed, but I would plan in a very repetitive, single-minded way, not seeing the next possibility.

It is a narrowing down of his consciousness, even a state of confusion, accompanied by or leading to a massive form of denial, as if to say: "I go blank. When something is highly charged, especially when I feel helpless and humiliated, suddenly nothing makes any sense."

In that state, foolish decisions are made, very destructive actions committed—based on such massive denial that in turn had been prompted by intense anxiety about the conflict between aggression and guilt: the state of pseudo-stupidity.

Behind that the deeper conflict shines through: "I was angry at my mother for going to work in the evening and for having my sister. I remember whenever I went to bed or mentioned the word *sleep* I would start crying—the fear of being separated." And with that comes the memory of play or actions of throwing dolls into the incinerator. That and the reference to babies are remembered without feeling—thought severed from affect (isolation)—but it reemerges in displaced form as does the affect; or, even more important, the screen affect of sadness has to cover for the murderous rage. His sadness is anger filtered through guilt.

To repeat the sequence: (1) sense of loss, or humiliation, or threat; (2) anger, helpless rage; (3) guilt and shame about such "badness"; (4) attempts to undo and isolation; states of going blank, of confusion; (5) narrowing of consciousness with massive perceptual contraction, that is, denial; (6) acts of pseudostupidity; followed (7) by a return of the original aggressions in a pale affectless form. This sequence is almost automatically triggered by a situation of unfairness and humiliation that he can not rectify.

In this particular case, the dangers involved are denied—either not seen at all or at least not perceived as to their significance and importance for himself and hence self-punishment incurred in the form of physical or financial damage or of humiliation.

Part identities would make frequent appearances in dreams—an innocent child who shoots down driver and passenger going by in a car (mother and fetus!), or as vicious lions, tigers, snakes, and dogs (his own oral aggression), or as a prankster who would frighten his wife by jumping out of the closet (turning the tables so to speak), then in "those crazy ideas" of aggression, or in hours of temper tantrums where he resembles very much a 3-year-old, screaming, whining boy. During much of his professional and private life he feels detached and somewhat unreal.

He adds to that dream of the two selves—the adult doctor versus that innocently shooting child (really the helplessly angry, anxious, and guilty child!)—that it was *he* who "tied down" that child after the shooting. He describes how similar to the split in him between the good-looking facade and the childlike self, there is a split reality at home—a denial of all the unhappiness and strife and craziness, all hidden behind a facade of sweet bonhomie. And while he is talking about this he feels himself lapsing into a dreamlike state: "It is like cutting off a part of myself—that part that I tie down." He sees the image, it makes sense, but he cannot quite feel it. Yet each day we find palpable evidence for that other personality—particularly in his moments and acts of regression into "pseudostupidity." I believe that these brief dreamlike or contracted states largely operate with massive, unspecific denial of the present-day world: He eliminates the other rivals and becomes the baby himself—the wish fulfillment by identification and regression.

[Transactionally, to draw on Dorpat's valuable contribution,] in many ways even the children accepted the shared denial of their parents by submitting to a stereotypical role (the "doctor") regardless of their individual needs and interests. Such acceptance was interrupted by acts of episodic, yet abortive defiance—"pseudo-stupidity." Again such shared denial led to a split in each personality, a duplicity in every meaning of the word.

In this clinical vignette, we see the centrality of denial as well as its links to all other forms of defense. Denial, the mechanism, is analogous to the complex form of the affect shame seen in the adult; shame itself is inextricably interwoven with denial in this case as in so many others.

Because, broadly speaking, denial says: "I don't want to see—", we have the particularly intriguing connection to the affect *shame,* part of which may be expressed ("translated") as: "I don't want to see you anymore. Disappear!" Shame is, both in transaction and intrapsychically, the affective counterpart to the defense of denial. Both dictate a removal of parts of perception under the dictate of anxiety and conflict—shame mostly, though by no means exclusively, in regard to being seen, the *passive* aspect of perception, denial mostly, but again not exclusively, in regard to *active* perceiving.

DENIAL AND IMPULSIVE ACTION: CLINICAL APPROACHES

Recently, I have been struck by the role of impulsivity in the pathology of many patients. Some may fit what Fenichel described as "impulsive neurosis," for example, drug addicts or binge drinkers, or patients with bulimia and anorexia; but others clearly belong to other categories—phobic character, depression, hysterical syndrome, as-if personality with severe depersonalization, and especially masochistic personality. What links these cases for me is a marked tendency to deal with anxiety through the use of neurotic action outside, and acting out within the therapeutic relationship. Often it is possible in the therapy to discern some form of dynamic sequence leading up to, and following upon, the impulsive action, although not *all* the dynamic meanings of the steps forming each sequence may be recognized.

It is as if for a brief moment another personality, another consciousness, took over and steered all behavior in the direction of some primitive wish fulfillment. Many therapists are inclined to see in this above all a breakthrough of the id and a wild assertion of narcissistic omnipotence (a breach of the limits set by nature and culture) and thus recommend a sharp departure from the usual technique of psychoanalysis or psychotherapy, in the form of confronting and setting limits. So they often become quite judgmental, and on the assumption that they are dealing with a typical issue of "borderline" pathology—with "splitting," superego defect, and "projective identification"—they are then likely to proceed to a radical alteration of technique from that used with cases of "classical neurosis" and engage in consistent confrontation of such splitting, denying and transgressing; they impose "ego structures" and "superego strictures" from the outside in order to counteract the massive denial accompanying the supposed defense of splitting.

My clinical experience accords, however, better with that of a number of other authors, most recently Abend, Porder, and Willick (1983) in their excellent monograph from the Kris Study Group on borderline patients. I have come to view such pathology very much within the frame of the classical knowledge of (albeit severe) neuroses. Concretely, this means: There is not an absence or even weakness of the superego but rather a particularly severe problem about, and conflict with, self-condemnation and self-punishment. "Splitting" is not a separate defense but just another descriptive term for severe ambivalence; it is the phenomenological outcome of massive Oedipal and pre-Oedipal conflicts, involving as compromise formation a host of defenses. Denial, projection, and reversal are in themselves not more primitive as defenses than, let us say, repression or isolation. It is rather the *massivity of conflict,* the intensity of anxiety, and with that the greater problem of ego integration that creates the much greater clinical severity.

Another misunderstanding needs to be cleared up: that there is an antithesis of defense versus coping or adaptation. Defenses are not pathological; the compromise formations comprising them may or may not be pathological, that is, adaptive or maladaptive (not that this exhausts the definition of "sick" or "abnormal"; cf. Kubie's 1970 essay on this question, and my own chapters on this, both in the "The Hidden Dimension" [Wurmser, 1978] and "The Psychiatric Foundations of Medicine" [Balis, Wurmser, McDaniel, & Grenell, 1978]).

I address also the broader concern impelled by my experience with such patients. I have been disturbed by the currently widespread cavalier use of terms indicating severe psychopathology—psychosis, borderline, ego or superego defects, unanalysability, and the like. The effect of such sloppy and pejorative-judgmental diagnostic language on what we do and how we approach our patients can be drastically detrimental. In this context it is especially important to stress that denial is, as Basch (1974) wisely remarked, one example of a situation in which a ubiquitous defense against some aspects of perception has been almost automatically regarded as primitive and diagnostically ominous. In truth, denial can be part of the psychopathology of everyday life; it is a typical part of the neurotic process; it may be widespread even in easily analyzable cases—severe or not so severe though they may be—or it may, in certain specific forms, be one part of a profound psychotic decathexis (or rather, of the psychotic form of compromise formation).

In studying each individual sequence of impulsive actions one can discern the regularities and similarities of sequence in which denial plays a pivotal role. Yet what is being denied varies remarkably, not only from one clinical group to another, but from one part identity lived much of the time, to that shown manifestly during the impulsive action sequence.

Several groups can be discerned. Here I restrict myself to two types, in which we encounter opposite ways by which two superego parts dictate antithetical forms of denial and of manifest impulsivity. Thereafter some cases in which denial plays a role in preventing impulsivity will be studied briefly.

DENIAL IN THE SERVICE OF DEFIANCE

First a case is presented where the impulsive action consisted, among other things, of severe drug abuse that continued during treatment so that it was possible to study the sequence microscopically in *statu nascendi*. It may also illuminate the correlation between what Lansky

(1984) describes as the phenomenon of "lack" or "emptiness," preceding the impulsive action, and the dynamics of denial. Despite the fact that the patient was able to achieve control of these symptoms only after the initiation of treatment with Lithium and antidepressants (suggesting a biological predisposition to the pharmacological modulation of affect) I believe that much can be learned from the data gleaned during his therapy.

The patient is a male drug addict in his early 30s—mostly using heroin and cocaine; duration about 15 years. He describes a recurrent pattern: "Whenever I achieve any kind of success, I have to sabotage it. How can I allow myself to be successful, how could I deserve anything good, if I am so angry—or so competitive—or so greedy—or so pleasure seeking and selfish? Perhaps by failing I can attain forgiveness for those forbidden wishes." Parallel with this: "I am so afraid of failing that I rather give up *a priori*. I rather bring it about myself than to be caught by surprise."

Following a minor setback, he describes some of his impulsive actions—explosive rage, huffy arrogance, getting drunk or high as being initiated in this way: "I feel criticized or attacked. My self-esteem is so fragile, incredibly so. That led me into my problems: I would take heroin to give me a coat of armor against the world, so that I would not be bruised so easily. With heroin the hurt would still be registered and absorbed, it still would fester, but at the moment it is: 'I don't care!' But when I come out of it I am even more fragile than before. My basic sense is of avoiding emotions; I am scared of feelings. I have always been arming myself. When a relationship becomes really intense, I turn to the drugs. It has much to do with my defensiveness, with other ways of putting the armor up—my arrogance, my withdrawal, the lack of a real emotional commitment—to anyone or anything. Even when I am in a relationship, I always have to stress my independence, the transient nature of love or any intense emotion, to protect myself against commitment. I may stand at its brink, but I can never cross over and say: 'I love you.' I am terrified of commitment." He goes into details how, 2 years ago he had lost his last girlfriend because of this—what I have described elsewhere as a claustrophobic fear of commitment, of "entrapment," by any closeness or closure. He explains it as a fear of failure but is himself dissatisfied by that glib explanation. I ask: "But very concretely—why the heroin, day before yesterday?":

> I know exactly—a kind of immediate gratification and sensual pleasure. It is still so iffy whether L. [a girl he feels very strongly attracted to] is coming to visit me, and I am very impatient about the time to pass. The time was crawling, and with the high the hours drift by very pleasantly. It is *my old enemy "Time"*! I was impatient, wanted to call her, and did not want to wait.

He goes on reminiscing about the drug scene, the drug market, and how he, like many other drug addicts, tends to substitute a love relationship for drug use, "a relationship equally destructive, dangerous, clinging, sick, and with symptoms of withdrawal." He goes on describing his apprehension that the new girl might reject him:

> But when I am rejected, even if it is minor, I take it as a huge blow against my self-esteem. It proves that I am a 'geek'—unattractive, unintelligent, a nobody. And immediately: What did I do? What did I do wrong? Only *now* I begin realizing that it may not always have been my fault.

I said, "It is the inner voice that condemns you the whole time—" He interrupts: "'You are wrong, it's your fault!' That's my mother. Always: No, no, no!"

"The voice of conscience."

"And mine was overdeveloped. Always the chores my mother put on me! I felt I had to do more than all the other children, throughout the weekends; if I did something else it was wrong. It becomes more obvious with drugs: no, no, you should not do that; and I rebel against that voice within. It is an inner argument."

I said: "You mentioned the time, quite at the beginning of treatment," referring back to what he had described then as the *defiance against time* and its tyranny: by never wearing a watch and by consistently coming at the wrong time to his appointments: "The watch is part of the uniform of society. I refused to have time hanging over me. Just as I never was oriented towards a goal; that's almost a foreign concept for me. . . . Instead I retreated into a world of fantasy, into daydreams of heroes, villains and magic, of extremes of right and wrong, and where I defeated Evil."

The watch symbolizes for him the tyranny of time, hence bourgeois morality. Time stands for his mother's puritanical bitterness and austerity, yet also her hypocrisy in not only condoning "white lies" but repeatedly deceiving him—for example, making his security blanket disappear by cutting it down, piece by piece, ascribing its shrinkage to the wash.

Now—what role does denial play in this sequence? Our patient says: "What I don't want to hear is: that I am attacked. So I tune it out—with the help of heroin: I don't care anymore."

More broadly: "I can shut out time. I can make all obligations inoperative. I can avoid any commitment." As if to say: "I am not closed in by requirements of outer or inner authority." He continues: "Instead I can fly off into a world of daydreams where I am not helpless, but magically powerful and can triumph over Evil." The impulsive action is thus initiated by denial and is engaged in in order to deepen and to cement such denial: "I don't perceive frightening or hurting or shaming reality" and to help with the attendant affect blocking: "I don't feel the shame or the hurt anymore. I don't need to get angry. I don't have to kill myself." (Some patients actually stated: "If it had not been for heroin, I would have jumped out of the window long ago; heroin saved my life.") And it helps repressing one part of the wishes—namely the wishes to *please* authority within as well as without, instead of defying it.

During another severe binge with cocaine that forced his hospitalization, he aptly said: "I am so independent that any bit of structure I violently resist. I don't want to have to answer to anybody for anything I do."

The whole impulsive action sequence is thus set up to prove how independent he is from any outer and inner authority. It is a wild protest, built upon denial and leading soon enough to the acknowledgment and forcible submission to what had been so testily denied: his utter dependency.

The binge is triggered by severe anxiety about rejection and the depressed realization of his unworth and unlovability—the confirmation that his inner judge had been right and his flights into fantastic fulfillment just one more source of humiliation and self-ridicule.

The sequence here is therefore: (1) hurt by, or fear of, rejection and shame; (2) anger about, and revolt against, such weakness; (3) such manifest rebellion supported by a triple denial: that those feelings of hurt mean anything; that time has any relevance and sway; and that the acts of drug taking, dealing, lawbreaking, and breaking of all promises and commitments would have any long range consequences. Parallel with that triple denial there are two events I cannot easily subsume under denial: the pharmacogenic suppression or blocking of disturbing affects and the alteration of time experience. (4) The "crash" thereafter in form of contrition and remorse—a reassertion of the denied superego in the form of massive shame and guilt; followed (5) by acts of reparation, expiation, and grandiose fantasies of undoing the perceived flaws. At that point, the part identity of the defiant self is so far away indeed that it seems like belonging to a different person. In such aftermath, the denial is not that of the superego but of the "bad," that is, defiant self.

DENIAL AS PART OF MASOCHISTIC IMPULSIVE ACTION

In a large number of basically moderately to severely depressed patients, most of whom had no substance abuse problems, I noticed a characteristic sequence: Their more or less chronic depression and sense of emptiness and profound unworth, a depression often accompanied by periods of depersonalization, yet also most of the time by good professional functioning, is suddenly interrupted by a state of increased despair or agitation and an occasionally frantic search to find a way out. They may stand up for their rights and break their perceived external shackles in defiant anger and self-righteous indignation. They may attack a degrading partner in an outburst of wild rage, yell, scream, smash things, get drunk, have a car accident. Yet others (as the case next described) engage in acts of sexual union with reckless abandon, which are followed by rejection, then by deepest shame, then by defiant anger, and this again followed by renewed emptiness and desperate, near-suicidal loneliness, and thus once more leading to the search for the lover and his approval.

A successful professional woman noted a distressing split in her love life and sought treatment in hope of achieving a stable loving relationship. She deeply cared for one man to whom she seemed ideally matched in all regards but that of sexuality: Most of the time she was completely turned off by him and, during intercourse, "anesthetized" from the waist down. At the same time she would feel sexually attracted to, and engaged in a series of affairs with, men who patently stood below her in all respects: emotionally crude and withholding, if not cold, far less intelligent, insensitive, save for their physical appearance: very muscular, heavy, even fat, slow moving, and slow thinking. Several of them had serious problems with drinking, some clearly abused her physically and loved to humiliate her privately and publicly. Neither her friends nor she herself could comprehend why she would forsake her lovely, erudite, extremely bright and even athletically fit fiancée for a muscle-bound, "dumb jock exuding virility, who could answer only with grunts and whose handwriting and spelling was illegible" as one of her friends described the patient's lover, a "bump on a log," as she herself often called him.

Parallel to this split in her love life there was a split in her self-perception: Most of the time she felt detached, numb, almost without feelings—a clear state of *depersonalization.* In contrast, when she was with her lover, her reality could be painfully or ecstatically intense, and similarly it was during brief moments of (*hysterical*) *hallucinations* where she thought a man was waiting for her on the top of the stairs or hidden in her closet, ready to stab her, or where she woke up from a nightmare with the overwhelming sensation that the darkness was weighing in on her like an intruder or somebody smothering or throttling her; she could, therefore, not sleep without a light. There were nightmares that could be more vivid and real than her waking life.

She saw gradually, over the course of the analysis, how depersonalization and masochistic sexual involvement were two opposite, but complementary states, the former guarding her against the latter. Already on the surface of it, the first state was dominated by *disavowal* and affect blocking—virtually all perceptions of self and surroundings being stripped of their emotional significance, whereas her factual functioning remained excellent. The second state, that of manifest *masochistic perversion,* self-destructive acting, and *depression* (occasionally a kind of rageful suicidal tantrum) was introduced by some act of impulsive rashness and recklessness and looked as if it was simply the breakthrough of some masochistic impulse gratification accompanied by some condign punishment.

She describes the motive for her impulsivity again and again after each break returning to her lover: "It always came from inner agitation; I felt extremely uncomfortable, and the impulse was to try to end the uncomfortableness—that things were intolerable, and I had to do something to change them, and I had to do it *now.* Twenty-four hours would have seemed an eternity. Something seemed to be hammering at me and nagging at me." What? "The fear of abandonment, of losing his love, his approval, his body."

The impulsive action had the aim to merge with one who had everything that was forbidden or denied to her; and it thus could be used to circumvent and defy the prohibitions. With that, both her own separateness and the validity of those injunctions were denied. Such overriding of reality and its prohibitions had immediately to be followed by a vast assortment of self-punishing acts and a sense of profound contrition, repentance, and perhaps most of all of shame.

The repression of her aggressive wishes was accompanied by the denial of a large part of herself: "I am not this—envious, angry, cruel, vindictive. Rather I am like dead: wholly deprived of feelings, of pleasure."

Why? Because all pleasure, all sexuality had become tied to such a sadistic intent—especially that of robbing the man of his pleasure by castrating him—and had to be repudiated with strictest vehemence by her conscience: It is this sanction by the superego that effects such disavowal.

So the No is against her *wishes* (mostly aggressive ones)—*repression;* the No is against *feelings* in general, pleasure, envy, shame, and anger in particular—*affect blocking;* the No is against *seeing herself* as angry, envious, and defiant—the *denial* of an important part of her identity.

In turn, when the man is strong enough to "take" her aggression, respond to her sadistic impulses with a far greater retaliation, she could counter that triple *No* with a triple *Yes,* in a frenzy of love, surrender, orgastic pleasure, and outrage, followed by contrition and, eventually, a relapse into the triple *No,* with its depression, depersonalization, and near-suicidal rage.

Thus the doubleness of her life and of her self-representation could be understood as follows: She split herself into one figure who possessed asexual power, was detached, impersonal, efficient, could even be gentle and somewhat feminine, certainly caring—her *depersonalized self;* and a second person whose sexual sadism was projected onto, and safely experienced vicariously through, her lover under the guise of her sexual masochism—her *masochistic self.* In the first part identity, she disavowed any sign of weakness; in the second she denied that it was she who equated violence and sexuality and lived out such an equation. Instead: "Not I, but he!"

Because, in reality, she is anything but a weak personality, this explicit stress on masculine power and on her identification with her cruel, hard lover serves a much more relevant denial, namely of that side of her (that part of her self-representation), of which she feels deeply ashamed. It is the part identity of a *cheated* girl that wants to take *revenge* and would be *punished* for it—cheated by her exclusion from the union mother–infant brother, cheated because she was not a boy, cheated because she felt deprived of her mother's love throughout, cheated also because her individuality had so often been squelched—denied—by her mother.

The first part identity was ruled primarily by a defense against *perception*—disavowal; the second was under the sway primarily of a defense against *drive*—repression, specifically of sadism vis-à-vis the pregnant mother (the "heavy man").

The conflict was the same in both states but dealt with in radically different ways of defense.

One could also state it so: In the first, she *accepted* the aspects of phallic power of her sadism but not its cruelty, yet largely *denied* her own femininity; hers was then a powerful, masculine self, but safe, because her sadism was sufficiently sublimated to be of high professional value. In the second, she denied her own power but accepted sadism, provided it was not her own: It had to remain disguised (repressed)—projected, reversed in direction, turned against the self, simultaneously pleasurable and painful.

In terms of the superego: In the first state, the *shame* of being weak and "shortchanged" was wiped out—denied—by her being detached, different from that wishywashy, helpless girl of yore, strong and manly, though feelingless. In the second state, her *guilt* for her sadistic murderous wishes toward her mother and the castrating wishes toward the man was being atoned for and forgiven—accepted and canceled—by her suffering as a tortured victim.

Impulsive action was the switch and transition from the first state to the second. It is difficult to say what always triggered it: loneliness, humiliation, hormonal changes—all played a role in the rising sense of anxious agitation. I presume, anything that would touch upon the deep equation: "I am cheated = left out = castrated = humiliated" would act as a precipitant and lead to an increase of the unconscious aggression, hence of self-condemnation, hence of anxiety and depressive affect, and require the second type of compromise formation.

Her fiancée was ideally suited as pendant for state one—the asexual friend, admirer, supporter, and confidant, who made her feel strong, though guilty, but was unsuited for the aims of her sadistic side, "too weak to contain" her, meaning: unable to live that part safely out for her and with her. Exactly the reverse held true for her lover: With him she could project and vicariously satisfy her sadism; instead of feeling strong she succumbed to him; guilt she did not feel so much with him; he took care of that, but she felt humiliated and shamed instead.

The resolution of her neurosis lay in the acceptance of her disavowed weakness and shame of the first state—her being shortchanged and "castrated"—and in her acceptance of her (repressed) disavowed cruelty and vindictiveness and of the guilt of the second state—her being "castrating" or murderous, and thus in the integration of these two part identities. (The analysis has been concluded successfully).

What is it then that initiates the impulsive action in both cases, and how may we relate this to denial? I go back to Melvin Lansky's (1984) scheme: He sees the prodrome of the impulsive action in an experience of *disorganization* and disintegration, which the patients themselves express as "*lack*" or "*absence*" and treat therefore very concretely as a gaping hole and a defect, one to be filled by some consummatory act; this is undoubtedly an apt clinical description, and one that has led many to postulate a kind of "structural defect" that needs to be filled by some educational or otherwise supportive–suggestive measure. What is this lack, this absence, this sense of being empty, cheated, rejected, or abandoned? Is it just the memory trace of a traumatic occurrence, of some affect storm out of control? A derivative of some ego disorganization? A hallmark of some structural defect? Is it, as Lansky seems to imply, a structural breakdown that ultimately eludes the grasp of language—"an ego that is preoccupied with the threat of disorganization . . ."? I think not.

I hold with Rangell (1982) that there is no *separate fragmentation anxiety*. Every severe conflict involves issues of overvaluation of self and others and hence narcissistic aspects. Therewith it entails severe anxiety; all anxiety *eo ipso* encompasses a small- or large-scale experience of "falling apart," of "going to pieces," of being confused, bewildered, perplexed—all synonyms for weaker or more severe forms of fragmentation and disorganization. This is especially the case for shame—with its double nature as an affect of anxiety and as one of depressive realization that humiliation has already occurred—with yet more to follow (Brenner 1982; Rangell, 1968). I think it is the anxiety aspect that endows shame with its peculiar intensity of the sense of loss of cohesion and of inner discontinuity. Both, anxiety and depressive affect, prompt a panicky search for some thing or some action that could prevent or repair such a shameful defect and its exposure, still the raging feelings, soothe the fright, and expiate the wrong, or make up for the flaw. The *self-potentiating* quality of shame resides not only in the well-known circle of "shame about shame" (S. Levin, 1971) but in the secondary shame resulting from those impulsive acts that in the first place have been set up to counter the affect of shame. This self-reinforcing, self-confirming quality is, however, not only one of the paradoxes of shame conflicts but of neurotic symptoms in general. Freud referred to it as the "return of the repressed"; it is probably more accurate to see in it, with Brenner (1982, p. 113), simply the expression of compromise formation.

If my understanding is accurate—that is, that all such disorganization or fragmentation is part of overwhelming anxiety, or, more generally, part of all overwhelming affects—(rage, despair, shame, besides anxiety)—and not the other way around (i.e., that disorganization would lead to such archaic affects), then our therapeutic task would consist in finding out what *core affect*—especially what form of anxiety, of helpless exposure—is now consciously felt as fragmentation, therefore as lack and emptiness, and then warded off by impulsive action. When studied carefully, that prodromal feeling of emptiness is, like what follows, a complex compromise formation:

Most direcly, it is an *inner sense of condemnation:* "I am worthless, I am just an empty shell. I have nothing within—no substance, no value." Why this often frantic self-disparagement? Because of a vast array of damnable wishes, derogatorily called by the patient's inner voice and by the outer one of parents, social authority, and many therapists and counselors, "demands, greed, bad desires, unacceptable wishes disguised as needs, narcissism. . . ."

Language thus conspires with the superego within and with the authority without to condemn.

What this superego injunction really comes down to is this: Such condemnation is a needed restraint (Gray, personal communication) against very intense wishes and needs for love and power, for self-confirmation, for trust, for one's own identity, and the aggressions engendered by those impulses. They are accompanied, they call for, or stem from, the four great *anxieties* described by Freud—(1) of losing the other; (2) of losing the other's love and respect, that is, shame, often felt as contempt by the other or as the rape of one's identity, the denial by the other of what one feels, perceives, or wishes; (3) of being mutilated, dismembered, and castrated; and (4) of being punished by one's conscience. Or it is the depressive conviction that these four threats have already materialized (cf. Brenner, 1982).

Tactically I have found the work on the *anxieties* underlying the impulsive actions and especially those related to the *superego*—that is, shame and guilt, internal and reexternalized—particularly helpful for gaining the necessary leverage. Not only is it this superego anxiety that offers particularly valuable entrance, but the impulsive action seems always aimed at gaining some sort of *protection* against severe anxiety— ultimately all four anxieties mentioned. Such protection would come from a protective person, for example, as approval, love, closeness—or a protective, soothing, quieting substance, the drug—or a protective system, for example, the "buddies," the ambiance of the drug setting, the penal system, the program, the authorities, AA—or protection by forgiveness and renewed dependency on parent, spouse, and therapist.

So "lack or absence" is not the last level of meaning, in my experience, nor is this the impulsive "taking" to fill that emptiness. All this is rather the beginning than the end. Behind that phenomenology is the story of the unconscious conflict; and the more severe those unconscious conflicts, the more massive, that is, archaic (regressive or unmodulated) the anxieties and many other affects involved.

In both cases described (standing for entire groups of patients) we encounter impulsive action and denial together. In the first case, the impulsive action is used to *achieve the denial* of one part identity that obeys the part of the superego symbolized by Time's tyranny. In the second case, impulsive action is used to *break through* the stranglehold that massive denial has on an important part of the patient's self. It serves to assert her taking and envious, defiant and vengeful side, and, most deeply, her sadism. Yet both sequences result in the same: a temporary *defense against aspects of the superego* in the form of the impulsive action, followed by reestablishment of the superego's sway.

The impulsive action means to protest in the first case: "I am not wounded anymore, not hurt, not vulnerable. I don't have to submit. I am not ashamed for failing. Quite to the contrary: I am beyond time's strictures and reality's structures." *It denies the shame part of the superego.* The end point of the sequence is naturally guilt.

In the second case, the impulsive action means: "I am not aggressive—he is; I am not wounding, I am not castrating or destroying children—on the contrary, I am wounded and gladly submit to torment, and I want to have a child. He is defiant, not I. In the joyous suffering and self-destruction, I am at least not guilty anymore." *It denies the guilt part of the superego.* The end point of the sequence is factual humiliation and the sense of shame. The first is the "sociopathic" form of impulsive action; the second is the masochistic form.

In both instances, it is evident that the sense of lack or emptiness is itself the outcome of massive defense, whereby denial and affect blocking play a crucial role: "I don't feel anything; I am a nothing, an empty shell, without substance, value, goal, or fantasies"—a defense against overwhelming affects and hence a refusal to be aware of that part of the self that would be associated with, no, filled up by, such odious "demands" (quite concretely seen)—wishes that one or both parents had refused to acknowledge as part of their "good" child. *Their* denial is matched by the child's denial, and the child's defiance against such blindness still uses the same defense of denial—not only against drives and feelings as part of the self but also against authority, values, and commitments. The rebellion against conscience, ideals, and time enlists very prominently this weapon of not-perceiving—the defense of denial. It is supported and deepened by impulsive action (hence the defense mechanisms of turning passive into active, externalization, projection, identification with the aggressor) and may lead to a temporary numbing of the disturbing affects themselves (affect blocking), either by the intensity of screen affects, or by the use of drugs, or, as in the second group, by the suffering endured. However, this is followed by a deepening of the initial conflict and an intensification of self-condemnation (in the form of shame and guilt), hence by a yet-increased need for renewed denial, action, and numbing. This is the vicious spiral in compulsive drug use, in love addiction, in "compulsive honesty" (a kind of "Bekenntniszwang," a compulsion to confess or to be indiscreet, in order to find absolution), and quite generally, impulse neuroses and impulsive actions.

In both it is so, as I have written here, that denial is the weapon used by the one part identity against the other at the behest of one superego part against the other.

To go one step further still, eventually the denial is reinforced by the action in yet another and more encompassing way: "I don't have any inner problems. Everything is on the outside and can be corrected by manipulation there." Or: "If I only get rid of the drug use—or this or that noxious behavior—everything will be alright."

Inner conflict, inner reality all in all, is denied as having anything to do with life's problems (or there are no problems at all!). Most drug addicts show for a long time this vast denial. It results in what I have called *psychophobia,* a disregard for the importance of introspection of any kind and its resolute and self-righteous avoidance—in fact, not rarely a disdain for any approach to it.

The well-known denial of the alcoholic of having any problem with drinking at all is, of course, only the most superficial version of the many layers of denial.

PROBLEMS OF TECHNIQUES WITH DENIAL AND IMPULSIVE ACTIONS

The extent of denial and impulsivity, including substance abuse, may prompt many to view these patients as somehow close to the psychoses, as "borderline," and to alter drastically the therapeutic approach. In many instances, this proves, however, not to be necessary.

Technically it seems to me crucial to avoid a moralistic stand toward the impulsive actions. One has to realize that these represent both a momentary respite, an escape from *too much superego,* not a sign of too little, of a lack or a lacuna of the superego. Moreover, it is always done in such a self-destructive way that massive retribution is a built-in feature of the impulsive action—what Paul Gray (personal communication) calls a kind of "package deal." That is, of course, also a major part of the transference implication: to provoke the therapist into protection, rescue, and punishment and, in regard to the accompanying denials, into stating "the truth" or into pointing to "reality," and with that, into "setting limits" or "confronting." It has been my experience that it is better *not* to be placed into such a role of punisher and warner. A consistently analytic approach can be very effective if it remains grounded in, and compatible with, *a strong emotional presence* of the therapist, an attitude of warmth, kindness, and flexibility.

A good many patients with such severe psychopathology—usually classified as "borderlines"—can be treated quite well in psychoanalysis, with only minor modifications. I currently have a number of compulsive drug users and other patients with "severe acting out" and "impulsivity" in effective treatment of such nature. This nonjudgmental approach in regard to what may be looked at as ominous "acting out" sooner or later leads to the insight that precisely those impulsive actions hold the *key* to the comprehension of the deep unconscious conflicts and to their resolution.

Even if or when it is necessary to intervene, because of the massivity of conflict and anxiety ("acting out" in the common pejorative parlance), with more active measures like advice or brief hospitalization or a medication like an antidepressant or narcotics antagonist, this may often be only a temporary expedient, a form of crisis intervention; soon the attention can move back to a dynamic understanding, one that specifically deals with the superego side of the conflict, with the affects expressing such conflict, and with the specific defenses used.

DENIAL AS PREVENTION OF RAGE AND AS PART OF THE "BLINDING BY IMAGES" (SHARED DENIAL IN THE FAMILY)

Much of what I have described up to now has to be viewed against a family atmosphere that predisposes for the duality of impulsive action and of denial—especially of the several forms of blocking out certain aspects of the superego. There are two features I would think to be particularly important: One is severe *traumatization,* either by violence or by sexual abuse (as is, by the way, evident from the childhood history of the majority of patients with compulsive drug use). Again under the sway of the superego, the observation must be blocked: It cannot have happened because usually the child sees himself or herself as the guilty and shameful party, and such conviction is deepened by accusation, disbelief, and full denial on the side of the adults. In the child, there may not be full amnesia, only partial repression; but concomitantly there is a tuning out of perception: One does not hear, does not respond, has not noticed, does not want to talk about the details—not only about the traumatic experiences themselves but about a broad or broadest circle of derivative experiences, up to a full-blown form of psychophobia. Yet it is most prominently again a cutting out of all that could be seen as criticism (or rejection or ridicule) or could lead to it.

The other feature in the family background is *parental denial* of the *child's individuality*—his or her personal needs, wishes, fears, his or her autonomy—in favor of impersonal categories. Specifically I refer to what Schottländer, some 30 years ago, referred to as *"Blendung durch Bilder,"* blinding by images—the parental denial of the child's individuality in favor of some impersonal categories, resulting in a superego that mirrors such massive denial and a split identity.

In the case that follows, the family atmosphere led to a kind of character attitude of: "I cannot allow myself to see certain parts of the family reality" because it would lead to intolerable rage.

A former drug addict in his 30s, youngest of three, has in slightly modified psychoanalysis become an exemplary success in personal and social regards and deeply involved in the analytic work, in spite of 15 years of severe narcotics addiction (including a near fatal overdose) and abuse of most other drugs and alcohol. After being present when his mother was severely belligerent against a friend of his, he said: "I was not conscious of it until the friend and my wife made me aware of it. I tuned it out. I did not listen to it. Only later on did I realize it. For me it was: It did not happen. I shut myself out from it. I declared myself neutral and invisible. I have no connection with that woman. The feeling is: that I vanish emotionally. I have taught myself that for years, the ability to shut out. I cut myself off way back." Instead of those perceptions, he had noticed an unexplainable tension and restlessness, a driven overactivity and hectic pressure, "as if I am ready to pursue the prey." Behind that, there was the conflict of seeing his mother both as a friend in childhood and as a vicious, nasty, alcoholic tormentor who had no ability to see him as an individual.

The oldest brother of the patient had died of an overdose; the middle brother is an alcoholic, violent, and a social misfit (Wurmser, 1985).

Back to the scene at issue: His opposing feelings toward his mother, those of embarrassment and anger and those of allegiance, had been blocked while he had "tuned out" the entire scene.

Denial in regard to many details of his work is still, in spite of great success since his abstinence, a prominent part of his character, and it keeps leading to many small mishaps or to more serious accidents. It is as if he had come to say habitually to himself: "I have to shut out part of what I see and hear because it might be too angering, too frightening, too embarrassing, or too painful." Denial prevents the painful affects by blocking perception. The drugs played a role in it: "I was too blinded by the drugs to see the reality"—namely how he was neglecting his own child in ways similar to those he had seen in his parents.

He proceeds to develop the theme that he had been the favorite child but has never felt good about it. He finds it as frightening as all other success; more generally he feels competition and confrontation to be prohibited: "My fear is their power."

"It is a shadowy feeling of massive guilt, almost of mythical proportions," says this otherwise rather inarticulate farmer.

Another symptom of that ghost is his restlessness—an impulsive flight from being confined by any commitments, like our appointment schedule: "I am running away from my weakness—from facing issues; I am running away from what I should do." His guilt is projected onto those outer obligations he tries, impulsively, to avoid or break. His claustrophobia—"I fear to be confined"— rests on such projection of superego strictures; and his bursting out derives from the deep anger against such authority within and without, just as he was angry at the horribly self-centered, disappointing, alcoholic parents—"that lack of ideal and example. . . . I was despising them, and yet I longed for their love."

Such claustrophobic restlessness and the equation *claustrum* = *superego* can explain much impulsive action by drug addicts and alcoholics (Wurmser, 1984, 1987a,b, 1988).

In fact, while he had successfully conquered the impulsivity of drug taking and the dangerous outbursts of rage, another symptom took their place and created serious problems. I mentioned how he avoided all kinds of confrontation, but he went farther: He had difficulties saying no to the demands put on him by employees, friends, associates, and relatives, and he found himself suddenly in a mess caused by his "lack of prioritizing" and disorganization. At one moment, no less than 28 of his checks bounced, and his telephone was disconnected, whereas his wife kept bitterly complaining that he had restricted her outlays and shopping sprees. The sequence leading up to this (kind of) impulsive giving-in to the exigencies of the moment revealed itself: "It's a lack of self-discipline, of control, and something in me that does not let me succeed." But what is that? "I have too much going on, more than I can afford. I could have told M.: 'I cannot help you.' But I felt I owed him this." He could not say No. Why? "It is always the sense of guilt—anger and guilt colliding with each other—for having survived, for trying to succeed—anger at my predecessors, my family, my own weakness. A voice in me: you won't succeed, or it will come so hard that it won't be worth it. When I lay off somebody I feel: It should be me, not him! I blame myself." (He often expressed this also about his brother that had succumbed to an overdose, whereas he had been resuscitated).

Giving, bending over backwards, never to say No—all that was done in order not to hurt—to hide the intense aggressions.

The sequence: (1) feeling unloved, rejected, hurt; (2) vengeful wishes—largely unconscious; (3) self-condemnation: "You are a bad boy for entertaining such wishes"; (4) "A voice: Be good, or you will be rejected; don't do that, be a good son and friend, and never say No; don't be like them"; (5) "denial that there are limits in reality to what I can do," especially when being called upon to help; (6) chaos . . .

Basically: "The fear of not being accepted controls all of my decisions. Why cannot I accept myself but need the approval of those old ghosts?" Because there is so much unfinished business of hurt and anger! That's why! "I want to shut out my feelings about my parents. It is as if all the faces in the family were behind a glass plate—their lips are moving but nothing is coming out—that I am not one of them." So denial is a mitigated and muted derivative of his wishing them dead.

Relevant for this vignette is the effect of the experience of having been denied in one's self-expression by one or both parents—of *not having been seen*—and the replication now, in current life and the transference, of the active blocking out of perception by the patient, be it with the help of drugs or of fantasies of idealization. Parallel with such blocking of perception, dangerous impulses and unpleasant affects are being kept out. When those fantasies break down and denial of perceptions ceases, the affects of depression and shame, or of defiance, rage, and guilt can become overwhelming and may lead to some impulsive action. A strong "corrective emotional experience" of "being heard and seen" in the therapy has allowed a nearly complete ceasing of impulsive action and a piecemeal recovery of the denied perceptions.

One final remark about some of the terms used and the need for greater caution with that use of ominous labels. I have been much struck by the fact that those terms are being used to *judge* patients and, even more reprehensively, to judge co-workers and colleagues. "Borderline" has become, like "narcissism," one more category used to condemn someone else and to justify aggressive behavior under the guise of health care; such associated language as "defect" or "splitting" but also "projective identification" and "denial" has become an arsenal of weapons. When we remember that one of Freud's great insights was that we all have many of these problems, we all share in these conflicts, in defenses and solutions, so appear these new dichotomies and the judgmental attitudes promoted by them particularly lamentable, a regression in terms and spirit to Janet and Charcot.

Our preeminent task is not that of being the outer authority—of confronting, limit setting, or pointing to reality even with these patients. Rather we may do best in the long run by helping our patients to *analyze* their superego precisely in the transference, instead of their just obeying or overthrowing it, that is, by helping them to see through its duplicity.

Impulsivity is after all an attempt to break out of the confinement of the superego—an attempt doomed by its very nature to failure.

The study of denial offers convincing evidence for what I find to be an inescapable conclusion: The superego is still the sleeping giant of psychoanalysis.

REFERENCES

Abend, S., Porder, M., & Willick, M. (1983). *Borderline patients*. New York: International Universities Press.

Arlow, J. A. (1972). The only child. *Psychoanalytic Quarterly, 42*, 507–536.

Balis, G., Wurmser, L., McDaniel, E., & Grenell, R. (1978). *Psychiatric Foundations of Medicine*. Butterworth.

Basch, M. (1974). Interference with perceptual transformation in the service of defense. *Annual of Psychoanalysis, 2*, 87–97.

Basch, M. (1976). The concept of affect, a reexaminaton. *Journal of the American Psychoanalytic Association, 24*, 759–777.

Basch, M. (1983). The perception of reality and the disavowal of meaning. *Annual of Psychoanalysis, 11*, 125–154.

Beebe, B., & Sloate, P. (1982). Assessment and treatment of difficulties in mother-infant attunement in the first three years of life. *Psychoanalytic Inquiry, 1*, 601–624.

Brenner, C. (1982). *The mind in conflict*. New York: International Universities Press.

Dorpat, T. (1979). Is splitting a defense? *International Review of Psychoanalysis, 6*, 105–113.

Dorpat, T. (1983a). Denial, defect, symptom formation—and construction. *Psychoanalytic Inquiry, 3*, 223–254.

Dorpat, T. (1983b). The cognitive arrest hypothesis of denial. *International Journal of Psychoanalysis, 64*, 47–59.

Federn, P. (1952). *Ego psychology and the psychoses.* New York: Basic.

Fenichel, O. (1945). *The psychoanalytic theory of neurosis.* New York: Norton.

Freud, A. (1936). *The ego and the mechanisms of defense.* New York: International Universities Press.

Freud, S. (1915). Repression. In *Standard edition* (Vol. 14, pp. 143–158). London: Hogarth.

Freud, S. (1925). Negation. In *Standard edition* (Vol. 19, pp. 235–242). London: Hogarth.

Freud, S. (1940). An outline of psychoanalysis. In *Standard edition* (Vol. 23, pp. 144–208). London: Hogarth.

Kubie, L. S. (1970). The retreat from patients. *International Journal of Psychiatry, 9*, 693–711.

Lansky, M. (1984). *The explanation of impulsive action.* Paper presented at meeting of American Psychoanalytic Association.

Levin, S. (1971). The psychoanalysis of shame. *International Journal of Psychoanalysis, 52*, 355–362.

Polanyi, M. (1964). *Personal knowledge.* New York: Harper & Row.

Rangell, L. (1968). A further attempt to resolve the "problem of anxiety," *Journal of the American Psychoanalytic Association, 16*, 371–404.

Rangell, L. (1982). The self in psychoanalytic theory. *Journal of the American Psychoanalytic Association, 30*, 863–892.

Schachtel, E. (1959). *Metamorphosis.* New York: Basic Books.

Trunnell, E. E., & Holt, W. E. (1974). The concept of denial or disavowal. *Journal of the American Psychoanalytic Association, 22*, 769–784.

Waelder, R. (1951). The structure of paranoid ideas. In *Psychoanalysis: Observation, theory, application* (pp. 207–228). New York: International Universities Press.

Wangh, M. (1962). The evocation of a proxy. *Psychoanalytic Study of the Child, 17*, 451–472.

Wurmser, L. (1978). *The hidden dimension.* New York: J. Aronson.

Wurmser, L. (1979). *The sharing of defenses—The addict and his family.* Paper presented at the International Psychoanalytic meeting, New York.

Wurmser, L. (1981). *The mask of shame.* Baltimore: John Hopkins Press.

Wurmser, L. (1984). The role of superego conflicts in substance abuse and their treatment. *International Journal of Psychotherapy, 10*, 227–258.

Wurmser, L. (1985). Denial and split identity: Timely issues in the psychoanalytic psychotherapy of compulsive drug users. *Journal of Substance Abuse Treatment, 2*, 89–99.

Wurmser, L. (1987a). Flight from Conscience: Experiences with the psychoanalytic treatment of compulsive drug abusers. *Journal of Substance Abuse Treatment, 4*, 157–179.

Wurmser, L. (1987b). *Flucht vor dem Gewissen.* Heidelberg: Springer.

Wurmser, L. (1988). "The sleeping giant"—A dissenting comment about "Borderline Pathology." To be published in *Psychoanalytic Inquiry.*

13

Denial in Borderlines

Michael H. Stone

REMARKS

Denial plays so prominent a role in the psychopathology of borderline patients that it is probably nearer the truth to say *not* that "borderline patients use denial" but rather that patients exhibiting this mechanism to any great degree tend to get labeled *borderline*.

Little is understood concerning the factors predisposing to the borderline's use of this defense. In some cases, one can envision certain psychological sources; in others, neurophysiological factors appear operative. It may be that in the average case, both sets of factors interact.

With respect to constitution, it would appear that certain persons, carrying risk genes for manic-depression, are neurophysiologically miswired in such a way as to manifest inordinate intensity of their drives. Their capacity to defer gratification of various impulses is correspondingly impaired. Given the emergence of an impulse, such persons have little time to ponder, to weigh alternatives, to assess consequences. Life, themselves, and other people—are experienced in extremes. Some are regarded with blind hatred; others, adored. Or else, one sees oneself in an exalted and blameless image—or as worthless. In all these states of mind: adoration, blind hatred, grandiosity, or self-villification, there is awareness of one set of qualities, alongside denial (literally, a blindness)

Michael H. Stone • Beth Israel Medical Center/Mt. Sinai Medical School, New York, New York 10029.

regarding an opposite set of qualities—the whole sum of which are nevertheless seen as relevant to the person in question by ordinary people who know him or her.

Whereas manic-depressive tendencies foster denial through an abbreviation of the *time* in which the contrasting qualities of persons and situations might otherwise be permitted emergence into consciousness, schizophrenic tendencies may also contribute to the denial mechanism— perhaps by means of an impairment in the ability to make connections and associations, even when the pace of events is leisurely enough to allow the average person to recall the negative and positive images that pertain to the subject at hand.

Many manic-depressives and many schizophrenics develop a paranoid personality and are given to sweeping generalizations and oversimplifications. These mechanisms imply a lack of awareness; often enough, a lack of patience, with nuance, allusion, subtlety. Some attributes are seen, therefore, in bold relief; others are denied. Something similar is at work in racial prejudice.

For sake of completeness, one could add that organic damage to the central nervous system as well as seizure disorders—also is frequently accompanied by excessive degrees of denial, as though diminution of available brain substance somehow lowers frustration tolerance, limits reflection, and fosters oversimplification and denial.

On the psychological side, the tendency to denial may be augmented by overstimulation during the developmental years. In children, early seduction can heighten drive intensity, weaken the ability to postpone gratification, and, at the same time, intensify "splitting." All these factors pave the way toward denial. A parent or other, older relative who has an incestuous relationship with a child will, for example, be adored (to the extent that the child finds him exciting) but also despised (as the child becomes aware of having been victimized). It is difficult for most people to retain both attitudes in consciousness at the same time, so one or the other is denied at any given moment. This mechanism is common in borderlines and in patients with multiple personality—both of whom are more apt to have been incest victims than would be true of the general population.

Childhood brutalization can foster denial also and thus becomes another factor on the psychological side. Parents who inflict physical pain unduly and wantonly or who inflict verbal humiliation again and again—inspire a hatred that cannot coexist alongside the love that ordinarily accompanies the parent–child bond. Again, one or the other attitude tends to be denied. Misuse of this sort is common in the histories of borderline patients.

Denial may be constant, or, as already hinted, oscillating, in nature.

In the first instance, certain ideas are split off from awareness and remain unavailable (except to the extent that they can eventually be made conscious through psychotherapy). In the latter instance, the patient behaves as though there were a on–off switching mechanism in his or her mind: In the context of an ambivalent relationship, his or her moment-to-moment attitude is governed by the valence of the latest impression inspired by the ambivalently regarded other. In the case of a sexual partner, for example, if the most recent impression were favorable, all negative memories disappear from consciousness and the loved one is regarded adoringly. But if the latest interaction were negatively tinged, all the "good" memories go suddenly out the window, and the love partner is regarded with venomous hatred about whom "nothing good can be said." This mechanism is very common among borderline patients and would seem to correlate, if not to account for, the tempestuous, roller-coaster quality of their intimate relationships. Pathologically jealous persons, the majority of whom function (at best) as *borderlines* (in Kernberg's, 1975, psychostructural sense of the term), illustrate this latter mechanism *par excellence*.

SOME NEUROPHYSIOLOGICAL ANALOGIES

Before going on to the clinical vignettes that, it is hoped, will exemplify the various denial mechanisms encountered in borderlines, it may be useful to speculate, within the framework of a neurophysiological model, just how interpersonal relationships might be negotiated under normal circumstances.

Even a young child, to say nothing of an adult, behaves as though his or her responses to the most recent interactions with the key persons in his or her environment (and, by analogy, his or her responses to strangers *resembling* those persons) are *modulated* in accordance with the history of his or her relationships with these key figures.

Physically painful or otherwise adversive (humiliating) encounters with the external world tend, of course, to mobilize our internal comparison-making machinery more quickly than positive experiences, inasmuch as the former have meaning with respect to survival. One can afford fewer mistakes when one is about to be killed than about to be kissed. It is of critical importance, therefore, that one processes adversive stimuli correctly, or, failing that, at least conservatively. By "conservatively," I refer to the tendency to protect oneself even when it turned out not to have been necessary.

In Figure 1, I have portrayed schematically the situation in which a person has just experienced something unpleasant at the hands of some-

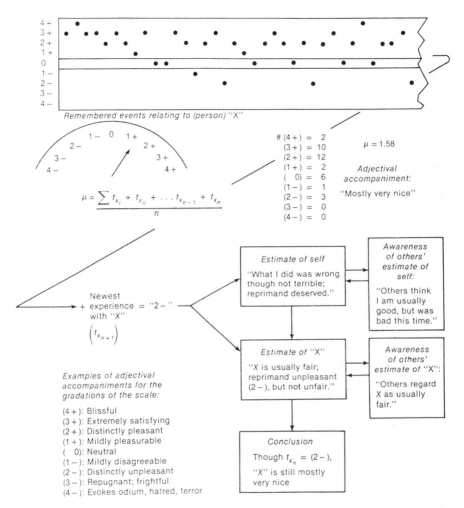

FIGURE 1. An example of an integrated response to an interpersonal event.

one familiar to him or her. To render the example less abstract, let us suppose the subject is a 6-year-old boy and that person "X" is his mother. He has just swiped a cookie from the cookie jar at 5 in the afternoon, and mother has just slapped his hand not too forcefully, and told him, raising her voice, "No cookies before supper!" The child's reaction will be shaped by the history of his relationship with mother—alluded to in the diagram in an unavoidably oversimplified way, via the dots on the memory band, where discrete events are not only recorded but assigned valences reflecting the intensity of positivity versus negativity. I have chosen a 9-point scale, ranging from blissful to terrifying—the latter signifying a threat to survival. The band in the diagram contains a mere three dozen dots; the average 6-year-old has spent, of course, some 2,000 days with his mother and has accumulated—and evaluated—thousands of separable memories of her. Those stemming from age 3 or so postdate the acquisition of language—enough to make many of the memories recollectable in a way we consider "conscious." The memory band in the example shows only a few (just over 10%) adversive instances, and of these, none descending to the level of terror. We assume these instances are "averaged," neurophysiologically, and not just in one way but in several. One can make an "average" reading, for example: In this case, amounting to about 1.6 on the scale, corresponding to a relationship that was overall quite pleasurable. Presumably, an average value of this level would be meaningful only to the extent that mother was consistently nice because a similar value derived from an erratic mother who elicited many "3+" and "4+" evaluations—but equally many "2−" and "3−" evaluations—would fail to reflect the disquieting unpredictableness of her behavior. The hypothetical mother of the diagram is, however, consistent. The child measures this by making what amounts to a kind of histogram, in which the frequency of "4+," "3+," and so forth encounters is quantified. A profile of mother's behavior emerges. Figure 1 shows a profile whose peaks would be in the "2+" and "3+" range and would lead to the child's experience of her as "mostly very nice."

The most recent, and in this case, adversive experience, as depicted in the figure, comes on the heels of, and is integrated with, a predominantly positive relationship. In addition, the child makes a number of other assessments simultaneously. He recognizes mother's reprimand as deserved; her punishment, not excessive. He has come to recognize that the outside world considers him mostly a nice boy and her—a mostly nice mother. His conclusion is, as a result of all this instantaneous and for the most part unconscious calculation, that nothing terrible happened. As he might say to himself, "It's no disaster!" Mother still loves him. Tomorrow will be a better day. Furthermore, mother is a reasonable person, from whom he need not fear an outbreak of menacing behavior without provocation. The mechanism of denial is not relevant to the normal situation we have been describing. There has been no life-threatening or ego-damaging trend in the mother–child relationship that would need to be denied in order to permit the child some love of his mother. Nor would there be a need to deny positive feelings in the interest of preserving a continuously alert attitude, for reasons of survival, such as might be prudent in the case where mother were frequently violent and abusive. Similarly, in the normal situation, we need postulate no damage to the child's own apparatus, in whatever this may consist, for making appropriate integration and differentiation (via comparisons) of the endless chain of interpersonal experience, or of the limitlessly long band of memory impressions that these experiences engender.

In patients at the borderline level, pathological forms of denial are the hallmark of their condition, viewed from the perspective of defense mechanisms, in the same manner that repression appears as the fundamental mechanism in neurotics. Splitting, projective identification, omnipotent control, devaluation, idealization, and the other defenses encountered in borderline patients—all may be seen as composed, in part, of an element of *denial*. Of the two oppositely valenced, contradictory attitudes involved in an example of splitting, one element is denied and removed from awareness, whereas the other is vigorously asserted, as though representing the patient's "only" attitude. In protective identification, one element—the recognition of which would ordinarily cast the patient in an uncomplimentary light—is denied and foisted on the shoulders of another person close to the patient. Thus the lover, the spouse, the analyst, is seen as jealous, unfaithful, repugnant, cheap, murderous, and so forth, instead of the patient her- or himself.

The quality of denial in borderlines is affected by a number of factors, some, alluded to in the introductory remarks; others, adumbrated in the discussion of Figure 1. These factors include: (a) the presence or absence of innate defect (the latter may be manic-depressive, schizotypal, or organic), (b) the nature of the actual early environment with the primary caretakers, (c) the memory of this environment, (d) the quality of enregistration of memory (are memories unduly amplified or not), and (e) the function of the neurophysiological mechanism(s) subserving integration and comparison making. Many combinations of these factors will be encountered clinically in various borderline patients exhibiting intense denial. Some of the more typical combinations are to be found in the following vignettes.

CLINICAL VIGNETTES

DENIAL IN A BORDERLINE PATIENT WITH MANIC-DEPRESSIVE TENDENCIES

A 36-year-old single woman sought treatment because of bulimia. In addition, her life was at a standstill: She was unable to work, had almost no friends, and had had no love relationships in about 10 years. Her day/night cycle was almost reversed: She could not sleep till about 5 in the A.M., awakened about noon in time to go to her exercise class. This was followed by selection of a spartan supper from the supermarket that she then prepared in her apartment. The latter she kept bare of eatables, lest she be tempted to "pig out." The evenings were spent either in frantic phone calls to the few people she had not succeeded thus far in alienating with her abrasive temperament or in going to certain fashionable singles bars where she hoped to win admiring glances from the men. Apart from that, she had no interest in the men and rarely dated. She lived off a large trust fund set up by her father, whom she periodically called for supplements—because she used up her funds very quickly in seeking consultations for various hypochondriacal complaints with specialists all over the United States.

She had been in "analytic psychotherapy" on several occasions in the past, though these exposures were really supportive in nature: She was immensely impatient for "results" and had no aptitude for psychological exploration. The strong narcissistic features she exhibited consisted of entitlement, demandingness, contempt of others, and an overpoweringly intense craving for praise of her "beauty." Her speech always came in a rush and was overly loud; she was so circumstantial as to permit no dialogue let alone "interruption." Although when conscious of needing something from another person, she could be momentarily obsequious, her usual stance was hostile. She reacted to each succeeding moment, within the context of any interaction, as though all previous moments did not exist. Thus during a (typical) conversation with her mother, who lived in a different city, she would start out tearfully pleading for some favor—to which, often enough, the mother acquiesced. But if her mother could not meet a demand—would be busy with her own life on a day the patient wanted her to come to the city, and so forth—she would explode with rage at her mother, call her a "useless fucking bitch" and slam down the receiver. A half hour later, as feelings of loneliness reasserted themselves, she would phone her mother again, beginning with a cheery introduction ("Hi, ma! . . ."), as though she owed no apology for her rudeness of a half hour before.

Although reconstruction of her past proved unusually difficult and unreliable, it appeared that her parents and brother were successful, emotionally stable, and reasonably affectionate people, whereas from the first moments of life, the patient was intense, demanding, and irritable. She had always experienced others in black-or-white terms and was far more prone to make negative than positive assessments. She would switch from positive to negative in a split second, given the slightest thwart to her wishes. In the transference, this tendency showed itself in her extreme intolerance for what she considered as lapses in my "attention." Unless I kept my gaze riveted at her continuously throughout the session, I was guilty of "inattention"—if, for example, I momentarily glanced at my tie or at the telephone. At such moments, even if the atmosphere had been agreeable beforehand, her tone instantly changed to one of murderous condemnation. She behaved as though unable to recollect that I had been generally attentive beforehand, let alone that I had spoken with her on the phone the night before for a half hour when she was in some kind of distress, and so forth.

Comment

The borderline patient in this vignette is best considered, from a diagnostic standpoint, as within the penumbra of manic-depressive illness; specifically, as an example of manic/irritable temperament (Kraepelin, 1921; Stone, 1980), or, as it was known in the nineteenth century, "sanguineo-choleric" temperament (Griesinger, 1871). Characteristically, patients with this condition "augment" or amplify reactions to stimuli both external and internal. The patient of the vignette overreacted to inconsequential bodily aches as though they were signs of fatal illness and to minor irritations in the interpersonal field, as though they were hostile gestures. She had great difficulty retaining impressions except of the immediate present, manifesting denial of whole segments of interaction with others. Denial of her offensive treatment of others, even of incidents from the previous hour or day, contributed to an uncompromising and accusatory attitude that alienated those with whom she came in contact. This heightened her aloneness, which she experienced as undeserved punishment from a hostile world, rather than as the inevitable consequence of her own hostility.

Denial in a Borderline Patient from an Abusive Environment

An unmarried woman of 23 had been hospitalized because of a suicide gesture. She had made a similar gesture, involving an overdose of aspirin, when she was 9, shortly after the breakup of her parents' marriage. Her family was chaotic, consisting of an alcoholic father, a depressed mother—who herself had been hospitalized for suicide attempts, and an alcoholic older brother. All three had been physically abusive toward the patient during her childhood, especially her brother. The patient was unable to complete college, having "fallen apart" after her sophomore year. Since then, she has remained locked in a symbiotic attachment with her equally dependent mother, rarely venturing outside. She has become, in effect, mother's new "husband," sheltering mother against loneliness and sheltered, in turn, by her mother, against the loneliness she would face if left on her own. She has developed a variety of socially visible symptoms that have the effect of safeguarding this cozy, albeit infantile, arrangement. Some of these she can barely acknowledge (handwashing compulsion, tics); others, she insists she "cannot talk about."

Interviewing this patient turned out to be a baffling task: As soon as one began to touch on an emotion-laden area (e.g., the brother's abusiveness, the father's abandonment, the immediate precipitants of her own suicide gestures), she began to look away and suddenly had "nothing to say." Her mind filled up with "scrambled" thoughts. She also pressed for early discharge as though she were "all right now," even though she had only been in the hospital a few days.

These abnormalities aside, she spoke coherently and at a moderate pace, related fairly well to her interviewer and showed no peculiarities in the formal aspects of her thinking.

Comment

One had the impression that this borderline patient exhibited a marked degree of denial, born not so much of constitutional predisposition as of extremely adverse factors in her early environment. She was an abused child caught between loyalty to her immediate family and conditions that would conduce to hatred of these same "loved ones." Whereas the patient of the preceding vignette denied love feelings by way of justifying a general attitude of outrage and contempt (at not having been "given enough"), this woman denied her outrage and hatred, as a way of making her dependency more tolerable. But she did not magnify her reactions as did the first patient: The terrible things she hinted at had really happened. Unable to integrate love and hatred toward the members of her family, she denied half the ambivalence and remained cognizant only of the positive feelings. The negative attitudes tended to express themselves symbolically via the behavioral symptoms. Many patients with multiple personality also (a) function at the borderline level and (b) have been the victims of truly outrageous physical and sexual abuse, which they have never been able to integrate into their internalized images of their beloved tormentors. Denial, in their case, however, takes on the peculiar form of compartmentalized, seemingly separate "personalities"—each one of which (usually) expresses one of the forbidden attitudes (lust, rage . . .) that dare not reach consciousness.

DENIAL IN A SCHIZOTYPAL BORDERLINE PATIENT

A schizotypal borderline woman with whom I have worked for some 18 years, thrice weekly, was reared by a frankly schizophrenic mother and a manic-depressive father, both of whom died in a mutual suicide pact when she was in her early 20s. During the patient's adolescence, her mother was often neglectful and punitive. Suffering a psychotic break when the patient was about 13, she became progressively more helpless and dependent, relying on her daughter for support and companionship as exaggeratedly as she had been rejecting earlier on. Ever since the suicide, over which my patient felt inordinately guilty (she lived in another city, and was not "there" for her mother in the final years), she became intensely preoccupied with a longing for the dead parent: Much of her mental life was spent in carrying on conversations with her mother or in trying to call up her image. She tended to experience others as carbon copies of her mother, denying, in the process, both the actual fact of the mother's death as well as the distinctions that might have served to differentiate her image of other persons from that of the irretrievably lost parent. In the process, she literally peopled the world with *replicas* of her mother (of which I was the most compelling "example"), often complaining *outwardly* because of the similarity of someone's gestures or comments to some of the more annoying qualities of her mother—but *inwardly* very glad that her mother was not "lost" to her after all. Cognitively, she is always aware that, behind her ambivalently cherished illusion, is the raw fact of my being—as she puts it—"only Dr. Stone." She is, in other words, not delusional. Her conviction never goes beyond the level of an over-valued idea—albeit it is one she clings to with the tenacity of a child clutching his teddy.

Her ability to see me as I am grows stronger, the longer I "stay put"; the weaker, just before and all throughout any separation. Though dimly aware of my distinctness at such times, she rails against *me-as-myself*—for having "re-jected" her as a woman. She invariably feels old and ugly before I go away—as if I were "ditching" her because she *were* old and ugly. While I am away, her denial takes on a somewhat different form: I am missed keenly as though I were her mother—not only the problematical and ambivalently loved mother she had in real life but the idealized "good" (and predictably available) mother she had always hoped for. When I return, she switches immediately into another state of being: Noticing herself having survived, she depreciates me, saying, "I got through the vacation OK, so what do I need you for, anyway?!" Here, there is a denial of the cooperative venture that the long years of her treatment constitute: It was as though my only purpose were to guarantee her survival.

Typical of many borderline patients, she cannot think of any flaws in my nature nor any ways I have disappointed her over the years, during those "good stretches"—yet cannot think of any kindness I bestowed upon her nor of any-thing positive ever to have grown out of our sessions, during the separation period.

Although her life has gradually improved since the beginnings of our work—she now has hobbies and a steady boyfriend, whereas her life was barren at the outset—she can be counted on to berate me as forcibly upon my recent returns as she did when I would come back from a week's absence many years ago. There has been such a history built up between us of my returning faithfully on the day I said I would—there cannot have been less than 40 such examples, if one includes lecture tours and vacations, since 1967—that I am regularly quite astonished at her outbursts upon my return. This, despite years of training and experience with borderline and psychotic patients and despite years of supervision by Harold Searles, who guided me in the treatment of this same patient in what may now be called "a generation ago." I know full well, that is to say, that in the porous membrane separating conscious from unconscious life in this woman, I will always be "mother" and mother will always be "alive" for her, no matter how many years she remains in treatment with me.

Having spotted the wedding band on my hand a few days before our last interruption, she realized I had remarried—at at first expressed a feeling of relief and contentment. As she mentioned: "Now I know I'm safe and that you won't try anything on me that way Dr. L. did with my mother" (whom, she felt, had been seduced by her last therapist). Negative feelings were denied until my return, upon which she promptly excoriated me for having rejected her in favor of my new wife. But even this admission was a thin coverup for the other set of previously denied feelings relating to the mother. These, too, she was able to express next, as she bitterly complained about the "abandonment." "You know you *are* my mother when you're away, don't you?!" is how she introduced the topic. I tried to point out to her the irony implicit in her experiencing me as her abandoning mother: As far as she could tell, she just hated me at such moments. But how much more reassuring it must be, I suggested, to envision mother alive—although rejecting, rather than not rejecting, but dead. "Of course," she replied, "but what can ever deaden the pain of her loss? I think of her every moment of the waking day." "Indeed," I told her, "this is part of why this year's vacation is as painful as last year's." "How can I ever get over my longing for her?," she then asked me. Only a lover can help with that, I told her—a remark I would have regarded as insensitive had she not recently acquired one. "So what good is therapy? You can't be one, and you can't give me one" was her next comment. To this, I replied that her *denial* of the difference between whoever she was emotionally involved with (me, in the transference; a boyfriend, in her outside life) and her mother was precisely what minimized the chances for a love relationship to flourish. So long as she personalized the brief absences of others—as rejections or insults, she would tend to remain hypercritical when they were about to leave or else excessively clinging, when they were with her. This behavior cost her nothing in the transference because it was just something for us to work on. But a boyfriend would ultimately tire of it and then truly reject her (as had occurred on dozens of occasions). Only a satisfying, real-life relationship could give her enough pleasure to outweigh the longing for mother. Such a relationship required of her that she overcome, more and more, her denial and along with it her ambivalent and alienating attitude toward others. It no longer seemed to be preaching something unattainable to speak to her in this fashion because she really had made measurable progress over the years. These days she could hold onto an image of me longer than was possible initially. Side by side with this improved internalization was a greater capacity to picture me as (a) clearly reliable about my promise to return and (b) more benevolent than malign.

The most difficult task for me has been to convince her that it is worth the effort she must expend—to envisage me as separate and benevolent even when I am absent. She tends to counter this with a question of the sort: "How dare I do that? If you're mother, I have a hold on you. If you're only Dr. Stone, I have none. Blood is thicker than water." I remind her that as mother I might be "blood" but am also unreliable and rejecting (as her mother unfortunately was in real life). As Dr. Stone, I may be "water" but water that is always there for her.

Denial in a Borderline Patient with a Manic-Depressive Illness and an Abusive Environment

A borderline woman in her mid-30s was seen because of marital difficulties culminating in a suicide gesture.

Prone to pathological jealousy, she suspected her husband of infidelity continuously since the beginning of the marriage. Over several years, the marriage deteriorated, and her husband—previously faithful—did begin to "step out" on her. When this was revealed, her behavior became erratic: She drove off to a different city under an assumed name, remained there for a week without telling anyone of her whereabouts, and seduced a number of men in various bars. Upon return home, she cut her wrists, albeit only superficially.

Her early years (ages 7 through 17) were spent in an incestuous relationship with her father, who would frequently punish her for some trivial "offense" (failing to bring him the newspaper, forgetting to pick up her clothes) by confining her to her room—and would then tell her she could "work off" the punishment by sucking his penis. On other occasions, fellatio would become the means of averting even worse punishment—because he was also given to beating her or to forcing down her throat the vegetables she may have left unfinished on her plate, etc. After the sexual encounters, he would become as tender and kind as he had been sadistic beforehand.

In relation to her father, she thus accumulated over the years two strings of experience, one highly pleasurable, the other, extremely negative.

She herself later developed bipolar-II manic-depressive illness, as had her mother and an aunt.

Her adult life was characterized by sharp mood swings and extreme unpredictability of attitude, the most minor disappointments serving to trigger an outburst of "psychotic" rage. In her love relationships, she fluctuated between the extremes of adoration and blind hatred, magnifying the valence of each interaction with husband or lover and reacting totally in relation to the quality (as she perceived it) of the last interaction.

Comment

In contrast to the patient of the first vignette, this patient had an early environment that was truly abysmal (the mother, for example, had abandoned her when she was not yet 2). She had never been able to form an integrated picture of either parent nor of the more recent significant figures in her life. She not only alternated between denial of affectionate feelings when in a transiently negative mood and vice versa but also denied her own strong tendencies to reduplicate the qualities of her father. In a subsequent marriage to a man who was faithful to her, she continued to make accusations of infidelity—which then served as the "excuses" for wild sprees of promiscuity on her part. The latter she denied as acts of infidelity, claiming that she "broke off" the marriage the day before, even though she would return to her husband a few days later as if nothing had happened.

In this case, there would appear to be a confluence of two factors contributing to pathological denial—an innate one, relating to her manic-depressive disposition, causing her to amplify mild experiences into major ones, and an environmental one, based on the realistically extreme nature of the positive and negative experiences of the relationship with either parent.

DISCUSSION

The tendency toward pathologic denial in borderline patients would appear to be exaggerated where either of two factors is operative:

(innate) neurophysiological defect affecting enregistration and appraisal of interpersonal experience; adversity of the psychosocial environment. I define the latter as "abysmal," where there has been physical brutalization, continuous verbal humiliation, transgenerational incest, or serious neglect (including abandonment). Many borderline patients have been the victims of such environments, although in the majority, the environment has been adverse, though not abysmal. A mentally disturbed but nonabusive parent (cf. the third vignette), early loss through death or divorce of a living parent, and the like constitute adverse factors, short of the "abysmal" level.

The reversibility of denial through psychotherapy will be most difficult where an abysmal environment has interacted with innate defect. The patient's basic equipment for developing a realistic appraisal of current and past relationships is so unreliable as to make it impossible, or nearly so, for the therapist to communicate effectively: What has become obvious to the therapist about the patient's life continues to be distorted and remains unintegrated by the patient. Persistent, compassionate, and accurate confrontations, however effective these are with less damaged borderline patients, fail to carry the day with the more damaged patients.

Absence (or relative mildness) of innate defect permits accurate reality testing even in the face of fairly serious environmental damage, whereas marked constitutional defect may render denial irreversible even when the reality of the nearly environmental situation was not overwhelming. In the first vignette, for example, the patient persisted in holding onto grotesquely overdrawn pictures of parents, who, as best one could determine, were no worse than average.

The stronger and more persistent the denial, the more the therapist may feel the need to resort from time to time to the impressions of close relatives and friends—interviews with whom may shed light on maladaptive behavioral tendencies, puzzling beliefs, and so forth in the patient—that could not otherwise be evaluated properly, so long as one had to rely solely upon the statements of the patient. Obviously, the more damaged a borderline patient is in this regard, the more the therapist must depart from the strict psychoanalytic model, where external communications of this sort would violate the rules of confidentiality.

A more complete discussion of factors bearing on the resolvability of borderline denial would require a much lengthier presentation. Briefly, one can add that evaluation of the patient's social and vocational assets is of central importance. Highly motivated borderline patients with good occupational skills, a pleasing social facade, and a reasonably intact capacity for intimacy may be able to overcome the effects of distinctly adverse environmental factors. Many of our most rewarding patients are of this sort.

To the thorny metapsychological issues surrounding the place of denial, disavowal, and splitting in the hierarchy of defensive maneuvers peculiar to our species, I have purposely given short shrift. This chapter is aimed more at clinical considerations. Besides, the metapsychological problems require a great deal of space to do them justice. Steingart (1983) has attempted to do so in his monograph on pathological play in borderline conditions. Steingart takes the position that denial and repression differ fundamentally in regard to how perception is used to construct meaning. In *denial*, certain thought structures are organized according to some "impelling, immediate, perceptual-like quality," whereas the more mature mechanism of repression involves "meaning-structures which possess an autonomy from such immediate, perceptual-like quality" (p. 52). In harmony with Lichtenberg and Slap (1973) and Lichtenberg (1983) and at variance with Kernberg (1975) and Kohut (1971), Steingart views denial/disavowal as necessarily pathological and not (as Jacobson had also considered it in her 1971 paper) part of "normal experience," however much it may be a part, transitorily, of the experience of most ordinary children. Here I speak of children particularly in their pre-Oedipal life, that is, before the solidification of the tripartite structure. Ordinary children, challenged for the most part by merely *manageable* as opposed to overwhelming stresses, utilize denial and splitting only infrequently. Children destined to become "borderline" are overwhelmed with great regularity (no matter whether on principally environmental or on principally innate grounds). A similar note was sounded by Lichtenberg (1983), writing about the unity of the self under certain circumstances:

> A different process may occur when moments of high intensity recur with such frequency that the integrative capacity is overwhelmed. . . . The unity of the self may become . . . endangered, giving way to separate [split] organizing of the experience along lines expressive of strong affective states. (p. 125)

The situation, though it involves a semantic question concerning "normalcy," may be analogized to certain common childhood physical conditions. All children have intestinal cramps on at least a few occasions. These may be the expression of constitutional abnormality, as in severe colic, or may be a "normal" reaction to noxious material. But the cramps are best understood as something pathological. Those who suffer them often, in the way that borderlines fall into denial and splitting often, are said to exhibit some definable and serious disorder. Those whom we call normal will have had no more than episodic and fleeting brushes with the pathological response because of their greater flexibility (enzymatic, in the one instance; psychological, in the other) and relative freedom from trauma.

Along a similar line of reasoning, Steingart argues that the disturbances in the realm of meaning that we characterize as denial and splitting, are, as I had claimed at the beginning of this chapter, the true center of borderline experience—and deserve pride of place over the issue of separation/individuation, as emphasized by Masterson (1982).[1] The transference relationships in borderlines are, by the same token, of the special, *not-real* yet not altogether delusional type, the latter being peculiar to the true psychoses. The excessive *aliveness* of the borderline patient's fears and cravings (the latter may involve drugs, sex, food), his or her experience of those close to him or her in larger than life terms— as either evil, adorable, murderous, irresistable, and the like—may also be seen as a persistence of the pathological play and engulfment in fantasy of a disturbed child and not the controlled make-believe of the healthy child.

REFERENCES

Griesinger, W. (1871). *Die Pathologie und Therapie der Psychischen Krankheiten*. Braunschweig: F. Wreden.

Jacobson, E. (1971). Denial and repression. In *Depression: Comparative studies of normal neurotic and psychotic conditions* (pp. 107–136). New York: International Universities Press. (Originally printed in 1957.)

Kernberg, O. F. (1975). *Borderline conditions and pathological narcissism*. New York: J. Aronson.

Kohut, H. (1971). *The Analysis of the Self*. New York: International Universities Press.

Kraepelin, E. (1921). *Manic-depressive insanity*. Edinburgh: Livingstone.

Lichtenberg, J. D. (1983). *Psychoanalysis and infant research*. New York: Academic Press.

Lichtenberg, J. D., & Slap, J. W. (1973). Notes on the concept of splitting and the defense mechanism of splitting of representations. *Journal of the American Psychoanalytic Association, 23*, 453–484.

Masterson, J. (1982). *Narcissistic and borderline personalities*. New York: Jaronson.

---

[1]Intense anxiety over matters of separation/individuation have, to be sure, played a rôle in the lives of many borderline patients. But the parents have not always been responsible for the adverse patterns (Stone, 1984). In some cases, a "good enough" mother (Winnicott, 1965) gives birth to a constitutionally vulnerable child, who cannot comfortably negotiate this phase even with warm and empathic handling. Bad parenting in this phase is thus neither a necessary nor a sufficient precondition of the borderline state. Denial and splitting, on the other hand, are part and parcel of all borderline pathology, by definition. Whatever factors contribute to these abnormal mechanisms constitute the "sufficient" causes. *Other* patterns, as well as poor handling of separation, are to be found in the histories of various borderline patients, some of which were indicated in this chapter.

Steingart, I. (1983). *Pathological play in borderline and narcissistic personalities*. New York: SP
    Medical Books/Spectrum Publications.
Stone, M. H. (1980). *The borderline syndromes*. New York: McGraw-Hill.
Stone, M. H. (1984). Critical and unresolved issues of borderline personality. *Integrative
    Psychiatry, 2*, 177–188.
Winnicott, D. W. (1965). *The maturational processes and the facilitating environment*. New York:
    International Universities Press.

14

Denial in the Development
of Homosexual Men

Richard C. Friedman

INTRODUCTION: ON SEX AND IDENTITY

In this chapter I discuss the role of denial in the development of homosexual men, a population different from others commented on in this book. Ideas about homosexuality have changed radically in recent years, both in the psychoanalytic community and the general public. In order to understand the psychodynamics of homosexual men, we must study the role of denial in their lives. Such a study may be taken as an example of the general importance of denial in psychological functioning.

In order to appreciate the importance of denial in the development of homosexual men, I must first present a brief overview of the relationship between erotic fantasy and activity and of the sense of identity in males. In this chapter, male sexual orientation is conceptualized as being a dimension of the psychology of boys and men. The discussion of homosexuality and heterosexuality that follows should not taken to apply to females unless specifically indicated. This qualification is necessary in light of extensive sex differences in psychological development known to exist (Friedman, Richart, & Vandewiele, 1974, MacCoby & Jacklin, 1974).

In the psychoanalytic, general scientific, and lay literature on homo-

Richard C. Friedman • Private Practice, 225 Central Park West, New York, New York 10024.

sexuality there is substantial variability with regard to the meaning of key terms. There is no accepted definition of the term *homosexuality* that has been used across studies. (Panel, 1983). The word *homosexuality* can refer to conscious erotic feelings and fantasies, unconscious erotic fantasies, sexual activity with others, or the sense of identity and social role. In this article, the terms *erotic fantasy* and *sexual fantasy* are used synonomously to denote consciously experienced phenomena. Erotic feelings are assumed to be associated with physiological changes involving the whole organism (Masters & Johnson, 1966). The limitations of space make it impossible to discuss fully the complex area of unconscious homosexuality. In *The Problem of Ego Identity* (1959), Erik Erikson discussed the conscious and unconscious meanings of identity, and I have adopted his use of the term. *Social role* simply means the public advertisement that one belongs to a specified social group. In light of the widespread modern recognition that "homosexuality" refers to multidimensional aspects of behavior, I have elected not to define it in this article. The meaning of the term *homosexuality* will depend upon its context. It is, however, particularly important to the clinician that we discuss the relationship between erotic fantasy and activity and identity and social role.

The importance of the relationship between *erotic experience* and cognitive social phenomena (i.e., identity/social role) requires particular emphasis at this time in the light of the enormous influence of Kinsey's formulations in the field of human sexual behavior. Kinsey, Pomeroy, and Martin (1983) stressed that people should *not* be described as *being* homosexual or heterosexual. "We have objected to the use of the terms heterosexual and homosexual when used as nouns which stand for individuals" (p. 657). Kinsey described erotic experience and activity along a 7-point scale. He reported that a large group of men was exclusively heterosexual, a large group bisexual to some degree, and a small group exclusively homosexual. Kinsey *et al.* (1948) stated the following:

> Males do not represent two populations heterosexual and homosexual. The world is not to be divided into sheep and goats. Not all things are black nor all things white. It is a fundamental of taxonomy that nature rarely deals with discrete categories. Only the human mind invents categories and tries to force facts into separated pigeon holes. The living world is a continuum in each and every one of its aspects. The sooner we learn this concerning human sexual behavior, the sooner we shall reach a sound understanding of the realities of sex. (p. 639)

It has subsequently been generally accepted that the *erotic dimensions* of sexual orientation do indeed lend themselves to meaningful description according to Kinsey's elegant notational system.

The furor that was associated with the publication of the benchmark

Kinsey volumes (1948, 1953) was in good measure due to the fact that the Kinsey Scale made it more practical to collect and summarize large numbers of sexual histories than had previously been the case. This led to data that were at variance with prevailing myth–belief systems about human sexual behavior. The denial mechanisms of many people were stressed by the realization that, contrary to popular belief, an enormous number of men were found to have experienced homosexual fantasies and/or engaged in homosexual activities. Dissemination of these results may have somewhat countered widespread discrimination against openly homosexual individuals because it made it more difficult to conceptualize them as belonging to an eccentric "outgroup" fundamentally different from other people. The results of the Kinsey investigations indicated that most people who experienced homosexual fantasies or engaged in homosexual activity really were part of the mainstream of society, differing only in degree but not in "kind" from a very large number of other people.

Kinsey's emphasis on erotic experience and activity, rather than identity/social role, limits the use of this scale to describe sexual orientation. Systematic description of the history of the relationship between erotic fantasy/activity and identity/social role must supplement data pertaining to erotic experience. Thus individuals who sort themselves into subgroups on the basis of sexual orientation (gay, straight, bisexual) often have sexual histories that are incongruent with the stated identity/role. Many gay men have experienced heterosexual fantasies and engaged in heterosexual activity, and many heterosexuals have experienced homosexual fantasies and engaged in homosexual activity (Friedman, 1974). Research comparing gay men to heterosexual "straight" men may be confounded by overlap in history of erotic experience/activity between groups, if assignment to research cells is simply made on the basis of self-assessment as gay or straight. This phenomenon is sometimes due to denial of the significance of erotic experiences that are incongruent with a person's identity and group affiliation. In many instances, men who would actually be described as bisexual in fantasy and activity (i.e., 2–5 on the Kinsey Scale) label themselves as gay or heterosexual/straight but not bisexual.

Although erotic experience and activity may be conceptualized along a continuum, labeling individuals as gay or straight involves assignment to categories, just as we do when labeling as male or female. It is largely because of the complex determinants of identity/social role that human sexual behavior has no adequate model among lower animal species. Many people apparently seem to *feel* like "sheep or goats" even though Kinsey apparently thought that they should not.

In an effort to simplify this difficult conceptual problem, some sex researchers have discussed homosexuality and heterosexuality as if these terms represented equivalent psychological constructs differing only with regard to the type of sexual object associated with or triggering the psychophysiological changes of the sexual response cycle. This minimizes, *denies* if you will, the difference in *meaning* of homosexual and heterosexual imagery and the importance of that difference to a wide range of people. In evaluating clinical dimensions of homosexuality, it is necessary for us to recognize that the unconscious meanings of homosexual and heterosexual imagery differ not only in psychopathology but also in broad areas of nonpathological human psychological functioning.

In Western industrialized society, heterosexual identity is the cultural norm and is assumed to be present unless there are specific indications to the contrary. When a stranger is introduced, it is generally assumed that he is heterosexual even though his sexual orientation is not noted in the introduction.

In discussing the social-psychological differences between homosexual and heterosexual social roles, I have commented elsewhere as follows:

> The gay person, like the heterosexual "straight" person experiences "being gay" as a cognitive-social phenomenon, not a sexual phenomenon. The strangers to whom the gay person is introduced however, are forced to attend to his *sexual* behavior *at the moment of introduction*. Direction of attention towards a stranger's inner sexual life leads to direction of attention towards one's own. Given the way the human mind works, focus is directed at imagistic concrete experience (the fantasy of the stranger engaged in sexual activity). The gay social role therefore functions in a manner analogous to undressing. The introductory situation itself becomes sexualized, thereby violating a social taboo. This distinction between heterosexual and homosexual social roles is important both with regard to the determinants of identity in the individual, and the response to the individual by the social unit. Irrational anxiety may occur in individuals who are threatened by their own homosexual impulses, but also in anyone whose aggressive and sexual feelings are barely repressed. Every potentially homosexual individual must take this into account in deciding whether to advertise or hide his homosexual identity. (Friedman, 1988:87)

CLINICAL AND DEVELOPMENTAL ISSUES

In the DSM-III-R, homosexuality is not considered a mental disorder. This is due to the fact that, in adulthood, homosexuality is not necessarily associated with distress, social or vocational impairment, impairment in vital psychological functions such as the capacity to love, care, play; or indeed in impairment in any psychological functions at all. The primary behavioral difference between lifelong exclusively homosexual and heterosexual men may be limited to sexual orientation itself. I have described a vignette of a highly integrated gay man as follows: (The term *sex print* in the quotation refers to consciously experienced stable erotic fantasies that are analogous to a fingerprint).

> This 40-year-old engineer, with homosexual sex print and identity, was seen in a research and educational context. He had never experienced an erection in association with a consciously perceived heterosexual fantasy, nor could he recall ever having heterosexual dreams. Homosexual dreams, with orgasm, had occurred from time to time during his life. From mid-adolescence to young adulthood, this person dated girls, hoping to become sexually aroused by them. Sexual activity was attempted a few times, but never could proceed because of an absence of a feeling of sexual desire or any of the changes of the sexual response cycle. This man's sex print emerged prepubertally, years before he knew what a homosexual was. His first sexual activity with another person occurred during young adulthood, more or less coincident with the recognition that he "must" be homosexual. Some people in this person's interpersonal network knew of his homosexuality, some did not, depending on his assessment of their attitudes and values. He had regular sexual activity with a few different partners, but never exhibited "cruising," nor did he visit any bars, or baths. He did not belong to a gay organization. As an adult, this man had a stable, productive work history. He had loyal, caring, durable friendships with men and women, and found pleasure in many aspects of his life. He had demonstrated the capacity for appropriate grief, and appropriate feelings of depression during his life. (Friedman, 1986, p. 66)

Recent research in the area of sexual orientation has demonstrated that just as men at opposite poles of the homosexuality–heterosexuality spectrum may be similar with respect to healthy ego functioning, they may also be similar with respect to severity of psychopathology.

Parallel types of psychopathology occur in men at different points on the Kinsey spectrum, but whose ego mechanisms operate at roughly the same levels. Thus a person may be exclusively homosexual, or heterosexual in activity and experience, or bisexual and also suffer from a psychotic disorder, character neurosis, borderline syndromes, and so forth. The data presently available indicate that neither a specific personality type (i.e., obsessive, schizoid, etc.) nor level of character structure organization (i.e. borderline) is found more commonly along one point on the Kinsey Scale than along another. Clinical situations require therapists to evaluate homosexual phenomena in their patients in a multidimensional manner.

A conceptual framework for describing sexual orientation in adults that I have found helpful involves description of three parameters of personality functioning: Kinsey Scale Number, Personality Type (i.e., obsessive, schizoid, etc.), Level of Character Structure Integration (neu-rotic-borderline, etc.). This model was borrowed from Stone's well-known diagnosis cube for describing borderline pathology (1980). Stone suggested that character pathology can be described according to a cuboidal model in which one axis depicted personality type, one axis level of character structure integration, and one axis predisposition to affective disorders or schizophrenia. I have modified Stone's model by replacing the third axis with history of erotic fantasy and activity: the Kinsey Scale number (Friedman, 1988).

Before moving on to discuss psychological development, it should be noted that there *is* one difference in psychopathology between groups of men who are predominately homosexual and predominately homosexual. If one restricts the comparison to men with severely compromised ego functioning (borderline and psychotic men), then gender identity disturbances occur more frequently in the predominately homosexual group (Bieber *et al.*, 1962). Although predominately homosexual men are not more likely to be borderline or psychotic, those who are globally impaired are more likely to have Gender Identity/Role Disorders.

FURTHER DEVELOPMENTAL CONSIDERATIONS: THE ROLE OF DENIAL

It is clear from the preceding brief overview that there are many varieties or subgroups of homosexuality. In trying to adopt a reasonable conceptual model for psychopathology, it is important not to condense the different behavioral components that together constitute the entity "homosexuality" in a particular individual. This becomes dramatically illustrated when one adopts a developmental view about sexual phenomena.

The sense of identity normally consolidates during late adolescence (Erikson, 1959). This is not the case with regard to erotic fantasies. In most men, the fundamental aspects of erotic fantasy begin during child-hood and remain unaltered for life. This is obviously not the case for *all* men. Some people do experience meaningful and lasting change in erotic fantasy during adulthood, sometimes in response to life stress, or to psychoanalysis, or for reasons that are not well understood at this time. The determinants of postpubertal plasticity in erotic fantasy are not known. In my view, men with this type of plasticity are much less common than those for whom erotic fantasies function as stable traits (Panel, 1983).

Regardless of sexual orientation, childhood erotic fantasies often precede the first orgasm, by months to years. The first orgasm most commonly occurs as the result of self-masturbation. When erotic fantasies are homosexual, they are likely occur to individuals who have never met a gay person and who know little (if anything) about homosexuality (Friedman, 1974; Friedman & Stern, 1980).

Although aspects of the sexual histories of predominately homosexual and heterosexual men are similar, homosexual and heterosexual fantasies affect psychological development in quite different ways (as might be expected). To illustrate this, I describe next a developmental track that commonly occurs among males with lifelong predominant or exclusive homoerotic fantasies and/or activity. The fantasies often begin during Oedipal years and possibly even earlier. The child who experiences homoerotic fantasies tends to be secretive about them. They are often disavowed and not acknowledged as being part of the self-system. With the androgen surge of puberty, lustful feelings become more intense and are often accompanied by guilt and shame. This type of early and midadolescent continues to believe that he is on a developmental path leading to heterosexuality, marriage, fatherhood, despite the experience of constant homoerotic fantasies. As he gets older the disparity between his own erotic inner life and his heterosexual role behavior becomes more of a source of concern. With progressive worry, he engages in heterosexual role behavior (such as dating girls) often with the hope that heterosexual fantasies will emerge. This hope is futile; heteroerotic fantasies are never experienced.

The homoerotic fantasies are disavowed. The significance of these fantasies for the sense of ego identity is denied. Many such men marry and are able to function heterosexually to the degree that they can father children. Heterosexual activity, however, is experienced as unnatural and alien. This is so despite the consciously experienced wish to "become" heterosexual. In midlife, a number of men with this type of developmental profile give up their denial of homosexuality and become openly gay. The reasons for this are several. Often awareness of the durability of the homosexual sex print coincides with the full recognition of one's mortality and the limitations of ambition that come with middle age. In any case, surrender of the defensive stance of denial/disavowal is sometimes associated with a sense of anguish. Optimally, this is followed by a feeling of pride at living up to the ideal of honest self-expression if the movement from heterosexual to gay identity/social role occurs in a healthy, adaptive fashion.

Enough data have been accumulated by now to suggest a biopsychosocial spectrum model for the factors influencing the development of homosexual fantasies. Biological predisposition toward homosexuality is hypothesized to be strong in one subgroup characterized by the specific influence of deficient hypothalamic exposure to androgen during a critical prenatal phase. (Dorner, Rohde, Stahl, Krell, & Wolf-Gunther, 1975) The most recent empirical support for this theory was published by Gladue, Green, and Helman (1984). These investigators observed that homosexual males showed a luteinizing hormone response to Premarin infusion midway between that of heterosexual men and women. In other subroups (Friedman, 1983), direct biological factors are hypothesized not to be important when contrasted with traditionally postulated psychodynamic development factors (Fenichel, 1945). Both sets of influences might operate in some people, in sequences yet to be determined.

Early in development, during the years that the boy experiences exclusively homosexual fantasies, denial operates in many ways. Intense rigid denial often allows the parents, as well as their son, to preserve a pseudonormal facade in a family with significant difficulties. A common clinical configuration involving denial in all family members is illustrated in the following vignette:

A 55-year-old construction worker and his wife, a 50-year-old secretary, had one child, a son of 18. The initial designated patient in this family was the mother, who sought consultation for depression when the father lost his job. On initial interview, the mother described her family as entirely "normal." Initially the father and son also stressed both their own normality and that of the entire family. Follow-up interviewing, however, revealed that the parents' marriage was full of strife. Each person had long given up hope of intimacy with the other. Each related to the other with hostility, criticism, detachment, and vindictiveness. The father had established a pattern of going to a local pub after work only to come home after his son was asleep. His wife would watch television most evenings, turning to the son for companionship. She would often take him with her when she shopped for the families supplies; often he cooked dinner when she was fatigued. The son was temperamentally closer to his mother than his father. He shared her interests in reading and music and hated his father's favorite activities—bowling and woodworking. This son had exclusively homosexual fantasies since age 5. He had become sexually active with others at puberty and had a number of relationships with lovers. Not only was his homosexuality unknown to his parents, but he himself believed that he was (as he put it) "basically heterosexual" despite never having experienced an erection to a heterosexual stimulus. This young man "assumed" that later in his development when it came time to marry, he would "naturally" become sexually interested in women. The likelihood of this actually happening of course was slim. In this family system, the father appeared often to displace hostility from his wife to his son. He would criticize aspects of his son's behavior that he labeled sissylike. The mother appeared to turn to her son for the emotional intimacy that she was unable to experience with her husband. The parents had not engaged in sexual activity with each other for years and attributed the reason for this to their age (another example of denial).

In presenting this vignette, I have intentionally selected a boy and his family as they presented clinically. This type of family situation has long been familiar to clinical investigators (Bieber *et al.*, 1962; West, 1959). Here the boy denies the significance of his erotic fantasies for his evolving self-concept. Global denial of marital dissatisfaction is also often present among caretakers in such families as is often noted when a son has symptoms of gender identity disturbance (Bieber *et al.*, 1962; Saghir & Robins, 1973), symptoms denied by his parents and reenforced in various ways.

A few points about the consequences of denial in the type of family system described previously deserve emphasis:

1. Researchers should not take the initial, manifest judgments (of family members) about various issues as being literally true. Responses to questions about intimacy, caring, sexual experience are likely to change as denial is interpreted in interview situations.
2. Triangulated families such as this are extremely common among homosexual *patients*. In this large group, a certain type of history occurs with great frequency. Typically, a boy with gender disturbance is estranged from his father and emotionally allied with his mother in the family system. (Often this pattern extends to siblings as well. The boy is distant from bothers and close to sisters).
3. This type of family system should not be taken as representative of all predominately or exclusively homosexual men, however (Siegelman, 1974, 1981). Many gay men, with high-level psychological functioning, never consult psychoanalysts. Relatively little is known about their background, and much more data are needed before valid generalizations can be made about this population.
4. Finally, secretiveness about homosexuality should not be confused with denial. Secretiveness is often adaptive because the cultural and familial climate in which gay men live is frequently homophobic. Communication to others about homosexual activity might lead not only to rejection but to outright persecution.

In the case presented before, an 18-year-old boy assumed that he was really heterosexual despite the fact that his fantasies and activities were exclusively homosexual for years. This type of history is common. Many of these young men go on to develop a stable sense of homosexual identity later in life. Many, however, internalize negative attitudes and values from the general culture and are consumed with self-hate because of their sexual orientation (Leavy, 1983). Here denial is also at work. The men deny the possibility of being masculine and worthwhile because of homosexual fantasies. Therapy is often difficult because of the many years that these patients have been exposed to devaluation of homosexuality by revered authority figures including teachers, clergy, and parents.

As I noted before, much needs to be learned about the backgrounds of homosexual men with normal or superior general psychological functioning. It should be noted, however, that not even all boys with gender-identity disorders and pathological family situations grow up to become neurotic, psychotic, or borderline men. Rather, they seem to become men who are distributed across a wide spectrum of functioning from the extremely pathological on one hand to superior on the other. The determinants that lead some of these men to *retain* childhood pathology and others to leave it behind require further study.

CONCLUSION

It is becoming increasingly appreciated by the analytic community that there are many subgroups of homosexuality. This fact in itself is sometimes denied, probably because of our own countertransference difficulties. Whereas homosexual phenomena appear to function as symptoms in some subgroups of patients, this is not always the case. At some point in their development, for reasons that are also not well understood to date, homosexual fantasies that are virtually exclusive may become a fixed, irreversible part of the mental apparatus. The significance of this irreversibility may be denied both by patients and by analytic consultants. As Isay (1985) has observed, when working with such individuals, analysts should maintain an empathic neutral posture and should not adopt an open stance favoring heterosexuality.

We psychoanalysts have little actual knowledge about human sexual behavior, despite assertions to the contrary (often manifestations of our own denial systems). Remaining open are fundamental questions about the effect of psychoanalysis on the consciously perceived sexual fantasy life of individuals at various points on the Kinsey Scale and at different levels of character integration. Much more information is needed in the key area of the effect of psychotherapy and psychoanalysis on the sexual fantasy life of adolescents and preadolescents, particularly those with gender-identity disorders. We must ascertain the point in life when sex-

ual fantasy becomes truly fixed. The contemporary psychoanalyst is required to maintain the capacity *not* to deny and to tolerate ambiguity
stemming from questions yet unanswered, all while maintaining an appropriate psychoanalytic posture. The attitude of openness is the best
antidote to denial.

REFERENCES

Bieber, I. *et al.* (1962). *Homosexuality: A psychoanalytic study of male homosexuals.* New York: Basic Books.

Dorner, G., Rohde, W., Stahl, F., Krell, C., & Wolf-Gunther, M. (1975). A neuroendocrine predisposition for homosexuality in men. *Archives of Sexual Behavior, 4,* 1–8.

Erikson, E. H. (1959). The problem of ego identity. In *Identity and the life cycle: Psychological Issues* (Vol. 1,1, pp. 101–164). New York: International Universities Press.

Fenichel, O. (1945). *The psychoanalytic theory of neurosis.* New York: W. W. Norton.

Friedman, R. C. (1974). Male homosexuality. Chapter in *The electronic textbook of psychiatry and neurology.* New York: New York State Psychiatric Institute.

Friedman, R. C. (1986). Male homosexuality: On the need for a multiaxial developmental model. *Israel Journal of Psychiatry and Related Sciences, 23*(1), pp. 63–76.

Friedman, R. C. (1988). *Male homosexuality: A contemporary psychoanalytic perspective.* New Haven: Yale University Press.

Friedman, R. C., & Stern, L. O. (1980). Juvenile aggressivity and sissiness in homosexual and heterosexual males. *Journal of the American Academy of Psychoanalysis, 8*(3), 427–440.

Friedman, R. C., Richart, R. M., & Vandewiele, R. L. V. (Eds.). (1974). *Sex differences in behavior.* New York: Wiley.

Gladue, B. A., Green, R., & Hellman, R. E. (1984). Neuroendocrine response to estrogen and sexual orientation. *Science, 225,* pp. 1496–1499.

Isay, R. (1985). On the analytic therapy of homosexual men. [Presented at panel entitled Toward a further understanding of homosexual men. American Psychoanalytic Assoc., New York, 1983.] *The Psychoanalytic Study of the Child, 40,* 235–255.

Kinsey, A. C., Pomeroy, W. B., & Martin, C. E. (1948). *Sexual behavior in the human male.* Philadelphia and London: Saunders.

Kinsey, A. C., Pomeroy, W. B., Martin, C. E., & Gebhard, P. H. (1953). *Sexual behavior in the human female.* Philadelphia: Saunders.

MacCoby, E. E., & Jacklin, C. N. (1974). *The psychology of sex differences.* Stanford: Stanford University Press.

Masters, W. H., & Johnson, V. E. (1966). *Human sexual response.* Boston: Little, Brown.

Panel (1983). Toward a further understanding of homosexual men. R. C. Friedman, reporter. Presented at Winter Meetings of American Psychoanalytic Association, New York. Summary published in *Journal of the American Psychoanalytic Association,* 1986, *34,* 193–206.

Saghir, M. T., & Robins, E. (1973). *Male and female homosexuality.* Baltimore: Williams & Wilkins.

Siegelman, M. (1974). Parental backgrounds of male homosexuals and heterosexuals. *Archives of Sexual Behavior, 3*(1), 3–19.

Siegelman, M. (1981). Parental backgrounds of homosexual and heterosexual men: A cross-national replication. *Archives of Sex Behaviors, 10*(6), 505–512.

Stone, M. H. (1980). *The borderline syndromes.* New York: McGraw-Hill.

West, D. J. (1959). Parental relationships in male homosexuality. *International Journal of Social Psychiatry, 5,* 85–97.

15

Denial as a Central Coping Mechanism in Counterhypochondriasis

HERMAN MUSAPH

Patterns of illness, influenced by ideologies, by culture, and by the fashions of an era create for us a world of constant change. In a children-oriented society, elderly people try to dress youthfully. In a military-oriented society, people care more for body building. I should like to draw the attention of the reader to a group of perimenopausal women seen in my private practice of psychotherapy and in the outpatient Department of Medical Sexology of the Academic Hospital in Utrecht.

Complaints associated with the perimenopause are to a great extent dependent on the cultural pattern that colors the perception of menopause. Moaz, Antonovsky, Wijsenbeek, and Datan (1977) and Datan, Antonovsky, and Moaz (1981) studied differences in adaptation to the climacterium of several ethnic groups in Israel. Notwithstanding the success of the international women's movement in improving the self-esteem and the real living situation of women, goals certainly egosyntonic with those of psychoanalysis, one must recognize some unfortunate "side effects" of this period of change. Although many of the uncomfortable symptoms of the menopause can be reduced in severity by hor-

HERMAN MUSAPH • Private Practice, C. van Rennesstraat 30, 1077 KX Amsterdam, The Netherlands.

monal treatment and although most women seem quite able to manage their lives with or without treatment, there exists a sizable group of women who deny entirely the existence of the climacterium and its associated symptomatology. In my clinical experience, these women are frequently married to men who are themselves intolerant of illness, and whose expectations of their wives do not take into account normal physiological changes accompanying aging. Linn (1977) has described a group of families in which the need for independence on the part of the wives is seen as complementary to such illness intolerance on the part of the husbands; thus both the illness intolerance and the need for independence are supported by the extensive use of denial in the family system.

In the cases I have followed, it seems as if the most important determinant of perimenopausal symptomatology is a woman's understanding of her mother's experience of this phase of life. If a mother feels that perimenopausal symptoms are normal and thus complains little, 35 years later her daughter (by a process of social learning and perhaps identification) will accept her own symptoms as normal.

So much may the natural path of aging be denied by some women that the denial itself fits into the pattern I described elsewhere in "The Negative Illness of Not Being Able to Fall Ill: Counterhypochondriasis" (Musaph, 1979). There are people who never allow themselves to fall ill. They distort their own symptoms much as will the hypochondriac (Lipsitt, 1974) but in a manner that precludes disclosure, rather than amplification of symptoms. These women will hardly notice bodily changes normal to the aging process, while protecting their fragile sense of self by the purchase of clothing and cosmetics characteristic of younger women. The vasomotor instability known as "flushes" or "hot flashes" is interpreted as an expression of fatigue; the general picture presented by these patients is one of "pathological health." We know little about the psychological roots, the infantile and early childhood experiences that determine the predisposition to pathological health, which I suspect may be an expression of identification with a key figure who, during a childhood disease, precipitated an emotional conflict and later counterhypochondriasis. In the passages that follow, I will attempt to sketch some of the reasons patients may wish to defend against the experience of symptoms.

THE SYMPTOM AS NARCISSISTIC INJURY

Patients who view the symptom as narcissistic injury ward off illness simply by devaluing and denying anything that might be perceived as a complaint. In our achievement-oriented society, many people cannot allow themselves to be ill, for they are afraid to lose ground in what they experience as global competition with others. To some women, this competition is joined at the level of the battle of the sexes, where having symptoms means to be inferior to their male partner in family or work settings, to be counted out, to be a loser. Although some people may utilize this defensive strategy as a spur to great achievement, rarely does it assist in the formation of a stable interpersonal relationship.

PERIMENOPAUSAL SYMPTOMS AS A HARBINGER OF PASSIVITY

Some very active women fear that illness may force them to renounce an energetic way of life and thus place at risk their self-esteem, self-confidence, and their entire psychic balance. Fear of passivity may be connected with the experience of sexuality, which is interpreted in the language of male dominance and female submissiveness. Passivity may also represent loss of control as when the ego is overwhelmed by emotion; such women may resist the loss of control inherent in orgasm. Where anger, hatred, vengefulness, sorrow, rage, or anxiety are modulated only by the superego, falling ill becomes a metaphor for loss of control—a metaphor that extends into the areas controlled only by the superego. Thus the perimenopause, with its normal concommitant of physiological symptoms, is considered as an illness that threatens the woman with decompensation and the fear of madness.

ILLNESS IMPLIES THE RISK OF DEATH

Death carries for each of us a wealth of meaning (Freud, 1913), for the aging process forces confrontation with loss. Contemporaneous with the perimenopause are such events as the death of parents, uncles, aunts, and the older relatives of our friends. Indeed, the departure of children from the home may be experienced as loss, often called "the empty nest syndrome," which itself is an indicator of the passage of time and therefore a sign of personal aging. So the perimenopausal period often is one of mourning, and the symptoms associated with it can trigger awareness of these other losses and deaths. Each and every physical complaint, whatever its nature, is experienced as a violation of the shield provided by denial.

ILLNESS IS SHAMEFUL, HEALTH IS PROUD

Pathological health offers an opportunity to be superior to sick people, who are rejected and condemned. In some families, such wellness allows the "healthy" member to maintain dominance, even tyranny over all others. To be sick in such a family means to risk attack and failure. Often we see physicians who refuse to acknowledge the presence of illness in any member of their families, who by counterhypochondriasis neglect every physical symptom of wife and children. One patient, whose mother tyrannized her family with rages and sulks that she attributed to hot flashes, developed a reaction formation to this behavior in the form of pathological health. In this case, as in so many others, counterhypochondriasis functions as an expression of unconscious aggressive feelings in an ambivalent conflict situation toward beloved and hated members of the family.

ILLNESS AS THE EXPRESSION OF DENIED MOURNING

There are people for whom falling ill has the specific function of commemorating an anniversary. Instead of lighting a candle or reciting a prayer to the memory of the beloved, these patients become sick each year on the anniversary of their loss; this illness is best treated as an homage to the deceased. Some fall ill on their wedding anniversary or on the occasion of the wedding of a child (Musaph, 1973). One root of the anniversary reaction is an undigested emotional conflict situation in which an ambivalence conflict, mainly in the aggressive sphere, plays a crucial role. One has to atone through this reaction for aggressive, mostly unconscious drives toward a key figure who must be commemorated. In this way, one tries to solve an unbearable conflict through symptom formation.

There are patients who, each year, fall ill in the period of commemorating the victims of the war—clearly a manifestation of survivor guilt—but only for a day or so. Most of the time, the true meaning of such illnesses is immediately apparent when the patient comes to the doctor for evaluation; the defense by denial and medical symptom formation is so successful that the patient rarely makes the diagnosis unaided.

CONCLUSION

In 1925, Freud gave a splendid example of Abweisung by projection in his paper called "Die Verneinung."

"Der Patient: Sie fragen wer diese Person im Traum sein kann. Die Mutter ist
es *nicht.*"

"Freud: Also ist is die Mutter." (p. 11)

[The patient: You are asking who may be this person in the dream. It is not
the mother.

Freud: Therefore, it is the mother.]

In the language of Melanie Klein (1948), this would be called
scotomization. "One of the earliest methods of defense against the threat
of persecutors, whether conceived of as existing in the external world or
internalized, is that of scotomization, the denial of psychic reality." In
this chapter, I have tried to emphasize the important meaning of the
defense mechanism of denial in the working relationship between doctor and patient, as well as its significance in the lives of perimenopausal
women.

In the Talmud, Berachot 45, it is written that

כְּשֵׁם שֶׁמַּפְתֵּחַ לַבַּיִת כָּן מַפְתֵּחַ לְאִשָׁה ·

—"Just as there is a key to a house, there is a key to every woman."
Denial is a ubiquitous defense; yet understanding its particular role in
the life of the perimenopausal woman can provide a key of wondrous
utility and wide general application.

REFERENCES

Datan, N., Antonovsky, A., & Maoz, B. (1981). *A time to reap. The middle age of women in five Israeli subcultures.* Baltimore: Johns Hopkins University Press.

Freud, S. (1913), Trauer und Melancholie. *Gesammelte Bande,* X, pp. 428–446. London: Hogarth.

Freud, S. (1925). Die Verneinung. *Gesammelte Bande,* XIV, pp. 11–15. London: Hogarth.

Keep, van, P. A., & Kellerhals, J. (1974). The impact of sociocultural factors on symptom formation. In H. Musaph, (Ed.), *Mechanisms in Symptom Formation* (pp. 253–261). Basel: Karger.

Klein, M. (1948). *Contributions to psycho-analysis 1921–1945.* London: Hogarth Press.

Linn, L. (1977). Basic principles of management in psychosomatic medicine. In E. Witt-kower & H. Warnes (Eds.), *Psychosomatic medicine. Its clinical applications* (pp. 2–14). New York: Harper & Row.

Lipsitt, D. R. (1974). Psychosomatic considerations of hypochondriasis. In H. Musaph (Ed.). *Mechanisms in symptom formation* (pp. 132–138). Basel: Karger.

Maoz, B., Antonovsky, A., Wijsenbeek, H., & Datan, N. (1977). Ethnicity and adaptation to climacterium. *Archives für Gynekologie, 223,* 9–18.

Musaph, H. (1973). Anniversary disease. *Psychotherapy and Psychosomatics, 22,* 325–333.

Musaph, H. (1979). The trigger function of the menopause. In H. Musaph & A. A. Haspels (Eds.), *Psychosomatics in perimenopause* (pp. 83–100). Lancaster: M.T.P. Press.

16

Beyond Denial
Replacement Fantasies in Patients with Life-Threatening Illness

LEA BAIDER AND E. L. EDELSTEIN

INTRODUCTION

During the past decade, research on the psychological aspects of cancer has produced some challenging ways of understanding the mechanisms by which patients may adapt to their illness, coping mechansms that may influence the process of survival (Greer & McEwan, 1985; Weisman, 1979; Wortman & Schetter, 1979).

The wide range of psychological and psychiatric reactions to the diagnosis of cancer, including denial, anger, depression, and anxiety has been described by many. In a recent collaborative study of the prevalence of psychiatric disorders among cancer patients, 47% of the subjects were found to have symptom complexes warranting a DSM-III diagnosis. Of these, 68% consisted of adjustment disorders, 13% of major depression, 8% organic mental disorder, 7% personality disorders, and 4% anxiety disorders (Derogatis, Morrow, Fetting *et al.*, 1983). Several investigators have proposed that certain psychological factors seem most

LEA BAIDER • Department of Clinical Oncology and Radiology, Hadassah University Hospital, Ein Karen, Jerusalem, Israel. E. L. EDELSTEIN • Department of Psychiatry, Hadassah University Hospital, Ein Karen, Jerusalem, Israel.

often to be associated with psychiatric problems. Prominent among these are the psychological meaning of cancer to the patient and concerns about the future. It may be especially important to consider psychological factors when evaluating the cancer patient because at any assessment, 50% of their emotional distress can be attributed to nonmedical causes (Goldberg, 1983; Holland *et al.*, 1986; Weisman & Worden, 1972–1976).

This chapter is an attempt to describe the phenomenology of the defense mechanism of denial in a group of seven cancer patients, and the way in which these patients went beyond our usual definition of denial to defend against the reality of their illness by a process of delusional thinking and/or sporadic hallucinations that we will define as an adaptive process. These patients, drawn from the oncology department of Hadassah University Hospital (see Table 1), all diagnosed as having malignant tumors and most with metastatic disease, had constructed for the specific experience of their illness a fantasized system of attributional meaning that gave an adaptive, gratifying meaning to their lives.

According to several authors (Pyszczynski & Greenberg, 1981; Taylor, 1983; Thompson, 1981), by understanding the causal attribution of a perplexing event, one may gain insight into its significance for one's life. Cancer patients develop theories about the causes of their disease from which they may infer beliefs about the extent to which it can be controlled, and by such control give meaning to their lives. Some of these perceptions and meanings are based on prevailing sociocultural stereotypes, and these are reinforced whenever such perceptions provide a source of internal gratification and/or a feeling of control. Spilka, Shaver, and Kirkpatrick (1985) explains that the attribution process is motivated by a need to perceive events in the world as meaningful; a need to predict or control events; or a need to protect, maintain, and enhance one's self-conception and self-esteem.

All attribution theories begin with the assumption that people seek to make sense of their experiences and to understand the causes of the events they witness (Kelly, 1967). Spilka *et al.* (1985) indicate that an event or experience has many possible and perhaps compatible causes, in which case the person's task is to choose among them and rank them in terms of personal importance or causal impact. If attributional processes are motivated by challenges to one's beliefs, sense of control, or self-esteem, the particular attribution selected should reflect its ability to restore these variables to satisfactory and gratifying levels.

The seven patients discussed here had exchanged the negative implications of their illness for a positive and meaningful conceptualization of their lives and a motivation for survival. Their distorted thought process seemed, at first, bizarre, dreamlike, and almost psychotic in

TABLE 1. Patients' Sociodemographic Data

Patient	Age	Sex	Marital status	Religiosity	Country of origin	Diagnosis	Treatments
1. K.	37	F	Married	Religious	Israel	Breast cancer (metastatic disease)	Surgery, chemotherapy, hormonal
2. A.	72	M	Married	Nonreligious	Germany	Rectal cancer colostomy, Dukes B.2.	Surgery, radiotherapy
3. T.	75	M	Married	Nonreligious	Germany	Lung cancer (Stage 2) (metastatic disease)	Surgery, chemotherapy
4. D.	22	M	Single	Nonreligious	Israel	Osteosarcoma	Surgery, chemotherapy
5. R.	42	F	Married	Religious	Iraq	Breast cancer	Surgery
6. B.	50	F	Married	Nonreligious	Austria	Ovary cancer (Stage 1)	Surgery, abdominal radiation
7. E.	26	M	Married	Religious	Turkey	Testicular teratocarcinoma (unilateral, Stage 2)	Surgery, chemotherapy

nature. Yet the distortion was encapsulated and integrated with a more or less normal role functioning, without disturbing the patients' sense of reality. The style and content of their delusions left an impression similar to that of a dream in its most primary process. From dreams, we return daily to reality, and it seemed as if these "daydreams" helped the patients to cope by providing an escape whenever necessary from their painful reality. These fantasies, as described by the patients, filled the void caused by the denial of the threatening reality of their illness. These mechanisms of attributional thought ranged from simple fantasies and delusional thoughts to visual hallucinations.

PATIENT CLINICAL DESCRIPTIONS

PATIENT 1: Ms. K.

Ms. K. was a 37-year-old Israeli woman raising one child in her second marriage. She was a high-school teacher of ancient history, with a strong religious sense and an extensive social and family support network. At age 35, 8 months pregnant, she underwent a radical mastectomy for Stage 2 breast cancer. She was in psychotherapy for a period of one month, which constituted her second and final relapse; the pain and suffering of extensive metastatic disease and pleural effusion were immediately apparent. She died soon after these sessions ceased.

The presence of the therapist was requested by the patient. She consistently tried to function in all her family roles without sharing her thoughts and fears with anyone. She always appeared very calm, composed, and extremely friendly. Feeling increasingly ill, Ms. K. began sharing what she called fantasized dreams, or imaginary daydreams in which her illness was given a coherent place within her life. She revealed that within her chest was the mythological figure of a child who blew clouds out of her lungs, cleaning them out and helping her to breath. She knew that nobody would believe such a description, that her mythological child could be seen as a product of her imagination or as a fairy tale, but she also knew that it could neither be proved nor disproved to her. She believed in what she felt, in what she described as the meaning of her illness and a source of her strength, and she was certain that through it, she could stay alive and be rescued. She felt safe and secure; she was not alone, and, merely by closing her eyes, she could feel and touch the clear breath coming from inside, from the strength of the child. She felt that she would not need this reinforcement for very long; that after being in control of her body and knowing that her lungs were totally clean, she would be able to continue a fulfilling way of life.

PATIENT 2: Mr. A.

Mr. A. was referred by one of our oncologists who suspected an underlying emotional conflict for his inconsistencies in keeping appointments for regular checkups. The initial visit was due more to the imposition of his wife's will than to his own decision. He entered the office alone, saying very politely to his wife that he did not need a guardian. During the next six sessions he was seen alone. Mr. A. was 72 years old, German born, and had been diagnosed as suffering from cancer of the colon for which, 2 years earlier, he had undergone a colostomy. After 46 years of a very happy marriage, his first wife had died of metastatic breast cancer 6 years before the appearance of his own malignancy. Since her death, the patient had complained of so much abdominal pain and discomfort that he was practically bedridden. A retired accountant, while at home he continued to indulge in what he called the hobbies of his life: gardening and stamp collecting. He believed that the only person who could help him was his dead wife, through their silent dialogue because only she knew his body well enough and their secrets and had shared all his illusions and frustrations. Mr. A. trusted the therapist and wanted to share things that he could discuss with no one else. He was a Holocaust survivor and felt the urgency of fulfilling an important mission in life, without having known the meaning of it until his severe illness. For months after his colon operation, he was preoccupied with his ability to distinguish the different smells of which no one else was aware. He felt totally cured of the cancer, but his illness had brought the most important meaning to his life and a new sense of life rather than a death sentence. His feces would be collected and used as fertilizer throughout the country, which would result in a more abundant and better quality crop production. This was his purpose and mission in his present life. He shared every detail of his fantasy, explaining how he controlled the use of his various fecal products. There were eight therapy sessions within a period of 3 months. During the last two sessions, he no longer talked about his fantasy. He only said that he had come to understand and to control his illness and that he had great hopes that he would be able to complete his mission before becoming too old.

PATIENT 3: MR. T.

Mr. T. was a 75-year-old artist who had survived the Holocaust and 2 years earlier immigrated to Israel from Argentina with his wife in order to dedicate his best creations to Israel. Once in Israel, Mr. T. received an invitation to participate in the Biennial Art Festival in Venice. However, after his arrival in Israel, he became ill, suffering from weakness, loss of appetite and fatigue, and was later diagnosed as having lung cancer. He was operated on and treated with chemotherapy and died about a year and a half after his surgery.

He was referred by his oncologist, who was surprised that the patient did not seem at all concerned about his health and refused all diagnostic radiology. He was seen for nine psychotherapy sessions during a period of several months. That his therapist spoke Spanish, was familiar with his work, and could understand other things he had suffered in his past produced an immediate positive transference. He said that he wanted to explain something that had been given to him as a unique miracle: what he called "universal grace." He did not know what form this "grace" would take, but he had realized its presence and meaning after his operation. The revelation of God was obvious and clear, and he could talk about his secret only within the therapeutic relationship. All his life he had wanted to paint the most perfect piece of art, something that would explicate life with absolute harmony and precision. It would be something that people would look at and through which they might appreciate the total integration of life. He said that his fingers had started painting without the need for external paints and colors; paints had traveled to the tips of his fingers from his lungs in unique color combinations. He knew that the operation had to have a meaning and that chemotherapy by intravenous administration was stimulating further the creation of these colors. He needed only a certain period of time to complete this work: the work of his life. He was partly concerned that he was "cheating" by not using "real" colors but justified it by explaining the need and temporary nature of this unique revelation. He knew that, after this creation was completed, he would return to painting in his traditional and habitual way and that this finger-painting episode would remain only as an internal symbol of fortitude, strength, and the conquest of life over death.

During the sixth session, he confided that the work was ready and prepared to be sent to Venice. He never mentioned this or any of his other fantasies again. After his death, his wife disclosed that for months before, he would shut himself in his studio, and while he was not actually painting, he believed himself to be creating his masterpiece and would come out in the evening exhausted, as if after strenuous work.

PATIENT 4: MR. D.

Mr. D. was a 22-year-old Israeli dancer with a diagnosis of osteosarcoma. His left leg was amputated above the knee, after which he had received chemotherapy according to several different protocols. He was without evidence of disease for about 1 year, but this period of hope was followed by several relapses and subsequent periods free from disease. He was referred by an oncologist because of a negative attitude toward treatment, and his mother's interference. He was the only child of a widowed mother; his father had been killed in the 1967 war. Mr. D. was seen for 10 sessions while hospitalized during his first relapse. During the first several sessions he ignored the therapist entirely. During the fourth session he began talking, but asked that these conversations remain confidential. He was concerned neither about his illness nor about the amputation, saying that it had been done specifically to readjust the shape of his leg. Even before his illness, he had suffered weakness and pain in his left leg. His new implanted leg was in reality his own natural leg, only stronger and more beautiful in comparison, and would benefit his dancing by allowing him to perform better. He wanted to surprise his mother, a ballet instructor, by being the best dancer with this new leg. He wanted to accomplish his best performance so that he would be remembered forever as a great dancer. He hated his hospital room because he did not have the space and the privacy he needed to rehearse.

His illness was the justification for getting the new leg he needed to attain his goal, even though he still appeared to others to walk with the aid of crutches. The day before he left for home, he called and said that he would send an invitation to a special preview performance, to which only his mother and the therapist would be invited. After another relapse, his family decided to take him to the United States.

PATIENT 5: MS. R.

Ms. R. is a 42-year-old religious woman of Iraqi origin, married to her cousin at the age of 16 by parental arrangement. After being ostracized by her own family for her decision to circumvent her husband's sterility by the use of artificial insemination, a malignant tumor was discovered in her breast. She underwent a radical mastectomy for Stage 1 carcinoma and was warned by the oncologist against becoming pregnant for at least 5 years. Already stigmatized by her family, the loss of her breast made her feel as if she was no longer perceived as a woman. At this point R.'s "Dybbuk" made its first appearance. She described it as her possession, yet it controlled her thoughts and deeds. She held dialogues with it and became certain that the Dybbuk would offer her the gift of impregnation. She understood her cancer as a divine retribution—to create a child from a death sentence. The Dybbuk would not kill her but rather give her the chance to exchange her current life for one more pure, healthy, and beautiful, after which her cancer would disappear forever. After more than 4 years, Ms. R. is still disease free and waiting for the miracle of her pregnancy.

PATIENT 6: MS. B.

Ms. B., a 50-year-old woman born in Austria, emigrated at a very young age to Latin America and came to Israel several years before her illness. She had undergone an ovariectomy and a subtotal hysterectomy a year and a half before the initial psychotherapeutic contact. She longed for her childhood environment of forests and hills and fantasized that during her operation, seeds had been planted in her abdomen, from which a small plant would start growing during the months following surgery. The plant would be of the purest quality; she called it the tree of health, and its leaves would protect her from any other infertile and devouring growth. She refused any kind of physical treatment (including chemotherapy and radiotherapy), which she believed would "poison the plant." Her illness had the explicit purpose of procreating life not only by creating her own internal protection but also by making available the seed to whomever needed it.

PATIENT 7: MR. E.

Mr. E. was a 26-year-old man, married with three children. He had undergone surgery for a testicular teratoma, after which he became impotent. He developed a fixation that inside his scrotum was an egg in which a bird was gestating; the egg would ultimately break, and the bird would emerge and fly out to sea. He believed that, in this way, the operation would be undone, like a dream, that he would once again possess both testicles and be fertile forever. He had to wait 9 months for gestation until which time his body would be the recipient of life, potency, and health. Life had chosen him to have a magical recuperation.

DISCUSSION

We are dealing here with a group of patients suffering from life-threatening disease, most of whom had undergone mutilating operations and similar intensive treatment. The dreamlike fantasies and delusional thoughts described before, although isolated and encapsulated, had followed successful denial of the anxiety-producing reality of the illness. The catastrophic fear of annihilation was then temporarily eliminated by denial, which was suplanted by the fantasized meaning given the disease and the associated imagined sense of control.

In his classic formulation, "The Two Principles of Mental Functioning," Freud (1911/1958) attempted to explain the possible acceptance of painful events. The deluded person perceives reality but has a need to disavow or deny this perception. Thus Freud asserted that the basic problem is not only the awareness of reality but the ability to accept the sometimes painful nature of this reality.

Jaspers (1968) emphasized the phenomenological experience of reality in which delusions provide a "world of new meaning." Delusions may be described as an altered experience of reality in which sensed objects are invested with new significance.

The qualities of omnipotence and regression with which the patients colored the experience of their illness demonstrated attempts at adjustment and adaption and at restoring a sense of internal control, power, and the ability to cope with the frightening ambiguity of the unknown. The patients' fantasies helped foster an enhancement of self-esteem and independence. This process inspired a search for meaning in which events were not seen as random occurrences and that therefore helped them endure future threatening events.

We can assume that such fantasies will be at the service of the ego, thus reinforcing denial and filling with meaning the psychic vacuum created by the denial of reality. These delusional fantasies are specifically related to the damaged organ; imagining a reversal of the illness that makes the organ healthy once again, compensating through regeneration, as a symbolic resurrection of life. These fantasies also created a sensation devoid of fear and anxiety, perhaps because a creator does not fear mortality.

Several studies of cancer patients have taken up the possible relationship between meaning and adaptation (Baider & Sarrell, 1983; Gotay, 1985). Silver and Wortman (1980) have argued that psychological adjustment may be influenced by the individual's ability to find meaning or purpose in his or her misfortunes. Sutherland (1967) has noted that the impact of experience depends largely on the meaning to the patient of the specific experience in his or her total life adaptation. Hinton (1981) presented data suggesting that patients who reported having a sense of fulfillment in life had better adjustment to terminal cancer. More difficult to deny than the diagnosis of cancer was the impairment of body scheme and body image caused by the disease and the treatments aimed at palliation or cure.

It is an accepted notion that different degrees of vulnerability are expressed clinically as variations in individual ego strengths. For some people, the expression of physical vulnerability is likely to occur under almost any circumstance, whereas for others, there must be a specific interplay between a physical vulnerability and a specific and significantly threatening intrapsychic stress (Asaad & Shapiro, 1986; Kroll & Bachrach, 1982).

Several studies have suggested that certain people are predisposed to hallucinations and delusional thinking as a result of an impaired ability to make clear perceptual distinctions, that is, boundary confusion (Richardson & Divyo, 1980). Horowitz *et al.* (1980) argued that some forms of hallucination may be understood as the common pathway of several determinants in the information-processing system—factors that cause a subject to interpret an image of internal origin as an external perception.

Alternatively, hallucinations and delusions may be regarded as symptoms of a basic major impairment of the ego. These observations suggest that hallucinations reflect the cognitive limitations of patients, who may choose different ways to describe and appraise a stressful internal experience (Kolb & Brodie, 1982; Zigler & Levine, 1983). The specific forms of cognition, appraisal and interpretation by which patients react to the threat posed by their illness may matter less than the functions served by these interpretations. These functions fulfill the individual's fundamental need to reconcile internal and external realities and thereby maintain a coherent and integrated sense of self (Engleman and Craddick, 1984). Patients may need to weaken the threat and to redefine impending death by a reaffirmation of life. Their sense of annihilation, of disintegration, and of being surrounded by a void is denied completely. From this negation emerges a meaningful sense of life. Our patients fought disintegration by filling the void with self-created golems that they saw as a meaningful recreation of life (Baider & Abramovitch, 1985).

The compensatory experiences themselves are held back in a selective and private manner. They are kept as a bond with the therapist only, as a symbol of continuity, as a link with reality, and as empathetic understanding. Sometimes the visual experiences appear like eidetic memories and thoughts; often they have the quality of fantasies in that they can be switched on and off, more or less at will. Sometimes the fantasies function much as do real hallucinations in that the patients have a strong conviction that the fantasies have replaced reality.

Terminal patients, alone in their deathbeds, often hallucinate and speak of long-forgotten memories, and of new, revealing meanings interpreted from these memories. Most studies of psychic trauma suggest that isolation and sensory restriction are important determinants of hallucinatory experience. Stress, a familiar concomitant of many isolation-related hallucinations, may be such a condition (Asaad, G., & Shapiro, B., 1986; Kroll, J., & Bachrach, B., 1982; Richardson, A., & Divyo, P., 1980).

Stress sufficient to threaten life itself will often produce hallucinations coupled with dissociation—feelings of unreality and attentional dysfunction. The psychological life space of these patients is therefore a strange amalgam of reality and illusion. We are thus dealing with a wide spectrum of intrapsychic experiences ranging from obsessional thoughts to the fixed idea, from fantasy to delusional thoughts, and from a temporary exchange of the reality of death for the perceptual world of illusion and compensatory fantasy.

SOME FINAL REMARKS

What we have described here are preliminary impressions that lack adequate follow-up. It would be improper to state a generalized conclusion on the basis of such a small, heterogeneous sample lacking homogeneity for the stage of diagnosed cancer or inferred psychopathology. Nevertheless, much can be learned from these clinical descriptions. In all our patients, the compensatory mechanisms we have discussed are directly related to and follow here upon the mechanism of denial. Denial manifests itself as a *gradual* dynamic process moving from the partially conscious to that of the completely unconscious. Patients will deny that portion of reality that includes the diagnosis itself, by denying the name of the disease or the kind of intervention involved; but, for the most part, by the mechanisms reported herein, they will have denied the meaning of the illness and the mutilating procedures to which they have been subjected.

Beyond denial, after the energy-savings deferment of relating to the disease, is the second mechanism that we have described. This compensatory mechanism has at least two basic functions. First, it fills the void. Denial becomes a meaningful creation; it is the positive that follows and reverses the negative. Second, it fulfills the need for hope, for a sense of life in the face of the catastrophic experience of cancer. Prospectively, it will be essential to understand if and how these elements of hope and invested meaning can help the patient cope and adjust to the disease more successfully (Pettingale, 1984; Pettingale, Morris *et al.*, 1985).

Although denial is common among patients with life-threatening disease, understanding and breaking through denial has been viewed as a means of facilitating health. Denial may be a healthy aspect of coping behavior in some patients, and it is important to understand the specific role of denial in order to achieve a total understanding of illness as it is experienced by certain highly creative patients (Beisser, 1979; Breznitz, 1983; Haan, 1980; Weisman, 1972).

What therapeutic implications may be drawn from our experience with these patients and the interpretation offered in this chapter? Our instinct is, of course, to replace illusion with reality, delusion with truth. Yet such behavior would constitute denial on the part of the therapist, denial of the poetic beauty of the creative solutions found by these patients for conflict beyond the realm of normal human experience. The cancer patient for whom life would be a living death, and full conscious awareness a punishment rather than a blessing, cannot be judged by the same standards as the physically healthy person faced only with intrapsychic conflict. What would be delusional thinking in the latter is only the healthy manifestation of sound adaptive internal resources in the former.

The psychological evaluation of patients with such chronic and painful terminal malignancies is in its infancy. No authoritative formulation may be derived from the scattered, ambiguous data concerning the intrapsychic and coping mechanisms of cancer patients. For now, all we can offer is an unclear metaphor, the implications of which lie beyond denial.

REFERENCES

Asaad, G., & Shapiro, B. (1986). Hallucinations: theoretical and clinical overview. *American Journal of Psychiatry, 143,* 1088–1097.

Baider, L., & Abramovitch, H. (1985). The Dybbuk: Cultural context of a cancer patient. *The Hospice Journal, 1,* 113–119.

Baider, L., & Sarrell, M. (1983). Perceptions and causal attributions of Israeli women with breast cancer concerning their illness. *Psychotherapy and Psychosomatics, 39,* 136–143.

Beisser, A. R. (1979). Denial and affirmation in illness and health. *American Journal of Psychiatry, 136,* 1026–1030.

Breznitz, S. (Ed.). (1983). *The denial of stress.* New York: International Universities Press.

Derogatis, L. R., Morrow, G. R., Fetting, J., Penman, D., Piasetsky, S., Schmale, A. M., Hendrichs, M., & Carnickle, C. L. (1983). The prevalence of psychiatric disorders among cancer patients, *J.A.M.A., 249,* 751–757.

Engelman, S. R., & Craddick, R. (1984). The symbolic relationship of breast cancer patients to their cancer, cure, physician and themselves. *Psychotherapy and Psychosomatics, 41,* 68–76.

Freud, S. (1958). *Formulations on the two principles of mental functioning* In *Standard Edition.* (Vol. 12). London: Hogarth. (Originally published in 1911.)

Goldberg, R. J. (1983). Psychiatric symptoms in cancer patients: Is the cause organic or psychologic? *Postgraduate Medicine, 74* 263–273.

Gotay, C. C. (1985). Why Me? Attributions and adjustment by cancer patients and their mates at two stages in the disease process. *Social Science Medicine, 20,* 825–831.

Greer, S., & McEwan, P. J. (Eds.). (1985). Cancer and the mind. *Social Science Medicine, 20.*

Haan, N. G. (1980). Psychosocial meanings of unfavorable medical forecasts. In *Health psychology handbook* (pp. 113–140). G. Stone, F. Cohen and N. G. Haan (Eds.). San Francisco: Jossey Bass.

Hinton, J. (1981). Sharing or withholding awareness of dying between husband and wife. *Journal of Psychosomatic Research, 25,* 337–343.

Holland, J. C., Hughes, A., Tross, S., Silberfarb, P., Perry, M., Comis, R., Oster, M. (1986). Comparative psychological disturbance in patients with pancreatic and gastric cancer. *American Journal of Psychiatry, 143,* 982–986.

Horowitz, M. J., Wilner, N., Kaltreider, N., & Alvarez, W. (1980). Signs and symptoms of posttraumatic stress disorder. *Archives of General Psychiatry, 27,* 85–92.

Jaspers, K. (1968). Delusion and awareness of reality, *International Journal of Psychiatry, 6,* 25–38.

Kelly, H. H. (1967). Attribution theory in social psychology. In D. Levine (Ed.), *Nebraska Symposium on Motivation* (Vol. 15; pp. 192–238). Lincoln: University of Nebraska Press.

Kolb, L. C., & Brodie, H. K. (1982). *Modern clinical psychiatry.* Philadelphia: W. B. Saunders.

Kroll, J., & Bachrach, B. (1982). Medieval visions and contemporary hallucinations. *Psychosomatic Medicine, 12,* 709–721.

Pettingale, K. W. (1984). Coping and cancer prognosis. *Journal of Psychosomatic Research, 28,* 363–364.

Pettingale, K. W., Morris, T., Greer, S., & Haybrittle, J. L. (1985, March). Mental attitudes to cancer: An additional prognostic factor. *The Lancet,* p. 750.

Pyszczynski, T. A., & Greenberg, J. (1981). Role of disconfirmed expectations in the instigation of attributional processing. *Journal of Personality and Social Psychology, 40,* 31–38.

Richardson, A., & Divyo, P. (1980). The predisposition to hallucinate. *Psychological Medicine, 10,* 715–722.

Silver, R. L., & Wortman, C. B. (1980). Coping with undesirable life events. In J. Garber & M. E. Seligman (Eds.), *Human helplessness: Theory and applications* (pp. 279–340). New York: Academic Press.

Spilka, B., Shaver, P., & Kirkpatrick, L. A. (1985). A general attribution theory for the psychology of religion, *Journal of the Scientific Study of Religion, 24*, 1–20.

Sutherland, A. M. (1967). Psychological observations in cancer patients. *International Psychiatric Clinics, 4*, 75–92.

Taylor, S. E. (1983). Adjustment to threatening events. *American Psychologist, 38*, 1161–73.

Thompson, S. C. (1981). Will it hurt less if I can control it? A complex answer to a simple question. *Psychological Bulletin, 90*, 89–101.

Weisman, A. D. (1979). *Coping with cancer.* New York: McGraw-Hill.

Weisman, A. D. (1972). *On dying and denying.* New York: Behavioral Publications.

Weisman, A. D., & Worden, J. W. (1972–1976). Coping and vulnerability in cancer patients, Research Report, Harvard Medical School N.C.I. 14104.

Wortman, C. B., & Schetter, C. (1979). Interpersonal relationships and cancer: A theoretical analysis, *Journal of Social Issues, 35*, 120–155.

Zigler, E., & Levine, J. (1983). Hallucinations vs. delusions: A developmental approach. *Journal of Nervous and Mental Disease, 171*, 141–146.

17

Denial, Coping, and Cancer

Avery Danto Weisman

Cancer is certainly one of the most dreaded and fatal group of diseases to which humanity is subject. Despite many reassurances about imminent breakthroughs and periodic reports about successful treatment of a few malignancies, most people, professional and lay, would still regard the diagnosis of cancer as far more distressing than heart, liver, or kidney diseases, although in some respects, the actual prognosis of certain cancers may be far better.

Physicians, too, are likely to be no more optimistic about the ultimate outcome of cancer than are less educated people, and for good reason. Cancer may be operated upon, say, and after a period of relative health, recur, with far less success for subsequent treatment. Doctors who are patients will deny at least as often as lay people, even when the evidence is there before them. As a result, despite much ado about clear communication and informed consent in cancer treatment, we can easily find that patients either are not told about their illness or find it difficult to establish communication with responsible health professionals. Given the bleak prognosis and bare communication, cancer patients provide ample resources for studying denial.

Denial, negation, contradiction, avoidance, and illusion characterize almost every transaction between human beings. Language, perception, and the conveyance of meaning depend on being able to negate as well

Avery Danto Weisman • Department of Psychiatry, Massachusetts General Hospital, Boston, Massachusetts 02114.

as to affirm statements and reports about what we experience and observe. Aristotle's age-old dictum of the excluded middle, A or -A, is a fundamental principle of logic without which we could hardly make sense to each other. Reality itself may be relative, but language, as we know it, requires linguistic denial, about which I shall not have anything further to say in this chapter.

Nevertheless, it is important to recognize two major types of denial that have utmost clinical relevance and are found regularly in cancer patients and in those caring for them:

1. *Cognitive denial.* This is denial *by* a person about the *what* of events.
2. *Existential denial.* This is denial *of* individual uniqueness or separate reality of person or group.

Cognitive denial refers to meaning, existential denial to the being of parts of human experience. Existential denial points to *who* is being denied of what; cognitive denial denies the special copy of reality communicated by one person to another.

If a gang of youths approach me at night, asking for money, I would be a superdenier not to realize that I was about to be robbed, should I refuse. The shared reality is that in many American cities, walking alone at night is almost foolhardy. To dismiss the meaning of being asked for money by a group of young men is to exemplify cognitive denial. I have not taken precautions by taking another, better-lighted path to where I must go, and as a result, have pretended to be more secure than I am by neglecting danger.

It is, of course, possible that I could be approached by a group of young men who are collecting money for a neighborhood club or some other less hazardous cause than robbery. In this unlikely event, I would have categorized these youths as muggers, and, I suppose, denied them of the right to solicit funds.

Cognitive denial, no less serious, might occur when I ignore one of the major signs of potential cancer, such as bleeding from an orifice, swellings and lumps, discolorations of moles, persistent cough, and so forth. If, for example, I note fecal blood and decide that it is probably from a hemorrhoid, I may be right or wrong. It does not matter. The test is what I do about it, except that cognitive denial is more likely if the bleeding persists and I still avoid having the problem checked.

Denial and affirmation have exactly the same preconditions; the test depends on substituting a milder, more favorable interpretation or statement for what might be more intimidating. Denial preserves the status quo, whereas affirmation is open to change. Denial tends to keep things tightly intact, as they were, in terms of facts, relationships, well-being, and so forth. The potential problem is a nonproblem that, of course, requires no further coping.

This chapter extends the concept of existential denial presented at the symposium in Israel, where existential denial and the right to exist are living themes that occupy the full attention of every citizen—denial that refers to such matters as separate existence and distinct individuality in atmosphere of menace. Existential denial can be seen in less unmistakably forbidding forms elsewhere, even under the most well-meaning of clinical circumstances. Existential denial categorizes people into separate compartments, qualities, traits, or constructs that enable clinicians to maintain power and control, if not open subjugation. Existential denial can be benign, when, for example, people are designated according to demographic characteristics. No one is automatically deprived of rights by becoming a hospital patient, unless the sick role, "patienthood," consigns that person to a submissive state in which complaints and questions are outlawed and autonomy must be suspended at the hospital entrance.

If a patient with cancer becomes only a receptacle for that cancer and not a sick person whose existence has been compromised by disease, then someone has enacted existential denial. If a pathologist does an autopsy, knowing only the medical facts about an individual who has died, existential denial has simply been built into the professional cognitive system, so that any other information aside from what is disclosed by the prosector is irrelevant.

Existential denial is malignant when the patient is ignored as a distinct individual, an act leading to stereotyping, categorization, even scorn and neglect. That this may occur in assemblyline medicine can hardly be disputed and may in fact be the price paid for treating larger numbers of people. The central question, of course, is whether existential denial is consistent with good medical treatment.

People have a right to seek information and get reliable, coherent answers to questions. Sometimes, however, doctors unilaterally decide that they know best and therefore deal in complacent fictions for their own convenience. Even doctors who routinely report, "I always tell my cancer patients what is wrong," are also guilty of existential denial by depriving patients of the adjustment required by what portion of truth they are able to use. Moreover, the diagnosis may not be the whole issue; some patients are more concerned about the social consequences of being sick, say, and being unable to support their families. Lying or deception is seldom indicated, if ever, even if some patients might prefer it, but careful appraisal of who is being told what and how much that person can use it is necessary if denial is not to be misleading.

Cognitive and existential denial often complement each other at times by combining forces to offer a totally fictitious reality. Indeed, existential denial quietly creeps in when cognitive denial takes over, little by little, by successively misleading distortions and deceptions.

The *process called denying* has an outcome in *denial.* It has five steps: (1) acceptance of a common field in which meanings seem clear and unambiguous, (2) rejection of a portion of that shared reality by means of statements and reports, (3) revision or replacement of that rejected meaning with something more acceptable, (4) reorientation of the resulting behavior with respect to the "new" reality, and, finally, (5) judgment by another person sharing the original field that the primary person has unexpectedly misinterpreted or renounced an obvious reality. Note that the question of who is right or wrong on any ground except implied consensus is not relevant here. Step 5 is required because we do not ordinarily accuse ourselves of denial, except in retrospect. We tend to believe the best and to trust our own perceptions and judgments, against much resistance and rationalization.

Because the denial process usually involves more than one person and is apt to vary depending on the people themselves, denial may be considered an interpersonal transaction, even a coping strategy, in which one person judges that another person's statements, perceptions, and behavior are erroneous, egregious, or unexpectedly deviant. In very simple terms, for instance, some patients will report only minimal or very favorable signs to their doctors. As a result, their clinical status is judged to be better than it is. This encourages erroneous judgments by the doctor, based on existential denial of the patient ("I am not so sick"). Doctors in turn can readily *impose* denial on sick patients by inquiring, "Everything is all right today, isn't it?"

Denial has a wide range of manifestations. It can be so extreme as to qualify as a delusion. "I was perfectly well until I came into the hospital. Just being here makes me sick!" Most denial is far milder, even somewhat innocent, indirect, and disguised:

DOCTOR: Have you ever had bleeding like this before?

PATIENT: No, not really.

This is actually an example of affirmation by negation or denial.

It is easy to deny that denial is as complex as it is and to assume that we know all there is about the process. Good definitions are deceptive. I find that it is more useful to examine the various dimensions of denying than to seek an all-purpose definition that covers all cases.

It is not enough simply to diagnose that denial takes place. Its dimensions include such matters as who denies what to whom when and under what circumstances. Understanding the implicit context of denial enables us to find out the purpose as well as the form of denial and therefore to discover the explicit affirmation buried in the negation:

A 36-year-old married woman with terminal ovarian cancer was about to be discharged from the hospital and return home for palliative care. To its surprise, the gynecology staff found that the patient was elated, optimistic, and behaved as if she were going home to resume a more or less normal life, instead of awaiting certain death. She talked about fixing up, redecorating her home, making plans for seeing friends, and, most prominently, spoke very affectionately about living with the husband from whom she had been periodically estranged. Understandably, the staff believed that an unexpected, almost global denial had set in and called for a psychiatric consultation.

The consultant, who happened to be me, found a very intelligent and articulate youngish woman who, indeed, was pleased about going home, a mental state considerably in contrast to that of the staff who was quite discouraged about her failure to improve after long and harrowing treatment.

I found no evidence of denial. The staff had judged her statements, mood, and behavior in the context of terminal illness and decided that her attitude was consistent only with abrogating the facts. But which facts?

She knew that time was running out; she had tried every treatment, from multiple operations to the Simonton method. She had come to terms with mortality and was actually fairly free of discomfort. Her enthusiasm and anticipation about going home, however, stemmed from a new understanding achieved with her husband. Over the preceding few months, they had become reconciled; each felt a renewal of affection and loyalty that they had not known since the early years of marriage. Together, as life was coming to end, there developed a kind of bittersweet romance that she welcomed and even embraced. It was, in my opinion, an affirmation from this viewpoint, not a denial.

But to be more clinical about her plight, the positive expectation still depended on cognitive denial because her romantic hopes required a similar response by her husband. And I knew nothing about his actual thoughts. It might be, for example, that his responsiveness was a result of knowing that time was limited, anyway, and that a temporary arrangement based on compassion, but not exactly love, could be worked out. Thus, she ran the risk of self-deception and, to a degree, showed inflated self-esteem. It was the staff, however, that denied by insisting that she feel as dejected as they.

DENIAL AND COPING

Threads of denial are woven into the fabric of almost every coping strategy and into every defensive tactic. I want to emphasize, however, that coping deals with problems met with in the world at large; it consists of what one does in order to bring about relief and resolution in an open universe. Defensive tactics, on the other hand, fend off problems, closing off the open universe and resisting the change that coping encourages and accepts.

Table 1 is a list of common coping strategies, likely to be used by you and me. Denial, in my opinion, becomes a legitimate coping strategy, that is, something one might elect to do, when it dominates the scene. It is the antithesis of candid confrontation or honest search for guidance and information. Its aim is, as stated earlier, to turn a problem into a nonproblem, so that coping is unnecessary. A man, sick with advanced cancer, with enormous ascites and profound weight loss, claimed that all he needed was a strong cathartic to reduce abdominal swelling!

Few cancer patients adopt denial as much as possible for as long as possible without the complicity of those looking after them. In a sense, denial tends to run in families, that is when supportive others insistently avoid facts, patients are encouraged to remain silent and to ask no questions. In fact, one of the most important contributions that can be made by an outside caregiver who would hesitate to contradict family policy openly is to ask patients how much information they have received, whether this amount is satisfactory, and, if such patients ask questions, to suggest that they ask the doctor.

Existential denial is also brought about when denial as much as possible becomes a uniform policy. Patients become compliant objects

TABLE 1. Common Coping Strategies

1. Seek reliable information
2. Share concern with someone
3. Change the emotional tone
4. Put it aside or out of mind
5. Keep busy
6. Confront the issue and act
7. Redefine the problem
8. Resign yourself
9. Do something, just anything
10. Examine alternatives
11. Escape from it all
12. Comply with expectations
13. Blame or shame someone, something
14. Give vent to emotion
15. Deny as much as possible

who are often hesitant to give offense by asking questions or voicing misgivings.

Cancer patients tend to deny three main elements: (1) facts of illness or the diagnosis itself, (2) manifestations of cancer, including implications of symptoms and treatment, and (3) long-term prognosis or outcome, especially the sickness unto death, when decline becomes unmistakable. I term these elements, primary, secondary, and tertiary denial. The distinction is important when we are called upon to say what is denied at any phase of illness. Obviously, psychosocial ramifications can readily be denied when any of these elements is denied. And denial as much as possible need not only involve facts about illness.

Commonly, a cancer patient may admit to having had cancer at one time, that is, before an operation, but fail to note a possible connection between new symptoms and the old diagnosis. Over 90% of patients returning to the hospital for cancer recurrence report having believed themselves cured after the initial diagnosis and treatment. This does not mean, however, that every one of these patients coped by denying as much as possible. But it does suggest a closing off of perception as part of the restoration to health. Perhaps this much denial is absolutely necessary to get going again. Preterminal patients sometimes startle their caregivers by beginning to make unrealistic plans for a future that will never come. Tertiary denial often presents itself by refusing to believe that illness and dying can be fatal. Frequently, care givers and supportive others conspire to encourage this belief by exaggerating minor improvements and suggesting an unduly generous prognosis.

What is wrong with denying? Does it help to deny, and does it take away hope? These questions are often asked, and we have a few answers. First of all, patients who deny as much as possible are found among those more seriously distressed emotionally than among patients who are coping well. Secondly, hope is not contingent upon extensive denial, although some deniers feign a shallow optimism. Hope is a product of self-esteem, not the avoidance of a problem; good copers have confidence in their ability to cope, not in the nonexistence of problems.

I suppose that undue pessimism can be a form of denial, especially in the absence of extensive and deleterious disease. It is likely to call forth denial in the caregiver who rejects the notion that everything is hopeless, there is no use struggling, and treatment is an illusion. Acceptance of the inevitable is a strategy that is entirely different from active repudiation of treatment. Undue pessimism is as serious a blunder as unqualified optimism; both extremes absolve us from making efforts to deal with uncertainty.

TABLE 2. What Do Good Copers Do?

1. They try to be as specific as possible about a problem.
2. They set a goal with realistic expectations.
3. They picture various intermediate steps that might help reach a feasible goal.
4. Then, they act according to best judgment about the consequences.
5. In doing so, good copers acknowledge their emotional pressure points of vulnerability.
6. They keep a measure of emotional composure, because extremes tend to warp judgment.
7. They restrain themselves from undue, imaginary, or idealized possibilities in favor of practical and reachable goals.
8. There are usually a number of choices and options between black and white alternatives.
9. They find that denial is a useful temporary distraction, and avoid self-pity, bitterness, or unwarranted optimism or pessimism.
10. They are ready to correct and monitor their own behavior, and seek guidance, knowing that belief in the capacity to cope competently fortifies morale and helps achieve good coping.

Good copers have more coping strategies at their disposal than denial. As Table 2 shows, they are more resourceful, flexible, practical, and, for that matter, consistently hopeful about their capacity to cope well enough under most circumstances.

Denial can be useful up to a point but, like any other strategy, may be overdone and used to excess. That point is marked by *bad faith*, to adopt a term espoused by Sartre. It means, as I construe the concept, self-deception and deception of others. It advocates a role, not a reality. Cancer is far too serious to be left to physicians; it is also mistaken to ignore the psychosocial problems imposed upon significant others who stand to lose and be lost by cancer and its ramifications.

Satisfactory coping with cancer demands more than militant, long-term denial on all fronts. All is not well and may not be well; but then, it might be better than bleak pessimism may insist. Good coping requires courage, enlightened perceptions, not foolhardy avoidance and docile submission. And we can acknowledge the uncertainty and hazards of existence without being crushed by their potential for demolishing us.

Patients who cope well enough and yet are finally forced to yield to

TABLE 3. Appropriate Death

1. Comfort and care for others and oneself
2. Control and collaboration in all important decisions
3. Composure with compassion
4. Communication with significant others, forthrightly and in truth
5. Continuity with valuable aspects of earlier life, even in token form
6. Closure on remaining problems so that time is not a pressing issue

mortality can achieve an appropriate death, the characteristics of which are given in Table 3. These are not people who deny our potential for dying but those who accept and live with a foreshortened future. It is not a passive or propitious death but often an active effort to maintain significant control, without denial, as long as possible. No one opts for misery and a painful death; the impairments of dying make limitations far worse than the fact of death. It is here that denial, coping, and cancer come together. Denial detracts from the appropriate death, that is, one that we might choose, had we a choice. Instead, coping conveys the full significance of being alive and still to be dying. Denial dehumanizes death.

SOURCES

Ahmed, P. (Ed.). (1981). *Living and dying with cancer.* New York: Elsevier.
Burkhalter, P., & Donley, D. (Eds.). (1978). *Dynamics of oncology nursing.* New York: McGraw-Hill Book Co.
Moos, R. (Ed.). (1984). *Coping with physical illness 2. New perspectives.* New York & London: Plenum Medical Book Co.
Sartre, J.-P. (1956). *Being and nothingness: An essay on phenomenological ontology.* New York: Philosophical Library.
Stoll, B. (Ed.). (1979). *Mind and cancer prognosis.* Chicester and New York: Wiley & Sons.
Weisman, A. (1972). *On dying and denying: A psychiatric study of terminality.* New York: Human Sciences Press.
Weisman, A. (1979). *Coping with cancer.* New York: McGraw-Hill Book Company.
Weisman, A. (1984). *The coping capacity: On the nature of being mortal.* New York: Human Sciences Press.

18

Denial in Patients with Myocardial Infarction

DIETER OHLMEIER

In an effort to prove to themselves, to their environment, and of course to their physicians that they are healthy and fit, many patients will attempt to deny both the existence and the significance of their acute myocardial infarction by performing deep knee bends, by jogging, or by the execution of other physically demanding tasks. Such attempts to "conquer" pain and thereby to ward off acceptance and understanding of this life-threatening illness may be understood as behaviors based on the defense mechanism of denial but serving to preserve the continuity of the patient's very concept of self and the position of that person in his or her perceived interpersonal network.

That any illness might have its origin in intrapsychic conflict is inconceivable to these patients. More often, one encounters an attitude of uncomplaining pride and (as phrased by many of those we studied) the sturdy fantasy that they had been "wounded" or that they had "died on the field of honor." Psychoanalytic treatment, with its inherent implication that fault may lie within the person rather than the outside world, is viewed as demeaning and therefore insulting; it is rejected summarily. Central to the character structure of the patients described herein was the need to maintain at all costs the appearance (to self and others) of

DIETER OHLMEIER • Sigmund Freud Institute, Myliusstrasse 20, D-6000 Frankfurt 1, Federal Republic of Germany.

normality, conformity, efficiency, and healthy functionality, despite the temporary dissolution of such an identity during the acute phase of the myocardial infarction. The tenacity with which these patients cling to such illusions and their blindness to inner reality and inner conflict has led us to think of them as "patients of denial."

This situation is doubtless responsible for the fact that psycho-analysts seldom see myocardial infarction patients, much less analyze them in the classic setting. Myocardial infarction patients rarely consult psychoanalysts of their own accord; if anything, they are referred by a cardiologist (although usually reluctantly), "in order not to neglect any treatment possibility."

It is also possible that psychoanalysts are not attracted by such "un-motivated" patients, feel themselves afflicted with a sense of helplessness in regard to psychoanalytic work with this clientele, and—perhaps as a form of "counterresistance"—succumb to an attitude of denial with re-spect to these patients' potential for development. This is reminiscent of the long-standing reluctance to treat psychotic patients with psycho-analytic methods.

Over the past few years, a total of approximately 15 patients under the age of 45 have been referred to me by a cardiology clinic for the purpose of conducting a psychoanalytic interview. In one instance, this contact resulted in a psychoanalytic psychotherapy lasting 18 months. Six patients were willing to participate in a psychoanalytic group therapy during their brief hospitalization following the infarction. My psycho-analytic experience with this clientele is therefore quite limited—it would constitute a denial not to realize this; but this clinical experience appears to me to be nonetheless suitable for drawing some conclusions, particularly concerning the aspect of denial.

PSYCHIC STRUCTURAL CHARACTERISTICS OF MYOCARDIAL PATIENTS

In summarizing a number of structural characteristics of myocar-dial patients, I will touch upon some aspects pertaining to the etiology and pathogenesis of this syndrome as seen from a psychoanalytic standpoint.

First of all, I would like to stress the *role* and *psychological implications* of the patient's *occupation*. Therapeutic experience with myocardial pa-tients—as I will demonstrate with a case example—show that *work*, usu-ally in the sense of feeling chronically overworked, offers a unique form of protection as well as an opportunity to attain a form of rational "control" over their human environment. In this context, therefore, work is not only a considerable burden and obligation, but offers, above all, a firm frame of reference that provides a certain measure of security within which human relationships have a preconceived place.

An incapacity to work, on the other hand, fosters insecurity and a loss of identity among these patients, often up to the point of feeling, for all practical purposes, "already dead." The myocardial infarction itself and the resulting incapacity to work—including the experience of being forcibly removed from the work process and the possibility of becoming permanently disabled—constitute an existential threat. In the eyes of these patients, the loss of their capacity to work as well as the well-regulated occupational framework is even more crucial than might be the loss of a partner. The significance of situations involving loss prior to the onset of heart disease has been stressed by Köhle and Gaus (1979).

What does this exaggerated role of the occupational framework mean with reference to the patient's perception of superiors, co-workers, and colleagues? These individuals tend to be more than willing to submit to the dictates and demands of their superiors. They identify with them. Fear of an emotionally charged disagreement tends not to arise as long as identification with or rather incorporation of the superior, including his demands, his work mores and ideology, is possible as long as conscious, or openly expressed differences of opinion can be kept to a minimum. The superior, finally, is no longer perceived in the form of a living person; in his place one finds an "organization" with all its "supraindividual" mechanisms and regulations.

As far as the earliest psychological origins of this illness are concerned, it appears that the "threatening father" never really materializes, at least not in the form of a tangible human object against which one has to assert oneself in direct confrontation during the process of developing one's own pattern of living. Instead, the "father–object" is all but eliminated through the processes of identification and incorporation mentioned previously. In addition, our experience has shown that these patients demonstrate a tendency to anonymize and depersonalize father figures (superiors, persons of authority, etc.) who are perceived not on the basis of their own identity, as human beings, but rather in functional contexts such as "the company," "the hospital," or "the state." The system, *the institution*, replaces the human being.

As long as this manner of perception and functioning can be maintained and the patient continues to identify with and conform to it, he or she will be able to derive from it a considerable amount of security as well as a feeling of power, significance, and acknowledgment of his or her own self. The forced removal from these institutional contexts, on the other hand, means a loss of identity and feeling of self, and is experienced by the patient as a powerful source of insecurity. Our therapeutic work with myocardial patients has demonstrated that one prominent feature of their psychological profile is such a profound fear of loss of identity. The patient, therefore, suffers from a lack of awareness of his or her own distinctive personality. This we find to be a typical characteristic of the personality structure of myocardial patients and of those considered to be cardiac risks.

Complementary to the anxiety just described, the patients tend to protect themselves against a loss of identity through compulsive control of self and others. Here one frequently encounters disguised sadistic tendencies in the patient's dealings with others, which is to say a tendency to control, to torment, and to force others into predicaments—much as they do with themselves—but in a "cultivated," rationally justifiable manner and with reference to circumstances beyond their control.

Patients with this personality structure must find it especially difficult to be immobilized by a life-threatening infarction, whereas, at the same time, "catapulted" out of their vital personal and occupational contexts. The identity crisis that becomes manifest along with the illness nearly always results in a severe depression combined with a sense of loss of all of one's occupational and life contexts.

CLINICAL EXPERIENCE WITH A GROUP OF MYOCARDIAL PATIENTS

In view of the structural characteristics of myocardial patients just outlined, it must be assumed that follow-up treatment and psychological rehabilitation depends at least in part on the degree to which a psychic reorientation of the pathological personality structure can be attained.

In considering group therapy with a group of these patients, we initially proceeded from the very general theoretical premise that the earliest phases of personality development occur within a group, namely the family (or a group resembling a family) into which an individual is born. These group influences lead to the development of not only an individual but also a group identity—thus, as a result of the conditions surrounding psychosocial development, a person is not only an individual but also a member of a group. Our hypothesis was that when dealing with myocardial patients, with their excessive problems in the area of social conformity and achievement as well as their fear of loss of identity and passive submission, the group situation (with its tendency to activate group functions) should prove to be of considerable value in the therapeutic process. Clinical experience in analytic group therapy with myocardial patients has confirmed this premise. It is hoped that the following clinical report on the course of a group of this nature will offer some insight into the therapeutic group work with these patients and clarify the aforementioned psychodynamic features.

The group consisted of six patients (five men, one woman), each of whom had experienced a myocardial infarction 4 to 6 weeks prior to entering the group and who were in the process of being discharged from a hospital (and not from a rehabilitation center). We decided upon a brief group therapy of only five sessions (once weekly, 90 minutes each), and chose the method of psycho-analytic group therapy as described by Bion (1961), by Grinberg, Langer, and Rodrigué (1960), by Argelander (1972), and by myself (Ohlmeier, 1975). In this method, the group is viewed as a whole, as a homogeneous organism that interacts with the therapist, and not as a mere congregation of individuals. Transference, resistance, and mutual unconscious fantasies are interpreted as a product of the entire group and not as those of the individual members. The contributions of individual members are understood to be representative of the group process. It is assumed that any specific individual conflict, the unique conflict situation of an individual group member, assumes a representative role in the sense that anything an individual says that is dwelt upon for any length of time by the group, thereby receives that group's unconscious consensus. In this manner, a culturally ego-dystonic process of self-revelation was made ego dystonic by defining it in terms of group process.

In the *first session*, the group began by expressing intensely aggressive emotions that then increased in a nearly explosive manner. The therapist was hardly able to say a word and felt as if he were being "forced into a corner." The group members complained in a fearful and angry manner about the loss of their capability to work and of their physical strength, whereas at the same time denouncing as lazy and demanding today's younger generation of "hippies."

Psychological problems were either completely denied or at least not mentioned. The infarction was described and rationalized as a purely physical episode. The participants joked about being together in a group and referred to the meeting as "group sex." The suggestion that such an attitude might constitute defensive behavior led to a depressive reaction with strong symbiotic undertones. Feelings of being neglected and of a sense of helplessness were then expressed by the group. The group's present "incapacity" gave rise to feelings of shame; these feelings were more pronounced by the male group members. At the same time, there became apparent a desire to, if possible, be in harmony with their environment and family on the basis of mutual trust and understanding. Nearly all interpretations attempted in the period following this phase of the session were met with resistance. The group was obviously not in a position to deal with them, and the session concluded with the grandiose fantasy that the "men of the house" had been expected to entertain the analyst by analyzing the analyst. It appeared as if their intense feeling of helplessness had been inverted to a grossly overinflated sense of grandeur.

In the *second session*, disappointment and depression were dominant, though often subject to resistance in the form of laughter and rationalization. Oral-symbiotic fantasies and wishes were mobilized, particularly whenever I attempted an interpretation, thus causing the group to feel threatened in its identity. At the same time, paranoid fears emerged—"What are they doing with us here? He's eavesdropping. What will become of the things we say here?" The group situation was now viewed by the group as a superego situation, as a difficult and demanding task, roughly comparable to the situation at home when the husband does not do as the wife wishes and, as a result, has to listen to her complaints. The only woman in the group was becoming more and more an outsider: "When men get together, it's easier for them when there are no women around." Homosexual wishes arose, viewed here as a defense against demands of a superego origin, namely against an object that (like the analyst) is endowed with a capacity for providing "maternal comfort." This must be resisted for the simple reason that it gives rise to a feeling of being pressured into helplessness.

The group then began behaving in a pronounced narcissistic manner regarding its work capability and its moral integrity. Nonetheless, an underlying atmosphere of depression could be sensed, which, however, the group found necessary to avert. Orderliness and punctuality, in other words, narcissistically cathected anal attributes, were mobilized in order to protect against a sense of being exploited by others. External regulations and principles—"law and order"—had to be maintained. My interpretation to the effect that the group found it necessary to ward off any free associations not compatible with "law and order," thus forestalling any potential activity, was met with an aggressive outburst directed toward today's youth (which also implied modern therapy methods). The group's behavior, as well as the fantasies and associations they expressed, became increasingly anal sadistic in nature. The fear of "not making it," of losing control and being helpless, was quite evident. However, at the same time a considerable amount of narcissistic gratification could be observed in the group's constant rationalized control of instinctual desires (drinking, smoking), namely in the anal-sadistic rejection of these "sins."

During the *third session*, the anxiety rose to a level that could hardly be contained by rationalization and denial. On the one hand, the value of therapy was deemed questionable, whereas on the other hand the oral-symbiotic desire to be nurtured increased. A fear of death, of being disabled, of complete loss of identity surfaced. The analyst was urgently requested to protect, to help, to indulge. And at the same time, the group's perception of its own helplessness and deprivation gave rise to feelings of humiliation. The fact that one is the recipient of help, of treatment, that one faces the prosect of being dominated by one's wife following the impending discharge, is experienced as a narcissistic wound. Nonetheless, rebellious and even furious remarks could be heard, such as: "Our being so ill is exactly what they deserve." These remarks were accompanied by paranoid fantasies: "We can't afford to be ill and vulnerable, otherwise someone might try to prove that we are useless." Some patients even had fantasies about being slandered after death. However, the fear of suffering a complete loss of identity through the disintegration of their very existence remained the group's dominant theme. Routine medical examinations, such as an electrocardiogram, began to take on the character of a test, and the group felt that such tests had to be passed with flying colors. The patients' relationship toward the analyst was imbued with ambivalence: On the one hand, he represented to them a protective and indulgent mother, whereas on the other hand they saw him in the role of what one patient described as a threatening and demanding "dentist." Every attempt to overcome this rather alarming view through rational discussion proved futile. The anxiety increased to the point that thoughts began to surface relating to the approaching "end of the world," or of feeling left on their own with their heart disease and abandoned during the rehabilitation phase. Finally, there emerged a fantasy of soon having to die alone without a doctor around to help.

This wish for care and assistance directed toward the analyst was maintained throughout the *fourth session*. However, the group was now in a position to accept the interpretation that excessive activity serves to protect from a fear of death and abandonment. In this session, the therapist was experienced as both demanding and achievement-oriented but also as helpful and indulgent. The group expected him to provide "milk from the mother's breast to give them the strength of a lion." This oral fantasy is also discernible in the notion that one must drink medications in large quantities in order to be fed strength and endurance by the doctor.

The *fifth session* saw a resumption of numerous oral fantasies, concealed to a degree by the new tendency of the group to view itself increasingly as *one* group, namely in the sense of a protective and indulgent mother, a role that the group as a whole had begun to assume. Fears of being isolated and left out receded, and the sphere occupied by superego mechanisms of a controlling nature gradually decreased in significance and nearly disappeared. Work within the group now began to convey a sense of security; in contrast, their incapacity to work continued to represent a threat of identity loss and death: "Anyone incapable of working must die." In the face of anonymous, inaccessible and unassailably authoritative fathers and bosses, one can nearly expect a reaction of both aggression and submission: "The moment I submit to the demands of my superiors, I no longer have to fear anything." In psychoanalytic terms, such a reaction constitutes identification with the aggressor, combined with pronounced oral-regressive characteristics.

Once an attempt had been made to interpret these meanings, the group suddenly found itself in a position to recall and express more memories from early childhood. However, the "threatening father" remained anonymous and depersonalized. Features of individual, "personal" fathers could not be drawn from the material; instead, there was talk of the Wehrmacht, prisoner of war camps, and the Nazi era, for these social or political or, as it were, suprapersonal phenomena were utilized as substitutes for personal parental figures. Finally, the group explained to the analyst that he, as a younger person, could not really comprehend the pressure under which they lived and live. Through this means, even the analyst became depersonalized within the group and transformed into an anonymous object fantasized as incapable of truly understanding the situation experienced by each individual. By defining the analyst as one who "doesn't understand us anyway," the group evaded and disavowed its conscious and rationally comprehensible fear of him.

CONCLUSIONS

This fragmentary material drawn from a psychoanalytic group situation confirms the opinion of Moersch *et al.* (1980) that denial constitutes the most pronounced defense mechanism in myocardial infarction patients. Of particular importance in this context are the strong oral-symbiotic wishes for dependency, observable in the transference that developed even in these few analytic group sessions. Superego demands and their representations are introjected by the patients in a manner reminiscent of the behavior of addicts, who, after temporarily having satisfied their needs, experience a feeling of security, much as the infarction patient feels "strong" and "fit" following the introjection of his omnipotent father and superiors and his overprotective mother. The strength and security gained through introjection, indeed through fantasies of incorporation, become threatened the moment this steady flow of introjections is interrupted. The result is a profound fear of loss of identity, of deterioration and death.

Arlow (1945) once stated that failure is synonymous with "being unmasked" or exposed: In this instance, a sense of helplessness, or in other words a devastating fear of worthlessness, can be perceived beneath the feelings of omnipotence and the manipulative control of objects. Realization or perception of a state of powerlessness must be averted, and this is accomplished through denial. Thus it has been observed that such patients generally resort to extremes of denial regarding all forms of dependency (Bahnson & Wartwell, 1962; Kits van Heijningen & Treurniet, 1966), including denial of an unconscious need for dependency.

Dependency creates profound anxiety, above all in the form of a fear of death, and can be overcome only through a gross denial of both inner and external realities. Consequently, grandiose fantasies of immortality are often reported by these patients (Moersch *et al.*, 1980). The circumstances leading to the disturbance or breakdown of this "homeostasis of denial" usually include humiliation, loss of prestige within one's occupation, and above all, separation.

Objects introjected in an addictive manner often become depersonalized or deindividualized in the process. From the patient's perspective, by transforming himself or herself into an institution or a system, or a part thereof, a mere human being conveys a sense of greatness and strength, as long as one conforms to and is at one with the perceived demands of the system.

In this context, the psychoanalyst becomes a transference object denied individual human features. The group's perception focusses on an asexual yet always dominant object, discernible mainly due to his or her functions and his or her "competence." This depersonalization and desexualization, the dehumanization resulting from denial mechanisms, are indicative of a considerable amount of destructive, nearly annihilating aggressiveness. If, as in Freud's (1924) opinion, denial is a form of defense consisting of the subject's refusal to acknowledge both the external and the inner, psychic reality of a traumatizing experience, then, with infarction patients, denial must be considered an additional "risk factor" (Moersch et al., 1980).

At this point in our work, denial among myocardial infarction patients can be observed in the following forms:

1. It is an important element of the personality structure and is mainly egosyntonic. Perhaps one can even speak of a "denial personality."
2. These patients exhibit a tendency toward denial of external reality, most obvious of all being the denial of the infarction itself as well as the concomitant factors of helplessness, threat to life, and the fear of being disabled.
3. There is a tendency toward denial of the individual uniqueness and vitality of human beings, who are often perceived and treated as "functions." A form of "deindividualization" takes place.
4. Finally—and often this is related to a life situation preceding the infarction—we find a denial of experiences related to separation. This also means a denial of death, above all of one's own mortality. Immortality is pursued in the sense of a perpetual ability to function, which essentially is the equivalent of a form of "dehumanization." This fantasy of grandeur often amounts to a reduction of that which is human to the level of functional machinery.

We find it justified to speak of, as Lowental (1984) phrased it, a "furious defensive battle to categorically deny the death instinct"—and in the process a conscious attempt is made by these patients to absolutely avoid both self-destruction as well as the acceptance of illness, mortality, and death.

Perhaps it would be possible to view the infarction itself, or the conflict-laden life situation preceding it (humiliation, separation) as Freud once described—"the end of the world," the first and decisive phase of psychosis. But contrary to the mad restitution of the psychotic, the myocardial infarction patient resorts to a form of restitutive denial. The "restitution" referred to here consists of conforming to "ultranormal," socially extremely acceptable views, coupled with the widespread collective fantasy of soon being restored to one's former level of efficiency, similar to the process of repairing a defective automobile. Following an infarction, the heart becomes the weak point in need of management, and successful management, in the patient's eyes, promises satisfaction, pride, and security.

Consequently, among infarction patients, there can often be observed an incapacity to mourn, characterized by denial, but also by projection, deindividualization and a systematization of other human beings. A. and M. Mitscherlich (1967) employed this term—*incapacity to mourn*—to characterize postwar German society—as a specific form of dealing with aggressiveness, destructivity, feelings of guilt, and loss of identity, or rather *not* dealing with them, not working through, but instead denying.

Of course, myocardial infarction is not a specifically German phenomenon but is one of the principal diseases of modern industrial society. It has become evident that in modern industrial society, there is a powerful tendency to attempt to overcome fear and aggressiveness—with their high potential for destructiveness—by means of technicalization and denial.

REFERENCES

Argelander, H. (1972). *Gruppenprozesse*. Reinbek: Rowohlt.

Arlow, J. A. (1945). Identification mechanism in coronary occlusion. *Psychosomatic Medicine, 7*, 195–209.

Bahnson, C. B., & Wardwell, W. J. (1962). Parent constellation and psychosexual identification in male patients with myocardial infarction. *Psychological Report, 10*, 813–852.

Bion, W. R. (1961). *Experiences in groups*. London: Tavistock.

Freud, S. (1924). Neurose und Psychose. *Gesammelte Werke* (Vol. XIII). London: Hogarth.

Grinberg, L., Langer, M., & Rodrigué, E. (1960). *Psychoanalytische Gruppentherapie*. Stuttgart: Klett.

Kits van Heijningen, H., & Treurniet, N. (1966). Psychodynamic factors in acute myocardial infarction. *International Journal of Psycho-Analysis, 47*, 370–374.

Köhle, K., & Gaus, E. (1979). Psychotherapie von Herzinfarktpatienten während der stationären und post-stationären Behandlungsphase. In T. von Uexküll (Ed.), *Lehrbuch der psychosomatischen Medizin.* München: Urban & Schwarzenberg.

Lowental, U. (1984). Psychosomatische Persönlichkeiten: Mehr als eine Dissonanz. *Fragmente, 12/13*, 160–175.

Mitscherlich, A. & M. (1967). *Die Unfähigkeit zu trauern.* München: Piper.

Moersch, E. *et al.* (1980). Zur Psychopathologie von Herzinfarktpatienten. Psyche *34*, 493–587.

Ohlmeier, D. (1975). Gruppentherapie und psychoanalytische Theorie. In A. Uchtenhagen *et al.* (Eds.), *Gruppenpsychotherapie und soziale Umwelt.* Bern, Stuttgart, Wien: Huber.

Ohlmeier, D. (1985). Gruppentherapie und Persönlichkeitsstruktur von Herzinfarktkranken. n W. Langosch (Ed.), *Psychische Bewältigung der chronischen Herzerkrankung.* Berlin, Heidelberg, New York, Tokyo: Springer.

V

Social and Political Implications

Often it has been said that reality is whatever belief is shared by two people. Belief formed through denial and shared by any two people becomes their reality; when denial extends from the intrapsychic realm into the interpersonal and further still into the societal, shared denial becomes culture. Just as denial can protect the individual from affect immutably linked to unacceptable perception, cultural denial can protect an entire people from understanding, from knowing the unbearable. For Israel the Holocaust has been the inescapable truth too extreme to be understood. Presented in any other context, the four chapters that complete this volume on denial might be overlooked as too close to the Israeli experience, too specific to one country or one people to warrant our full attention. Here in this volume, and now that we have learned so much about the mechanism of denial, such an attitude would be clearly apparent to us as a manifestation of our own denial, our understandable avoidance of what we cannot face in ourselves or in our view of humanity. Knowing the Holocaust sometimes means not knowing the Holocaust.

What we have presented as the first chapter in this section was actually presented by Wurmser as part of his discussion of another paper. We have elected to extract this portion of his remarks and offer them as an introduction to our consideration of denial in social and political process. Wurmser notes that the conference on which this volume is based took place at the university atop Mount Scopus, where Moses sent spies to reconnoiter the Promised Land; certainly, he says, no better place than the "Mountain of Perception" could be found to approach the culture of denial. What Freud encountered in his search for inner truth was not only the forces of resistance engendered by our embarrassment to reveal what lies beneath the surface we offer ourselves as well as our fellow humans but a cultural fear of knowing the psyche. To deny the existence of this psychophobia is to misunderstand the human.

Drawing on his personal knowledge of many cultures and many languages, Wurmser describes China as a land where inner conflict itself is disavowed, and psychic tension understood as failure to conform. In an era of mathematical rationalism, in which computers translate the feelings and analogs of real life into models built with digital precision, Western culture has begun more and more to avoid its linkage with history. It is not that we are doomed to repeat history but that we may end the story that is our culture if we fail to learn from the past, if we disavow the past. Scanning Jewish history over many centuries, Wurmser demonstrates the theme of denial and sets the scene for the chapters that follow.

Rafael Moses discusses the function of denial in many life situations. Military bravery depends on disavowal of danger; people frequently react to bad news by discounting its implications. Denial in praxis was seen and studied by Moses and his group at the request of Israeli and Egyptian leaders when the inhabitants of the Israeli town of Ophira seemed unable to comprehend that (as a result of the Camp David agreement) it was to be transfered to Egypt as Sharm-e-Sheikh and that they were all to be moved elsewhere in Israel. "Maybe," said some inhabitants only days before the transfer, "we can continue to run our small businesses in conjunction with the Egyptians." Moses points out that denial of danger, of any unpleasant reality, is normative for an Israeli citizen. Living surrounded by enemies, in a land peopled by survivors of unthinkable horror, denial becomes a way of life. What costs are thereby incurred becomes the subject of his inquiry.

Klein and Kogan explain that in traumatic neurosis, there is a triggering *incident* against which the individual must defend, whereas "the oppression of the Holocaust is a long series of traumatic experiences aimed not only against the physical integrity or at the life of the individual, but also likely to impair self-representation, beliefs, mythology and basic trust in the inner world." They illustrate denial sustained by fantasy formation, by means of words, and denial in praxis. As they sketch the structure of post-Holocaust defenses, what they call "the pact of shameful silence," Klein and Kogan ask us to understand that "what appeared to be a moderately healthy and adaptive way of dealing with the Holocaust had been achieved only by massive denial of the emotional impact of this period on the individual as well as the group." Often the children of survivors "recall" in great detail scenes of pre-Holocaust ghetto life, events and places actually unknown to them but adopted to create the illusion of continuity. By acceding to this intuited parental need, this next generation both accepts the parental system of denial and interferes with it. For the therapists who work with survivors and their children, certain risks must be appreciated. So much death, so much horror, so much terror is opened to view in such therapy that it is not uncommon for the therapeutic community to conspire in the maintenance of societal disavowal—we too must share the deafness when sound evokes such pain. As Israel has grown, as the Israeli experience is defined increasingly in terms of knowing, rather than not knowing the Holocaust, the very concept of psychotherapy implies awareness of Holocaust experience.

Finally, Davidson discusses the current shift in focus from physical survival with obligatory emotional withdrawal and blunting, toward systems of thought encouraging open discussion of "the unbearable pain and horror witnessed and experienced daily in the ghettos and concentration camps." Frequently, survival depended on hope facilitated by denial; the motivation to continue life itself was provided by mutual support based on avoidance of reality. "Prisoner doctors in the concentration camps were able to alleviate suffering and to give important albeit limited medical help to fellow inmates merely by augmenting denial." Utilizing cognitive skills as a massive defense against a terrifying reality, the rabbis of Auschwitz discussed "Halachic questions, rationally working out how they would in the future determine such questions as the marital status of survivors whose spouses had been [executed] without there being a witness to the actual death, as is required in normal life for the declaration of widowhood."

It is easier to skip this section, to avoid the searing emotion evoked in us by our identification with those who died, those who survived, and those who daily must treat the survivors. There are many areas of psychiatry that resemble Holocaust psychiatry. Patients with multiple personality disorder frequently describe the terrifying experiences for which they devised their dissociative defenses. No war is without horror, but those who saw in Viet Nam horror beyond their imagination are only now beginning to find words to describe their experience. More to the point, it is the general field of Holocaust study that has allowed us ears with which to hear these patients. Therapists are people with defenses based initially on intrapsychic mental mechanisms, but we are people brought up in societies, in cultures with specific patterns of denial and of awareness. It is fitting that the conference on which this volume is based was convened in Israel, for the shift from denial to awareness necessitated by the increasing emergence of Holocaust memories and Holocaust-related psychopathology has allowed our field opportunity for growth.

The existence of denial is a fact. We have seen it operate over a wide range of situations and settings. The purpose of this volume has been to bring these observations to the attention of our field and to all who are interested in the workings of the mind.

19

Cultural Paradigms for Denial

LÉON WURMSER

In this brief philosophical presentation, I would like to expand the scope from the clinical view of the individual to the history of cultures.

I begin with observations of two trends that affect many of our patients. One is "society's" joining into the psychophobia shown by so many of our patients: Their families, proponents of various treatment modalities, politicians, and other physicians agree that the study of inner life is superfluous and even harmful, a form of sinful self-indulgence on a level with symptoms, like drug use, and "there is nothing wrong with these people emotionally" (e.g., alcoholics). Beyond this there is now an immensely powerful current in modern *psychiatry* that advocates an elimination of most that is intimate, personal, long-term in psychiatric treatment; it is, in fact, quite successful in its endeavor to dismantle the influence psychodynamic understanding has had upon shaping the treatment of all psychiatric patients. Biological treatments and behavioral manipulation are more and more used, instead of working with and listening to individual patients. Kubie (1970) spoke 20 years ago about the *flight from patients*. In the years since, that flight has become a rout; and there are even legal and social moves afoot to do away with intensive long-term psychotherapy and psychoanalysis altogether—unless they are just private efforts of self-education. With that, the denial of

LÉON WURMSER • Private Practice, 904 Crestwick Road, Towson, Maryland 21204.

what is individual, personal, and specific, which so many of our patients had experienced in their families, is amplified by the agents of treatment themselves.

The other observation refers to the large-scale institutionalization and bureaucratization of life. "Alienation" by modernity has of course been observed for the last century and a half. Still, it might be rewarding to study the extent to which the use of others only as a means to an end, not as ends in themselves, is based on that denial of individuality (hence of creativity, of originality, and of privacy), and to what extent it similarly leads to acts of anarchic rebellion and self-sabotage, as we see in our clinical experience. The degree to which a cultural code of submission, self-abnegation, and conformity is prominent will be proportional to the forces of revolt and the rage against the carriers of values; but also the more totalitarian will be the eventual victor over the original ethical restraints. We know this of course from Freud's *Civilization and its Discontents* (1930), but I think the fact that such a sequence involves denial of the superego, the magical fantasies accompanying such denial, and violent defiance in action, may illuminate otherwise senseless events of mass destruction.

Moreover, political administration in general and bureaucracy in particular must use denial of the individual and personal in favor of technical control. The logical consequence of this denial is the bureaucratic elimination of those whose individuality does not fit the system. It makes, as Rubenstein (1978) pointed out, the Holocaust and its repetition possible, if not logical, the unleashing of what W. Burkert (1972) called *"Homo necans,"* Man the killer!

The balance between the individual and the political and social organizations that govern has always been a precarious one. If too much power is given to the one or the other, there is illness in the state, as Aristotle remarked.

But now I would like to cite two historical examples of denial within systems of great stability and without those features of impulsivity seen in the clinical reports (see Chapter 12). Such a study presents a philosophical problem. When we speak about denial, we assume we know what the truth is. We can only state these observations as made from our own, relative vantage point: For us it is the vantage point of very broad cultural and clinical knowledge that we all share, thanks to the modern systems of communication and retrieval of the knowledge accumulated over the millennia.

The first example is the *denial of the passage of historical time* and of the *historical present* throughout much of *Jewish* history after the Biblical period. I quote from Yerushalmi's (1982) work *Zakhor—Jewish History and Jewish Memory*. He sees in talmudic and midrashic literature a

> . . . characteristic concern for the larger configurations of history, coupled with indifference to its concrete particulars . . . an invisible history that was more real than what the world, deceived by the more strident outward rhythms of power, could recognize. (p. 21)

In the ritual act of the Seder with its "Ha lachma anya"—"this is the bread of affliction . . . [there is a] a fusion of past and present" (p. 44), where the "ke" (*like* the bread) had to be explicitly disavowed (p. 118) in favor of the reactualization in the present of Biblical reality. This is as such not different from other religious and mythical experiences, were it not simultaneously coupled with outright contempt for all historiography. Reading of profane history was seen by Maimonides as "a waste of time" (p. 33). And when there finally was a resurgence of true historical writing in the sixteenth century, its value was questioned by the writers themselves:

> It is as though the historian were saying in the same breath: Dear reader, although both of us know that what I am writing is unimportant, nevertheless it is important . . . [Also] historical chronicles are to be read "when sleep wanders" [bi-nedod shenah], for otherwise such reading is a frivolous waste of time that could otherwise be devoted to the serious study of sacred texts. (p. 67)

A similar point is made—against Martin Buber—by Gershom Scholem (1971) in his understanding of Kabbalah in general, of Hassidism in particular as an antiexistentialist, utopian movement:

> For precisely in that act [uplifting the sparks] in which we let the hidden life shine forth we destroy the here and now, instead of—as Buber would have it—realizing it in its full concreteness. (p. 241)

Also the classical literature of Hassidism "consistently treats the individual and concrete existence or phenomenon quite disdainfully" (p. 243). The concrete historical presence of the Galuth (the diaspora) is devalued, if not denied altogether, in behalf of the true reality of timeless Biblical history in the anticipated coming of the Messiah, the redemption and the homecoming.

Let us now turn to China:

> Harmony was seen as the great norm of both the natural and social worlds; Confucianism and Taoism were equally philosophies of balance, whether man's counterpoise was society or the natural cosmos. Imbalance would have meant man against man, man against nature, in either case a separation between the self and the "other." But Confucianism and Taoism, each in its

way, meant union, oneness, the concord and stasis of the eternal pattern"
(Levenson-Schurman, 1969, p. 113)

Also: "Conflict between Confucianism and Taoism was abortive, (a) because they had a common theme, *harmony,* and (b) because that common
theme, harmony, implied a philosophical deprecation of conflict"
(p. 116). Why Chinese culture appears to be so peculiarly antithetical to
the core of psychoanalysis lies in my opinion in this deep antipathy
against conflict, specifically inner conflict.

In the Chinese world view, inner conflict simply does not seem to
exist. Yet I have to qualify this a bit: There may be many other excep-
tions of which I am unaware, but there is one curious exception I would
like to mention. The nature of Chinese writing is such that many of the
ideograms present beautiful metaphors or astute direct observations—
for example, the character for shame, chi, is heart + ear 耻 —heart
for feeling in general, but the ear: "because the ear reddens when a
person is ashamed" (Weiger, 1927, p. 179). The fascinating little aperçu
is that the word for "I, ego, self, my own person," is derived from the
sign for weapon, gē = 戈, a halberd; it is "two 戈 weapons in conflict, two
rights that oppose one another, my right, and, by extension, my ego, my
own person; personal pronouns, I, me": wô = 我 .

If the character for sheep, the symbol of peace, is added, you get the
sign for yì 義 "harmony, peace restored after conflict, 我." I presume we
deal here with conflict between "me and others," but the analyst, looking
at this symbol of personhood, wonders (Weiger, 1927).

But back to the explicit literature about the Chinese attitude vis-à-vis
conflict: Fingarette (1972) writes that the ethical "task is posed in terms
of knowledge rather than choice" (p. 22) and notes "the absence of a
developed language of choice and responsibility" (p. 18) and Confucius's
"failure to see or to mention the problem of internal moral conflict" (p.
24). Hence "the proper response to a failure to conform to the moral
order [lǐ] is not self-condemnation for a free and responsible, though
evil, choice, but self-reeducation to overcome a mere defect, a lack of
power, in short a lack in one's formation" (p. 35). And he concludes:

> . . . that the images of the inner man and of his *inner conflict* are *not essential* to
> a concept of man as a being whose dignity is the consummation of a life of
> subtlety and sophistication, a life in which human conduct can be intelligible
> in natural terms and yet be attuned to the sacred, a life in which the practical,
> the intellectual and the spiritual are equally revered and are harmonized in
> the one act—the act of lǐ [Holy Rite]. (p. 36)

How can this large-scale denial—there of history and its con-
creteness, here of individual and social conflict, especially of inner conflict—lead to such an enormously stable result, both being the most

conservative continuous cultures in history (with the possible exception of India)? In the individual, we saw how denial is supported by actions to bring about a protective outer reality capable of screening out the frightening, hurtful, or shameful set of perceptions already tuned out by denial. As long as those actions truly support and protect, denial can be maintained. Psychoanalytic investigation of individual pathology suggests that those impulsive actions fulfill their task for only a brief period, leading instead to a vicious spiral of deepening shame, guilt, and anxiety.

In contrast, what I have described in both historical paradigms as denial has been supported by a huge *system of actions and of forms*, known in Jewish tradition as "halacha," as "talmud" in the literal meaning of learning, as "tzedaqa" (charity), and as the formalities of the "derech eretz" (social form); in China as Lǐ (ritual), Rén (humaneness, benevolence and kindness to the other person), Xiào (reverence, piety towards older persons), and Xüé (learning), all supported by a more or less well-functioning bureaucratic system with high emphasis on objective examination. I believe that these large *systems of action counterpoised to denial* makes them an effective combination of protection that in both instances endured more than two millennia. It has collapsed only under the onslaught of the modern intellectual and technological revolutions.

Combined with this action system was a *belief system* that placed very high value on the community, an undying community as a metaphysical entity, as in the "Kĕnesseth Yissrael" for example, at the opening of the Zohar; or the community over huge periods of time as seen in the family organization in China and depicted as the large "xìng," the smaller "shì," and its smaller subdivisions "jiā." In both too, the past remained a living and enduring presence to a much higher degree than anywhere else— the presence of millennia. Each individual had his or her place of dignity as part of the community. What Fingarette (1972) writes about the Confucian concept is applicable to the old Jewish world, too:

> The *mere* individual is a bauble, malleable and breakable, a utensil transformed into the resplendent and holy as it serves in the ceremony of life. But then this does not deny *ultimate* dignity to men and to each man; he is not a meaningless ant serving the greater whole. His participation in divinity is as real and clearly visible as is that of the sacrificial vessel, for it *is* holy. (p. 78)

I may add specifically, in regard to Judaism, that a high value was placed on *defiance*, on stubborn resistance against all threats, in behalf of a very specific and anciently formed identity—a defiance even in the face of death: It was a subordination of the individual and his death to the survival of the whole community—Klal Yissrael, the mystical community that transcended time and space, and thus made profane power, peril, and history ultimately irrelevant—deprived of deeper meaning, a "waste of time," compared with the "Netzach Yissrael," the eternity of Israel. A shared reverence for that which is written also weighs on the side of timelessness. Both are interpreting cultures, involved in the exegesis and hermeneutics of ancient texts, both sacred and profane, with particular attention to the meaning and origin of the signs themselves—in China of the ideograms that represent ideas in dreamlike, primary process condensations, in Judaism of the magical, world creating, divine letters.

It is far more difficult to see what is so denied in our culture, and whether action and belief systems are similarly stable counterweights as in the two paradigms given—or whether this denial, action, and belief resemble that in our patients. Meyerhoff, quoted by Yerushalmi (1982, p. 79), writes:

> The sense of identity and continuity with the past, whether our own or history's, has gradually and steadily declined. Previous generations *knew* much less about the past than we do, but perhaps *felt* a much greater sense of identity and continuity with it.

It seems to me that such continuity and identity with one's past are precisely given by those actions and mythical beliefs put in the center by the two ancient cultures—the Jewish and the Chinese. So the question is: What distinguishes us? What have we lost, and what have we gained—in terms congruous with the thoughts of this chapter? (When I talk about "us" I mean what some have called the culture built by, and resting upon, the "scientific intellectuals.")

What are our myths? One, with the greatest dominance, holds that all that we perceive as reality can be comprehended with, and dissolved into, that form of *rationality* that has been embodied best in mathematics and physics—even now in large part a rationality rooted in the mechanical physics of the nineteenth century. That means the view that *truth* is the highest value; all our endeavors ought to be directed toward ever closer approximation to such a true reality. We tear off mask after mask to approach what is seen as the essence. Such a view—mostly positivistic in nature—is now vehemently opposed by a much more relativistic philosophy. "What would we lose if we had no ahistorical theory-independent notion of truth?", asks Rorty (1980, p. 281). He would probably answer: "the illusion of something absolute"; in fact his reply is indirect: "knowing" is a "right, by current standards, to believe," and "conversation [is] the ultimate context within which knowledge is to be understood" (p. 389). Similar views are expressed by other contemporary philosophers of science, like Kuhn, Polanyi, and Holton.

What is, however, still unshaken by that philosophical reversal (actually one anticipated, most of all, I believe, by Nietzsche) is, as far as can be seen, the *primacy of the mathematical world view.* The modern scientific pragmatism of a Rorty or a Kuhn can proudly point to the eminent usefulness of such a world view.

Why then did I call it a myth? Its eminent and evident usefulness not withstanding, the question remains: Can such an approach centered on mathematical physics ultimately explain everything? The totality of such a claim is, I think, at this point mythical.

Based on such a mathematical rationalism, the systems approach has in praxis gained full sway over all of our life, especially with the awesome perfection of computers. With that, *quantity* has all but eclipsed the concept of quality or excellence. Quality is, at best, reduced to numbers. Personal creativity, individual specificity, originality, have little space in the world of computing; they are values restricted by and large to the arts and perhaps to cuisine or dress codes—with one mighty exception; there remains one area where the idea of "better" and "worse"—the idea of the comparison of qualities—has found a powerful bastion: that is, in competition. Even there, competitive superiority and inferiority are not measured so much in terms of creation or even excellence of performance as in terms of technological mastery, skills, power, fame, and financial status. In that regard, too, there has been much of a shift over the last century.

Parallel with this *myth of mathematical rationality as all-encompassing* runs the basic democratic credo of the *numerical equality* of everybody and of decision by majority.

Wherefrom though this centrality of mathematics?

The great turn toward modernity came with Galileo's shift to the ideality of numbers as a main tool to explain nature. That meant a jettisoning of Aristotle's view of the things of φύσις, of Nature (which included man), as striving toward perfection, toward their own intrinsic best or perfection and the right form. Instead, the adoption of the explanatory value of numbers meant the acceptance of Plato's equation of Good = Being = Number.

Consequently, instead of continuing to study—in the Aristotelian tradition—those regular transformations of individuum, state, and cosmos, according to their specific plans and their good or incomplete approximation, science had to reorient itself toward the Number, "Trennen und Zählen," in Goethe's words. Hence Quality receded from its central place in the understanding of Nature first, then of society, and now of the human mind as well. More and more it was and is being subordinated to Quantity, until it—the question of the Good—disappears entirely into what can be measured and counted.

Turning now to the sphere of *action,* we notice that this sway of mathematical rationality has led to an ever more radical exploitation of the laws and forces of inanimate nature on behalf of our short-range needs and desires. All the magical practices of Faust have been implemented in an all-encompassing conquest of material (not only inanimate) nature. The ever greater power of technology requires, however, also an ever more pervasive submission of all that is individual and personal to those *rules and standards* that have made possible such supreme mastery. It dictates a conformity of action, a kind of new ritual and formalism that is in no way less exacting than Halacha and Lĭ. And just as the latter two had rather little regard for the individual *per se,* or his or her creativity, nor for anything that was concrete, specific, in the here and now—in short, the existential dimension—so does the regime of the scientific intellectual and his technological Mephistos.

A sequel of such denial is the treatment of human beings only as means, not as "Selbstzweck," as aims for themselves. The commonplace application of the same terms of alienation, estrangement, depersonalization, both for the social and the psychopathological phenomenon, since the middle of the nineteenth century shows the recognition of this very dangerous development, but the diagnosis has unfortunately not led to any suitable treatment. That Golem has developed its own superhuman dynamics and power, dragging us all along—whether we run along with it or stand against it.

So, what is then *denied* in the sphere of perception? Ultimately everything that cannot be reduced: (1) to mathematical physics, (2) to standards of computation and technological control, (3) to numerical and impersonal equality, and (4) to the (physicalistic) balance of forces.

What is denied is the special value of much that is individual and creative; what is lost from sight is the importance of quality and excellence. What is more and more shunned is the concept of conflict, inner or outer, except insofar as it pertains to the types of competition mentioned, because system, its complementary opposite, is given near-absolute rule.

Humanity used as means, humanity as tool, humanity dehumanized and deindividualized, as Ohlmeier describes (see Chapter 18, this volume)—such a human being senses his or her humiliation and responds with helpless rage to this dehumanization.

Something else that is lost, therewith, is the feeling for community, both in space and in time. Numbers bridge all distances, but they fail to establish the true sense of community, that had at least been postulated for the "Kehilla" and the "Jia" (and many other forms of communities in the past), nor the sense of communion with tradition so highly prized in those two cultures of learning.

Another cultural value that is diminished, by universal leveling, is the sense for hierarchy of purpose, of qualification, of merit, although I would add that the examination system that the West has taken over from China, together with the bureaucratic system (Creel, 1970), establishes some new form of technological–scientific hierarchy.

The one great mind of the Western world who remained fundamentally opposed to that wholesale shift to the mathematical was Goethe. We all know how deeply Freud was influenced by him. Even the term upon which the whole building of psychoanalysis rests—inner conflict—was coined by Goethe. It is less well known but stressed by Waelder that Freud viewed the ego more and more in teleological terms and, Waelder says, approached the Aristotelian concept of *entelechy*—the reaching of one's individually right form (Waelder, in "Psychoanalysis: Observation, Theory, Application," pp. 340–341). *Entelechy* is the perfection inherent in the individual—in contrast to the modern aim of general truth, that is, of seeking ultimate reality in what is general, not individual.

It seems to me that psychoanalysis in its essence has tried to remain faithful to what is qualitative; to the forms, the images and constellations, and most of all the tensions and paradoxes of our inner world and to resist the temptations of quantity—the world of objects around us. Thus it is one of the few forces still opposing that relentless torrent that drives, it seems inexorably, toward the denial of part of human nature by quantification and computation.

But for how long?

We have seen the role of denial in these two ancient cultures, standing in intricate balance as part of stable configurations. We have examined the current thrust of denial in our own culture. The questions we cannot answer are these: How stable is this equilibrium of belief, action, and denial? Does it follow the two historical paradigms given? Or is it more similar to the clinical prototype?

REFERENCES

Burkert, W. (1972). *Homo necans*. Berlin: de Gruyter.
Cassirer, E. (1922). *Das Erkenntnisproblem* (Vol. 2). Hildesheim, Olms, (Reissued 1971.)
Creel, H. G. (1970). *What is Taoism?* Chicago: University of Chicago Press.
Fingarette, H. (1972). *Confucius—The secular as sacred*. New York: Harper Torchbooks.
Freud, S. (1930). Civilization and its discontents. In *Standard Edition*. London: Hogarth Press.
Gadamer, H. G. (1978). *Die Idee des Guten zwischen Plato und Aristoteles*. Heidelberg:
Gadamer, H. G. (1980). *Hegel's Dialektik*. Tübingen: Mohr.

Kubie, L. S. (1970). The retreat from patients. *International Journal of Psychology, 9*, 693–711.

Levenson, J. R., & Schurman, F. (1969). *China: An interpretative history.* Berkeley: University of California Press.

Rubenstein, R. R. (1978). *The cunning of history.* New York: Harper & Row.

Rorty, R. (1980). Freud, morality and hermeneutics. *New Literary History,* 177–185.

Scholem, G. (1971). *The messianic idea in Judaism.* New York: Schocken.

Waelder, R. (1951). The structure of paranoid ideas. In *Psychoanalysis: Observation, theory, application.* New York: International Universities Press. 207–228. (Reissued 1976.)

Weinstein, F. (1980). *The dynamics of Nazism.* New York: Academic Press.

Wieger, L. (1927). *Chinese characters and their origin, etymology, history, classification, and signification.* New York: Dover Publications. (Reissued 1965.)

Yerushalmi, Y. H. (1982). *Zakhor—Jewish history and Jewish memory.* Seattle: University of Washington Press.

20

Denial in Political Process

RAFAEL MOSES

When one peruses the literature on the defense mechanism of denial, one cannot fail to be impressed with the difficulties we encounter with this concept. Like so many concepts in psychoanalysis, denial is too elastic a term, including too large a group of defensive operations (cf. also Carmi, 1984). However, this state of affairs also has its advantages in that it allows for a conceptual development of the mechanism, albeit in different directions (Sandler, 1983). Some of the problems particular to the concept of denial that stand out in the literature are the following: (1) Is the institution of denial a conscious or an unconscious process? (2) Is it directed toward a threatening internal or a threatening external reality? (3) Does it occur at an early, primitive, archaic stage of development so that therefore we find it used by very disturbed persons—psychotic or borderline? (4) Or, alternatively, does it belong to a later stage and therefore is found mainly in neurotic and normal persons? (5) And finally, does the defense mechanism of denial delete, as it were, the total existence of the percept to be defended against, for the person who uses it? Or, alternatively, does it erase only the impact, the meaning or the affective meaningfulness of what threatens him or her who thus defends her- or himself?

A related question is whether the use of denial is concomitant with

---

RAFAEL MOSES • Sigmund Freud Center for Study and Research in Psychoanalysis, Hebrew University of Jerusalem, Jerusalem, Israel and Austen Riggs Center, Stockbridge, Massachusetts 01262.

the split proposed by Freud (1927a) with regard to fetishism, namely that there exist, concurrently, two perceptions of the threatening material: one that is accurate but unconscious and another, the denial, that contradicts reality and is therefore less threatening and less painful? With such a split, there still exist two possibilities: Denial may be so complete that there is no accurate conscious perception of the reality to be warded off at all; or the denial may be partial, so that at times there is a conscious or partly conscious perception of the threatening reality (cf. for a variety of descriptions and points of view, the works of Altschul, 1968; Brunswick, 1943; Deutsch, 1922; Dorpat, 1983; Freud, 1910b, 1924a,b, 1926, 1927a,b, 1938a,b; A. Freud, 1936; Geleerd, 1965; Greenson, 1952, 1958; Jacobson, 1957, 1967; Katan, 1964; Kernberg, 1975; Klein, 1937, 1946, 1952, 1963; Levin, 1969; Lewin, 1950; Linn, 1953; Lipson, 1963; Miller, 1977; Modell, 1962; Rubenfine, 1952; Siegman, 1967, 1970; Smith & Danielsson, 1982; Sperling, 1958; Trunnel & Holt, 1974; Waelder, 1951; Zetzel, 1949).

Clearly, these questions are to some extent confluent. If denial is used by neurotic persons, such a defense will tend more to be unconscious, will be more directed against external rather than internal percepts. In my view, it will then result in the coexistence of different levels of awareness. If, on the other hand, denial is viewed as a primitive archaic mechanism (Klein, 1952) and is probably—therefore—used more by psychotic persons (Jacobson, 1957, 1967; Lewin, 1950), then it will be seen as taking place on a level nearer consciousness; as being directed mainly against internal percepts—that is, drives and affects. It will then be more likely to be viewed as totally eliminating the threatening stimulus from consciousness. These problems have been addressed by Carmi (1984), the Kris Study Group of the New York Psychoanalytic Institute (1969), Dorpat (1983), who presents a microanalysis of the steps leading from perception to disavowal, by Stewart (1970), and finally by Smith and Danielsson (1982), who outline the defenses as they evolve through childhood and adolescence.

So much for a bird's-eye view of the very complex and fairly divergent literature on this widely discussed defense mechanism. A brief sentence of warning: In order to examine the mechanism of denial in some detail, we must artificially remove it from the surrounding psychological soil in which it is naturally consistently embedded.

I view the mechanism of denial as one that is at first primitive, in that it is used by children at an early phase. As Jacobson (1957) says, it is a defense that originates in the child's efforts to rid himself or herself of unpleasant perceptions of the outside world. Indeed, for the child, denial is almost appropriate and adaptive (cf. Anna Freud, 1946), whereas, in the adult, its use seems to many authors to be an indication of much psychopathology. At the same time, most authors agree, as did Freud in 1900, that denial is also a normal mechanism in adults. When used in a limited way, it is also a remarkably widespread mechanism in adults, more so than we generally allow. In grown-ups, the degree of denial activated will be roughly proportional to the severity of the threat from external reality, the danger to one's physical or psychological existence. And yet, it is not then the same primitive form of denial used either at an early age or by psychotic or borderline persons. It does not clash as completely with reality or wholly eliminate reality testing. Here, it is used with more differentiation and applies to a more limited area of reality and of psychic functioning. This adult version of denial is set in motion, then, by relatively healthy persons; it is unconsciously activated; and it is directed mainly if not exclusively at external reality. This external reality must, at the same time, always be representative of an overpowering threat with inevitable internal psychic correlates. Jacobson lucidly describes how, when such a threatening precept is disclaimed and disowned and then projected onto the outside, it enables the person to handle intrapsychic conflict as if it were a conflict with reality (1957). It seems both evident and logical that, in a similar way, *outside dangers are perceived in relation to the inner conflicts that they mobilize or are perceived to represent*—external and inner realities are perforce always interrelated.

It is my experience, as I will try to show, that such denial leads most often to a concurrent multilevel awareness of what is denied; that the two levels are not completely separate; and that they are not so separate as Freud saw them many years ago when he postulated a split in the ego with relation to the perception of the threatening reality of the absence of the penis in the woman (1927a). To my mind, the different levels of awareness are, rather, coexisting. They are often in a state of flux; this means that denial has its ups and downs; that there are changes over time both in what is denied and in the extent to which it is denied (cf. Moses & Cividalli, 1966).

The type of denial on which I focus is the one used by the individual; only through its description will I approach my subject proper, the use of denial in political process. I proceed in this way because, in my view, it is this type of denial—the neurotic, adult, normal kind—which is in use by persons in the large group, in the community, and in the nation and which becomes evident when one views political process.

The use of denial as a clear and well-defined mechanism in the form I have described is found most obviously in individual responses to the painful impact of an external reality. Here in Israel we cannot fail to be aware of two areas in which denial is thus used: soldiers in battle and persons mourning for their loved ones. Soldiers in battle deny the danger to which they are exposed. This has been general knowledge certainly since World War II and has been described by many (Colbach & Parrish, 1970; Ferenczi, 1921; Grinker & Spiegel, 1945a,b; Stouffer *et al.*, 1949; Zetzel, 1949). It seems that man needs to disavow extreme danger to life and limb in order to continue to function effectively. In this form of denial, what seems most striking is the soldier's apparent *unawareness* of the direct danger to which he is exposed. And yet, when talking to soldiers about the battles in which they participated, the impression persists that they did, at the same time, also have some awareness that they *could* be hurt or killed—most understandably so. We have learned in Israel that the extent of such denial and the degree of awareness of what is being denied clearly co-vary with changing social mores—another connection, then, between the individual and society in relation to denial (cf. Moses & Cohen, 1984).

A very marked form of denial in soldiers seems to occur when blatant dangerous reality is pushed away by the use of feelings of omnipotence that replace fear with an emotion that is its polar opposite. Such evidently omnipotent denial can be seen in soldiers who subsequently break down in combat but also in soldiers who face danger in heroic ways and are often decorated as a result. To the hero, awareness of danger often seems even further diminished. Perhaps all usage of denial toward an external danger involves some use of omnipotent thinking.

A variety of forms of marked denial can be seen in the initial reaction to learning of the death of a loved person. These range from the immediate "No! It cannot be!" to a concern that the dead loved one is suffering from the cold and rains of winter in his grave. We could enumerate a large variety of forms of denial in response to death over a wide continuum from normal to pathological (cf. Moses, 1986).

In our clinical experience, denial of severe external dangers always involves and requires the use of varying degrees of omnipotent thoughts and feelings. We know well how feelings of omnipotence defend against those of impotence. It was Melanie Klein who stated that "the denial of psychic reality becomes possible only through the feeling of omnipotence." Yet, the same is true for the denial of external reality, an aspect of denial we will now explore. In April of 1982, Sinai was due to be returned to Egypt under the agreement signed at Camp David. Ophira, known to the Arabs as Sharm-e-Sheikh, was a small town due to be returned as part of this agreement. When a group of mental health professionals interviewed a representative sample of Ophirians during the 3 months prior to their forced evacuation, the widespread use of

denial was most impressive. Three months before the due date we talked
to Ophirians about their future plans and their feelings. They told us
that they did not know yet where they would settle after evacuation. 2½
months, 2 months, 6 weeks, sometimes 4 weeks before the date on which
Ophira was once more to become Sharm-e-Sheikh in Egyptian hands,
many of its inhabitants had no plans—of where to move, of alternative
housing. Still later they had not arranged for the arrival of the movers
who were to take their belongings back to Israel before the handover.
The answers to our probing questions were evasive. They did not know
yet. There was still time. They would see. When pressed further, most of
them would finally say—often somewhat shamefacedly: "Well, maybe
they [the government] will change their plans at the last moment." Or:
"Maybe we can continue to run our small business in conjunction with
the Egyptians." Or, as a final resort, "maybe we can come back here
afterwards—they will need somebody to be the Israeli consul here, won't
they?" In this example, the denial used by a number of individuals
became group denial; individual denial evolves into public denial, and,
as such, it must be seen as part of the political process. Israelis and
Egyptians alike observed this facet of the political scene, although it was
hard to see any resultant dysfunction. All Ophirians managed to sort
things out in the end—with the help of the unmistakable pressure of
outside events, possibly aided a little by our nudging (cf. Moses,
Hrushovski-Moses, & Rosenfeld, 1987; Rosenfeld, Hrushovski, Moses,
& Beumel, 1984).

A more frequent example of the denial of an unpleasant or dangerous external reality for Israelis and one closer to home in everyday
life can be seen in the attitude of many of us—for decades now—to the
daily dangers that face us. We would manage not to be aware of the fact
that in the round of our daily activities we were being endangered by a
variety of possible routes of attack: Terrorist attacks throughout the last
five or six decades; the fire of Jordanian snipers from the walls of the old
city between 1948 and 1967; the recurring danger of a new outbreak of
hostilities; the danger of Israeli cities being bombed or attacked by mis-
siles; or even of Israel being overrun and occupied by an Arab army—all
"unthinkable" dangers. Or the only nowadays much more "thinkable"
dangers to which our loved ones were exposed: those who lived here; or,
even more so, the sons in the Israeli army, who were—and are—exposed to possible wounding or death. As part of normal living, most
Israelis would not pay attention to these actually quite considerable risks.
You may say that they—we—needed to disavow them, to keep them out
of awareness in order to continue functioning. For how can one function
adequately when concerned at all times about very real threats to one's

life and limb? We all know that the same is true in other parts of the world where violence can suddenly erupt. In Northern Ireland, or in London when a bombing has taken place, or in New York when in danger of a mugging—or anywhere else in the world where such dangers exist—people do not continuously maintain conscious awareness of the risks they incur. We are all acquainted with the fact that persons with friends or loved ones in an area where such violence occurs will worry about them much more than do the subjects of their concern. Danger looms in inverse proportion to its immediacy when denial clouds perception. And this denial, too, has an omnipotent quality. In my view, the ongoing denial of continuously existing external dangers, such as those faced in Israel, becomes part of the public life of that society. It is part of the political process in that it has become part of a pattern of living for the majority of the population. As such, it is usually sanctioned and supported by the powers that be. People within a network will support each other in denying, that is, ignoring such dangers. Thus such widespread denial results also from political events, among other factors, and will in turn affect the political events, including decision making.

A further question needs to be asked: Is there a price paid for this type of denial? And furthermore, does the price paid for the denial of danger—facing the individual or the group—lie in a reduction of the urge to solve the basic problems that underlie these dangers? Is it appropriate to seek an analogy for widespread communal denial with that for the individual, for example, when he or she—by denying the existence of a fatal illness—in fact increases the likelihood of its being fatal? Or when an unwed young woman massively denies her progressing pregnancy, thereby making it difficult or impossible to have the pregnancy interrupted?

Let us return to that question later and look now at another form of denial used by Israelis. This is a denial of our own aggressive behavior in many situations of daily life. Whereas outsiders coming to Israel react strongly to the amount of aggression expressed, for example, while driving, either verbally or in the act of driving itself, or when standing in line, or when attending to various bureaucratic errands, Israelis will tend to be unaware of this phenomenon. Or at least they tend to be much less aware of it than outsiders (cf. Moses, 1983). It does strike them more when they return home from several weeks or months abroad. This use of denial does not, on the face of it, seem to involve external danger. However, when trying to understand the genesis of this aggressive behavior, we may wonder whether it is aroused in response to the very serious dangers that Israelis face, and if so, whether such aggressive behavior might serve to discharge excess aggression. Such denial might then be a part of the wider denial of the daily dangers that—perhaps—arouse such increased aggressiveness.

The use of the mechanism of denial by Israelis is also evident in relation to the Holocaust. The impact of the Holocaust and of the terrible experiences undergone by those who survived and by those who did not, had not been allowed full awareness by Israelis for many years after the facts of the Holocaust were known. Although the bare facts were certainly public knowledge by 1945, it took much longer for them to sink in, to be accepted, to be integrated into the Israeli psyche. This denial extended to the recognition of psychological reactions to the Holocaust, descriptions of which appeared in the professional literature only in the late 1950s or early 1960s—a time interval of 15 years! (cf. Moses 1984).

Similarly, psychological reactions of the children of Holocaust survivors should rationally have been expected, considering the immensity of the experiences undergone by their parents and given our knowledge of how psychological conflicts and disturbances in one generation influence the next. And yet, it was only some 10 years ago that we became familiar with the term and with the syndrome of the "second generation of the Holocaust." In all this, we are not alone: The same quality of denial can be discerned in people the world over: The immensity of the holocaust was pushed out of awareness all over the world; the psychological syndromes were not described earlier outside of Israel; the full taking-in of the awful facts was neither easier nor quicker elsewhere. And, in fact, tragedies of a lesser magnitude elsewhere in the world have been—and are being—pushed out of awareness, that is, denied, by people everywhere all the time.

You may ask me then, if that is so, what is so special about Israeli denial? Let us leave aside the question of whether, as Israeli Jews, we should have been more aware of the Holocaust, of its happenings and its impact, than others elsewhere.

The answer to the question of denial among Israelis is, of course, that its use is by no means special to our national group. I have presented to you examples taken from the Israeli scene because that is the scene I know best. But I firmly believe that the use of the mechanism of denial in political process is ubiquitous. In each nation and each society, denial will take on a form, a garb that is specific to those circumstances that elicit denial. Such a specific form would be akin to how the development of a given reaction pattern is shaped by the conflict of an individual. In the society, these circumstances presumably consist, among others, of something related to national characteristics and to the given external exigencies.

I believe that the use of denial can be observed not only in the inhabitants of Ophira as they were about to be expelled; not only in the average Israeli who denies the dangers of daily life or the not quite so daily dangers of the outbreak of war; not only in the history of the political Zionist movement, particularly toward the Arabs in Palestine and toward Arab nationalism. The same usage of denial can be found anywhere in the world—more particularly, more strongly so when and where there is acute conflict. We, most of us, push out of awareness whichever warning signal is presented to us. Most people in the United States, in Europe, and in Soviet Russia deny more or less continuously the dangers inherent in the possibility that an atomic war might be unleashed. Such dangers, too, are so appalling as to defy imagination and therefore invite denial. People in strife-torn areas of Ireland must similarly make use of denial to avoid the paralysis, the hopelessness, the anxiety that would accompany a realistic appraisal of the situation. Denial was also at work in those U.S. army officers who did not pull together the information at their disposal in 1941 to predict the Japanese attack on Pearl Harbor; and the scene was similarly set for denial for those Israelis who failed to use available information to predict the Yom Kippur War. And so it is also in individuals: in the soldier in battle; in those of us who suddenly lose a loved person; in those who face a fatal or serious illness—particularly of our own but also of those who are very close to us. Denial of this kind must be viewed as a ubiquitous phenomenon, denial used by adults, by neurotic and normal rather than psychotic persons, denial that wards off external rather than internal reality; denial that is an unconscious mechanism; denial that is accompanied by fluctuations over time in the degree of awareness within the person. At different times, on different days, in different circumstances, in different relationships, one is more aware of what is denied; at others less.

Scientific discussion that singles out one mechanism of defense permits us to isolate one aspect of psychological functioning despite the fact that, in life, it is intimately interwoven with other defenses and other psychological material. It is important for the assessment of the use of this particular mechanism of defense and perhaps of all such mechanisms to evaluate and to understand the quantitative aspects of denial. Even if we assume that some degree of denial at certain times allows us to cope more effectively than otherwise, such denial must clearly be limited both in the period during which it is used and in its extent. As soon as denial is used to too great an extent or for too long a time or at the wrong time, our ability to cope effectively will be impaired. Defensive mechanisms in humans often and easily overshoot their mark and extend beyond their prescribed goal.

Finally, I would like to return to the question of the price paid for this type of denial in political process? Bluntly stated, I believe that such denial brings about an impediment in the ability to face and therefore deal with the danger that is being partially denied. By not facing danger, the society, just as the person, is able to deal less efficiently than possible with the approaching threat. By the time denial has become a significant factor in political process, efficiency has already been considerably impaired. We can all give many examples of how this kind of denial hampers the individual in facing up to and, therefore, actively dealing with approaching danger. When passing the scene of an accident, we endanger our lives more than is necessary, by denying its impact and the lesson to be learned from it. The cancer patient who denies symptoms in this way thereby postpones diagnosis and treatment. The European, or American, or Israeli citizen who lives exposed to nuclear danger and denies the threat of extinction is thereby less able to work actively for change. Pearl Harbor and the Yom Kippur War could not be appropriately faced by those who were attacked because of denial. Similarly, I believe that we Israelis inhibit our ability to deal with dangers actively and successfully by partially denying the threats that face us, dangers with psychological as well as very real political implications.

One first step in combating denial in political process generally and its use in Israel particularly is to become aware of the widespread use of denial and through such awareness to begin to counteract its excessive usage.

REFERENCES

Altschul, S. (1968). Denial and ego arrest. *Journal of the American Psychoanalytic Association, 16*, 301–318.

Brunswick, M. (1943). The accepted lie. *Psychoanalytic Quarterly, 12*, 458–464.

Carmi, M. (1984). A critical discussion of the concept of denial (disavowal) in psychoanalytic literature. Unpublished master's thesis, Hebrew University of Jerusalem.

Colbach, E. M., & Parrish, M. D. (1970). Army mental health activities in Vietnam 1965–1970. *Bulletin of the Menninger Clinic, 34*, 333–342.

Deutsch, H. (1922). Ueber die pathologische Luege (Pseudologia fantastica). *Zeitschrift fur Psychoanalyse, 8*, 153–167.

Dorpat, T. L. (1983). The cognitive arrest hypothesis of denial. *International Journal of Psychoanalysis, 64*, 47–58.

Ferenczi, S. *et al.* (1921). *Psycho-analysis and the war neurosis.* London: International Psychoanalytic Press.

Freud, A. (1946). The ego and the mechanisms of defense. New York: International Universities Press.

Freud, S. (1900). Interpretation of dreams. In *Standard edition* (Vols. 4, 5). London: Hogarth.

Freud, S. (1910). The psychoanalytic view of psychogenic disturbances of vision. In *Standard edition* (Vol. 11, pp. 209–218). London: Hogarth.

Freud, S. (1924a). The loss of reality in neurosis and psychosis. In *Standard edition* (Vol. 19, pp. 183–187). London: Hogarth.

Freud, S. (1924b). Neurosis and psychosis. In *Standard edition* (Vol. 19, pp. 149–153). London: Hogarth.

Freud, S. (1926). Negation. In *Standard edition* (Vol. 19, pp. 235–239). London: Hogarth.

Freud, S. (1927a). Fetishism. In *Standard edition* (Vol. 21, pp. 149–157). London: Hogarth.

Freud, S. (1927b). Humour. In *Standard edition* (Vol. 21, pp. 159–166). London: Hogarth.

Freud, S. (1938a). An outline of psychoanalysis. In *Standard edition* (Vol. 23). London: Hogarth.

Freud, S. (1938b). The splitting of the ego in defensive processes. In *Standard edition* (Vol. 23, pp. 271–278). London: Hogarth.

Geleerd, E. (1965). Two kinds of denial. In M. Schur (Ed.), *Drives, affects and behavior* (Vol. 2; pp. 118–127). New York: International Universities Press.

Greenson, R. (1952). On negation and denial. Paper read before Los Angeles Psychoanalytical Society.

Greenson, R. (1958). On screen defenses, screen hunger and screen identity. *JAPA, 6,* 242–263.

Grinker, R. R., & Spiegel, J. P. (1945). *War neurosis*. New York: Blakiston.

Grinker, R. R., & Spiegel, J. P. (1945). *Men under stress*. New York: Blakiston.

Jacobson, E. (1957). Denial and repression. *JAPA, 5,* 61–92.

Jacobson, E. (1967). *Psychotic conflict and reality*. New York: I.U.P.

Katan, M. (1964). Fetishism, splitting of the ego and denial. *International Journal of Psychoanalysis, 45,* 237–246.

Kernberg, O. (1976). *Borderline conditions and pathological narcissism*. New York: Jason Aronson.

Klein, M. (1937). A contribution to the psychogenesis of manic-depressive states. In *Contributions to Psychoanalysis* (pp. 282–309). London: Hogarth and Institute of Psychoanalysis.

Klein, M. (1946). Notes on some schizoid mechanisms. *International Journal of Psychoanalysis, 27,* 99–110.

Klein, M. (1952a). Some theoretical considerations regarding the emotional life of the infant. In *Envy and gratitude and other works*. London: Delacorte Press. (Reissued 1975).

Klein, M. (1952b). Some reflections on the Oresteia. In *Envy and gratitude and other works* (pp. 275–299). London: Delacorte Press.

Klein, M. (1963). *Our adult world*. New York: Basic.

Kris Study Group. (1969). *The mechanism of denial*, Monograph III. B. Fine *et al.* (1969). New York: I.U.P.

Levin, S. (1969). A common type of marital incompatibility. *JAPA, 17,* 421–436.

Lewin, B. (1950). *The psychoanalysis of elation*. New York: Norton.

Linn, L. (1953). The role of perception in the mechanism of denial. *JAPA 1,* 690–705.

Lipson, T. (1963). Denial and mourning. *International Journal of Psychoanalysis, 44,* 104–107.

Miller, F. (1977). Denial: A contribution to psychoanalytic theory. *Journal of the American Academy of Psychoanalysis, 5,* 187–194.

Modell, A. H. (1961). Denial and the sense of separateness. *JAPA, 9,* 533–547.

Moses, R. (1983). Emotional response to stress in Israel: A psychoanalytic perspective. In S. Bresnitz (Ed.), *Stress in Israel* (pp. 114–137). New York: van Nostrand Reinhold.

Moses, R. (1986). Denial in non-psychotic adults, Samiksa. *Journal of the Indian Psychoanalytical Society, 40*(3), 77–93.

Moses, R., & Cividalli, N. (1966). Differential levels of awareness of illness: Their relation to some salient features in cancer patients. *Transactions of the New York Academy of Science, 125,* 984–994.

Moses, R., & Cohen, I. (1984). Understanding and treatment of combat reactions: The Israeli experience In H. Schwartz (Ed.), *Psychotherapy of combat veteran.* (Chap. 10, pp. 269–303). New York: Spectrum Publications.

Moses, R. (1984). An Israeli psychoanalyst looks back in 1983. In S. Luel & P. Marcus (Eds.), *Psychoanalytic reflections on the Holocaust: Selected essays* (pp. 52–70). Denver: University of Denver. New York: Ktav Publishers.

Moses, R., Hrushovski-Moses, R., & Rosenfeld, J. (1987). Facing the threat of removal— Lessons from the forced evacuation from Ophira. In E. Cohen (Ed.), The forced removal of settlements and towns from Sinai, *Journal of Applied Behavioral Science, 23*(1), 53–71.

Rosenfeld, J., Hrushovski, R., Moses, R., & Beumel, R. (1984). North of Eden: The evacuation of Ophira, Sinai. *Jerusalem Quarterly, 33,* 109–124.

Rubenfine, D. L. (1952). On denial of objective sources of anxiety and "pain." *Psychoanalytic Quarterly 21,* 543–545.

Sandler, J. J. (1983). Reflections on some relations between psychoanalytic concepts and psychoanalytic practice. *International Journal of Psychoanalysis, 64,* 35–45.

Siegman, A. (1967). Denial and screening of object images. *JAPA, 15,* 261–281.

Siegman, A. (1970). A note on the complexity surrounding the temporary use of denial. *JAPA, 18,* 372–378.

Smith, G. W., & Danielsson, A. (1982). *Anxiety and defensive strategies in childhood and adolescence,* Psychological Issues, Monograph 52. New York: I.U.P.

Sperling, S. (1958). On denial and the essential nature of defense. *International Journal of Psychoanalysis, 39,* 25–38.

Stewart, W. A. (1970). The split in the ego and the mechanism of disavowal. *Psychoanalytic Quarterly, 39,* 1–16.

Stouffer, S. A., & Lumsdaine, A. A. (1949). *The American soldier: Vol. 2. Combat and its aftermath.* New York: Wiley.

Trunnel, E., & Holt, W. (1974). The concept of denial or disavowal. *JAPA, 22,* 769–785.

Waelder, R. (1951). The structure of paranoid ideas. *International Journal of Psychoanalysis, 32,* 167–177.

Zetzel, E. (Rosenberg) (1949). Anxiety and the capacity to bear it. *International Journal of Psychoanalysis, 30,* 1–12. Also in *The capacity for emotional growth.* New York: I.U.P. (1970).

21

Some Observations on Denial and Avoidance in Jewish Holocaust and Post-Holocaust Experience

HILLEL KLEIN AND ILANY KOGAN

DENIAL AS A DEFENSE MECHANISM DURING THE HOLOCAUST

The Holocaust is the dark core of the twentieth century. It has assumed a place among those events that have permanently shaped our perception of humans. It has altered our vision of the present and of the prospects for the future. As time passes, the need to interpret its relationship within the whole fabric of human experience becomes more pressing, so that we neither blind ourselves to the aggressor/victim within us, nor ignore the human psychobiological capacity for recovery, healing, and revival (Klein, 1983). This chapter presents an analysis of the vicissitudes of denial during and after the Holocaust.

The mechanism of denial was prominent in the interplay of the complex network of defenses against the phantasmagoric realities of the

HILLEL KLEIN • Private Practice, 14 Tchernichovsky Street, Jerusalem, Israel. ILANY KOGAN • Private Practice, 2 Mohaliver Street, Rehovot, Israel.

apocalyptic world of ghettos and concentration camps. Denial through the cognitive processes of memory, fantasy, and words as well as through acts was one of the adaptive defenses used to escape from the timeless, arid wasteland to a world beyond the barbed wire.

Denial of what was happening in the outside and inside world of individual and family was sometimes part of the day-to-day fight for survival, whereas, at other times, when life was unbearable, it was an expression of the death wishes, as they were expressed in the Musselman stage.[1]

At the other pole stands the heroic fight of the Jewish Warsaw fighters, which we can understand as denial of individual physical survival in the service of the realization of self-ideal and fusion with something that is eternal.

There is an apocalyptic dimension of trauma in the totality of terror, in the psychotic cosmos of the concentration camp. Trauma, in the normal world, is defined by most authors by its economic nature, a disturbance of the usual distribution of psychic energy, the temporary overriding of the pleasure principle and regression to archaic fantasy level (A. Freud, 1967; S. Freud, 1920).

We have tried to redefine the characteristics of the trauma of the Holocaust in the following way: Whereas in traumatic neurosis there is typically a sudden single traumatic experience that destroys the defenses against excitation, the oppression of the Holocaust is a long series of traumatic experiences aimed not only against the physical integrity or the life of the individual but also likely to impair self-representations, beliefs, mythology, and basic trust in the inner world; it can bring fragmentation, doubts in the self and the world of ideas in which one was reared. In confrontation with these traumatic experiences, denial served as a defense mechanism. We will explore here three forms of denial: (1) denial sustained by fantasy formation, (2) denial by means of words, and (3) denial in act.

The concept of *denial sustained by fantasy formation* contains a paradoxical attitude to reality during the Holocaust. The world of fantasy was the only way to return to a world where the concept of true reality existed; this reality continued as a sense of love, normal relationships as they express themselves in group formations, forming a bridge from the past to the future. In order to conserve of inner reality and the con-

---

[1]Robert Lifton, in *The Nazi Doctors,* cites Langbein's *Menschen in Auschwitz* (Vienna: Europ-verlag), 1972, p. 114 as follows: "'Musselman' or 'Moslem' was camp jargon for the living corpses who were so named, according to Hermann Langbein, because "when one saw a group of them at a distance, one had the impression of praying Arabs." Thus, Musselman has come to signify zombie, or "the living dead."

sistency of one's own self, the survivors had to deny the chaotic external reality threatening them with annihilation.

During the Holocaust, denial sustained by fantasy served also to devalue the internal and external realities of ghetto and concentration camp by substituting in their place rescue fantasies, daydreams with ego-syntonic content. Yet, all the while, the knowledge that this was, alas, only fantasy remained unobscured. In "Civilization and its Discontents," Freud refers to this substitution of life by fantasy when he speaks of the intention to "make oneself independent of the external world by seeking satisfaction in internal pyschical processes" (Freud, 1930). At the time when the sense of reality emerges, the fantasy imagination is expressly exempted from the demands of reality testing for the purpose of fulfilling wishes that are difficult to carry out (A. Freud, 1946). During the calamity of the Holocaust, denial sustained by fantasy formation may be seen as one of the hallmarks of a still existing ego functioning. It serves as a screening instrument in the service of the ego: It was used to modify and elaborate the actual current external and internal experiences by illuminating the semirepressed memories of the good object representations of the past without removing them too far from reality.

It is our hypothesis that, during the period of prolonged traumatization produced by the Holocaust, denial sustained by fantasy formation functioned as a defense against traumatic overstimulation—as an attempt to get distance from the external "fantasylike" world of aggression and hopelessness (Klein, 1973a).

The *denial by means of words*—poems and prayers, singing of songs and psalms with highly pleasurable or supportive content, which contrasted strikingly with reality, was a repetitive coping mechanism to overcome anxiety and depression. By using psalms, people who had never been religious denied their hopelessness and the omnipotence of the aggressor. The longing for fusion of the individual and the group with a benign loving and holding God gave the feeling of hope in spite of the total destruction. For example, the song that one group of survivors sang after the destruction of their ghetto was "Our soul is waiting for God. He is our saviour, He is our helper."

Another example is the poem of Mordechai Gebirtig, "Es wird kummen a Tog von Nekumme"—"The Day of Vengeance Will Come" (Gebirtig, 1937) in which the poet denies his own anxiety and fear about annihilation, longing for vengence toward the tormentor on a universal level. Hope may be regarded as the condensation of the total reservoir of internal good objects and fantasies projeced onto the future, using relevant interpersonal experiences from past and present, denying other fragments of reality that could be devastating (Klein, 1973a). Hope, which was an essential resource in the tolerance of pain and painful affects during that period, has in it an element of denial.

The mechanism of *denial in act* was even more prominent in children than in adults. "Denial in act" was expressed sometimes in change of roles, children becoming parents of their own parents by helping or even rescuing them. Denial of extreme danger such as rescuing kind of activities, as smuggling food, were changed into playful activities connected with feelings of pleasure and vengeance toward the aggressor. In situations of separation and abandonment that awakened anxiety, the children's basic defense was denial. There was a similar tendency to deny conflicts of envy, guilt, and intrafamilial hostility and to express all of these toward the aggressor. Friendships and group formations helped the survivors to deny in act the loss of their beloved ones and build a new sort of family with cohesive libidinal ties of holding quality, wherein members were assigned different roles in fantasy and reality.

To sum up, denial in the face of danger is a part of the attempt by the psychic apparatus to hold on to the known and cherished parts of the self. Therefore, parallel to the denial of dangerous external and internal reality, a process of reindividuation takes place.

DENIAL AS A DEFENSE MECHANISM IN THE PHASE OF RECOVERY FROM TRAUMATIZATION

The Pact of Shameful Silence

In the post-Holocaust era, we can observe again the denial of knowledge, of acceptance of the Holocaust, as part of a complex defense mechanism interfering with memory and the work of mourning. What appeared to be a moderately healthy and adaptive way of dealing with the Holocaust had been achieved only by massive denial of the emotional impact of this period on the individual as well as the group.

Another reason for silence, apart from the need of the survivors to forget, had to do with the world's need to forget and deny. Eli Wiesel wrote:

> Had we started to speak, we would have found it impossible to stop. Having shed one tear, we would have drowned the human heart. So invincible in the face of death and the enemy, we now felt helpless. . . . We were mad with disbelief. People refused to listen, to understand, to share. There was a division between us and them, between those who endured and those who read about it, or would refuse to read about it. (Wiesel, 1977)

We have learned that the survivors' needs for a process of restitution and for love were often ignored by the German people, augmented by an inability to mourn, and amplified by a society overwhelmed with guilt, which denied, avoided, and shunned them. The survivors discovered that a guilty society was unable to respond to their needs for love, for rebirth, and restitution (Klein, 1983).

DENIAL IN THE PROBLEMS OF READAPTATION AND REINTEGRATION OF THE SURVIVORS TO SOCIETY

It appears that, for survivors of the Holocaust who live in Israel, daily confrontation with the problems of the Holocaust makes repression and denial of their own traumatic past very difficult. They are confronted with these problems through the media of communication, which bring detailed news about trials of war criminals, political discussions and decisions about relations with Germany. Especially since the Eichmann trial, crude denial, as it was used by political leaders, became impossible. Moreover, living together with so many people who have shared the same tragedy, experiences made current by the annual recurrence of Remembrance Day that brings reminscence of every destroyed community, complicates any attempts at denial and repression.

The special history of the survivors creates highly charged conflicts for these individuals and their families who live in Israel—a country surrounded by enemies. They deny identifying the Germans with the Arabs, but, in many instances, they reveal that they do associate the two enemies with each other, as illustrated by the remark of one man: "When I fought for the first time with a gun in my hands, I thought what a pity I did not have a gun then" (Klein, 1972).

The problem of the "second generation" involves the adaptation and integration of survivors to their new life. The second generation was seen by the survivors as confirmation of life and denial of their losses. This denial was connected with obsessive undoing, as when one gives birth to a child even when not prepared psychologically for parenthood. Paradoxically, the process of parenting regenerated the capacity for love and holding in the survivor–parents, helping to undo or repair the denial-based attrition of these human capacities taken from them in the enduring longitudinal process of destruction. The total preoccupation with the future of the child and the actual process of parenthood awoke in many survivors old resources and capabilities for holding and the capacity to be one with the child, as well as the more difficult processes inherent in the separation/individuation phase of development. Alas, however, many survivor parents had been injured for life by the terror that their children could be injured and destroyed. These parents often

developed a variety of obsessive-compulsive symptoms of overprotec-
tiveness in denial of their own aggressive wishes and as a defense against
a world changed into a traumatic millieu.

Notwithstanding the range of attitudes seen in individual survivor
families, each child born after the defeat of Hitler represented a victory
over the persecutor; at the same time, it also revived memories of the
children who had died, evoking guilt and shame. The complex and tense
emotions surrounding the arrival of an infant into any family are amplified so powerfully in these families of survivors that denial is overcome.
Memory floods consciousness and produces resonance between the terror of abandonment and loss and the joy of attachment.

Whether through shared dreams, shared fantasies, or intricate reciprocal acting out in fantasy, an illusion was created that parents and
their postpersecution children had been together before the actual birth
of these children (Klein, 1973b). One chid vividly and intuitively described the life of her mother's family, the street, and the house in which
they lived as if she were now living and acting in that world that had
perished. Yet, perhaps through this special bond, the child could replace
a mother, a sibling, or another child whose death had left the victimized
parent the misery of survival and guilt (Kogan, 1987). "Through my
children I live and through them I restore my dear lost ones"—children
may be a source of reassurance and confirmation of revival whereas, at
the same time, bearing the traces of unmourned loss.

DENIAL IN THE PROCESS OF THERAPY WITH SURVIVORS

Reluctance to seek treatment for psychological impairment is based
on large part on denial of injury. The feeling that they had "conquered
death" allowed the survivors to experience themselves as unique (in
having "been saved" from destruction in the midst of general catastrophe) and perhaps omnipotent. This form of infantile narcissism, rarely
verbalized, created a major therapeutic paradox (Klein, 1968).

In the process of psychoanalysis, we observe within both transference and countertransference many of the vicissitudes of the myths
of survival (Klein, 1981; Kogan, 1987). The person traumatized by Holocaust experiences or the child of a survivor tends to create personal
myths or fantasies different from those exposed to other types of traumata. Such myths will contain memories from the past and may serve to
preserve a traumatic screen (Kris, 1956), hiding massive amounts of
hostility unleashed by brutalization, anxieties, or personal symptomatology. The myth built up about his life in the Holocaust is intended to

solve the conflictual emotions and unconscious wishes about living or dying. We have followed these myths from parents to children through three generations (Klein & Kogan, 1986).

The development of the myths of survival is a longitudinal process beginning during the Holocaust, continuing its influence over the various phases of the life cycle. It influences body image, object relations, political views (of being a savior or a victim), and one's relationship to the problem of living and dying. Repressed and denied in the myths of survival are the negative aspects of one's experience antagonistic to the ideal self, such as lack of fidelity to one's own family or group when confronted with death; affirmative experiences were remembered again and again as islands of humanity that offered permission to live and to search for the ideal self. The personal myth affects the process of reparation for self, family, and future generations. Denial of "weaknesses," adaptive during traumatization, prevents intrapsychic solution and growth. The survivor may still be living in an internal world of apocalypse with a network of defenses inappropriate to the new, actual world. Denial interferes with the normal growth process—it is important that the survivors' children be influenced by reality, rather than by the myths of the omnipotent father or mother for whose acceptance and love they fight in an ambivalent battle their whole life. The child is trapped in an internal ambivalent relationship with either an omnipotent or a weak parent, one who failed to achieve his or her idealized self-image. An expression of the myths of survival in the survivor's life is the illusion, transmitted also to the second generation, that one can remain always young and omnipotent and thus avoid illness and death.

Psychoanalysis allowed the survivors to retreat from the world of external objects and assess their idealized selves as well as their own personal myths (including the myths of survival) with their full range of benign and negative aspects.

Another form of denial that we explored in the treatment of survivors was their need to deny the destruction of their families, which led to the searching activities characteristic of mourners: They not only tried to trace missing relatives in a reality-oriented way but also scanned crowds in unfamiliar environments in order to discover a face from the past (denial in act). This "urge to search for and recover the lost figures" (Bowlby & Parkes, 1970) stems from a rebirth fantasy connected with regression to magical thinking (Klein, 1973a,b).

The search through the inner world for lost faces and representations of the past is an attempt to reassemble the past inner landscape in the outer world. Only in a later stage of the treatment, when the need to deny takes a different form, might the patient grapple with the very fact of the death of his or her family and mourn properly. It was through this long mourning process that the survivors came to recognize the source of love within them and were thus made to be in touch with old sources of love allowed, capable of investment in new attachments.

In therapy with survivors, it could be observed that the largely verbalized and desomatized feelings of anxiety, depression, grief, and shame appeared when the patient–survivor overcame pathological denial and discovered within the ego adequate resources for tolerating pain and the painful affects connected with self-representation.

If this self-representation included modes of behavior acquired during the Holocaust by introjection and by identification with benign objects, the survivor was able to use defenses and actions as protection against becoming overwhelmed by painful affects of loss. On the other hand, when there was total denial of violent destructive impulses toward the idealized, but disappointing, dead love objects, resulting in rigid walling off of the object representation from the self-representation, there was disturbance in the handling of aggression and guilt toward the love objects, especially in situations of loss, separation, and guilt. The denied and repressed impulses returned and were experienced as depression (Klein, 1968).

Denial appears in the countertransference reactions of analysts in beginning to appreciate the facts of the Holocaust, for they too must defend against emotional turmoil. Williams and Kestenberg speak about a latency period that had to be traversed before one could give up the denial and repression of the unspeakable terror (Sonnenberg, 1974). Analyzing a survivor before a successful working through of denial and ignoring the patient's past led to countertransference problems that interfered with analyses of survivors and their children.

The wish of the survivor to find within the analyst a lost love object (for whose return the survivor waits) produces varying degrees of countertransference in the therapist, ranging from a wish to be the saviour to total rejection of the patient out of fear of complete engulfment and fusion. Yet another problem is the anxiety experienced by the therapist who feels required to make life and death decisions for a patient involved with projections of the persecutor. Benign interpretation, too, can have the quality of an ultimate verdict utterly dangerous to life because of the realness of one's past experiences. It is clear what far-reaching implications the sharing of death-imprinted experiences have on the therapeutic lines. The liberation of the denial in the analysis and the "sharing" of an atrocity event has a particular intimacy because it revitalizes intense, repressed affects and thereby creates powerful transference phenomena. Utter helplessness, the dissolution of one's world,

cruelty, all these interpenetrate with personal, psychosexual development themes—in the survivor who tells and in the therapist who listens.
Those powerful regressed affects have an additional stamp of realness to
them because of the actual historical event they represent.

Within the Jewish community, as in the world at large, there are
pressures to forget, even to deny the Holocaust, and to escape from the
burden of "survivor's guilt". We believe that there is a mistaken tendency to use the term *survivor's guilt* only in a pathological sense and thus to
give it a pejorative meaning. Survival guilt is adaptive when it links
survivor and offspring to the past, to those who died, to a sense of
belonging to the Jewish world (Klein, 1984). There are pressures, too, in
the opposite direction: One is enjoined to remember, to commemorate,
never to forgive or forget the trauma. An important task of the
therapeutic–educational community must be to discover ways of remembering the Holocaust without transmitting its traumatic potential.
Our message to the young generation is therefore: Do not deny but
remember in a life-affirming way!

REFERENCES

Bowlby, J., & Parkes, C. M. (1970). Separation and loss within the family. In E. J. Anthony
    & C. Koupernik (Eds.), *Child and his family.* New York: Wiley.
Freud, A. (1946). *The ego and the mechanism of defence* (C. Bains, Trans). New York: Interna-
    tional Universities Press. (Reissued 1966.)
Freud, A. (1967). Comments on trauma. In S. Furst (Ed.), *Psychic trauma.* New York: Basic
    Books.
Freud, S. (1920). Beyond the pleasure principle. In *Standard edition* (Vol. 17). London:
    Hogarth.
Freud, S. (1930). Civilisation and its discontents. In *Standard edition* (Vol. 21). London:
    Hogarth.
Gebirtig, M. (1937). *Meine lieder.*
Klein, H. (1968). Problems in the psychotherapeutic treatment of Israeli survivors of the
    Holocaust. In H. Krystal (Ed.), *Massive psychic trauma* (pp. 233–248). New York: Inter-
    national Universities Press.
Klein, H. (1973a). Delayed affects and after-effects of severe traumatisation. *Israel Journal
    of Psychiatry and Related Sciences, 10,* 118–125.
Klein, H. (1973b). Children of the Holocaust: Mourning and bereavement. In E. J. An-
    thony & C. Koupernik (Eds.), *Child and his family* (pp. 393–409). New York: Wiley.
Klein, H. (1981, September). Yale Symposium on the Holocaust. *Proceedings.*
Klein, H. (1983). The meaning of the Holocaust. *Israel Journal of Psychiatry Related Sciences,
    20,* 119–128.
Klein, H., & Kogan, I. (1986). Identification and denial in the shadow of Nazism. *Interna-
    tional Journal of Psychoanalysis, 67,* 45–52. Also *Psychoanalyse im Exil: Texte Verfolgter
    Analytiker.* Würzburg: Königshausen & Neumann, 1987.

Kogan, I. (1987). *Analysis terminable and interminable—Eros and thanatos at strife.* Paper presented at the 35th IPA congress, Montreal, 1987.

Kogan, I. (1987). *The second skin.* Paper presented at the 35th International Psychoanalysts Association congress, Montreal, 1987. In *International Review of Psychoanalysis*, 1988 *15*, 251–260.

Kris, E. (1956). The personal myth: A problem in psychoanalytic technique. *Journal of the American Psychoanalytic Association, 4*, 653–681. Reprinted in *Selected papers of Ernst Kris.* New Haven: Yale University Press, 1975, pp. 301–340.

Lifton, R. (1986). *The Nazi doctors.* New York: Basic Books.

Sonnenberg, S. M. (1974). Workshop report: Children of survivors. *Journal of the American Psychiatric Association, 22*, 200–204.

Wiesel, E. (1977). The Holocaust: Three views. *ADL Bulletin*, November, 1977.

22

Avoidance and Denial in the Life Cycle of Holocaust Survivors

SHAMAI DAVIDSON

> *What happened—really happened*
> *What happened—really happened*
> *What happened—really happened*
> *I believe with perfect faith*
> *That I'll have the strength to believe that*
> *What happened—really happened.*
> T. Carmi (1977)
> "Anatomy of a War"

> *Not everything that is faced can be changed: but*
> *nothing can be changed until it is faced.*
> James Baldwin

The widespread processes of avoidance and denial manifested in relation to the Holocaust are a reflection on the one hand of humanity's desperate struggle to survive physically in the face of the overwhelming threat of death and on the other of the attempt to ward off knowledge of inconceivable catastrophe that threatens its psychological survival. The subject is thus one of adaptation to death and disaster in our culture. It seems that the danger to life can be faced and attempts made to master

SHAMAI DAVIDSON • Late of the Shalvata Mental Health Center, Hod HaSharon 45100, Israel.

and overcome it only up to a certain level of intensity. Beyond this level and especially when the danger is unprecedented and inconceivable in terms of the individual's life experiences and system of values, avoidance and denial processes are mobilized as important protective and coping devices enabling the victims to carry on with the daily struggle for survival. The general pattern of denial was contributed to and reinforced by: (1) the lack of knowledge and information available to the Jewish masses isolated in ghettos and camps; (2) the secrecy and systematic deception practiced by the Nazis in order to conceal the perpetration of genocide; (3) the collective historical "memory" of modes of "living through" past experiences of persecution and pogrom; and (4) the lack of the possibility of escape or of physical resistance for vast majority of families trapped and helpless together.

DENIAL PROCESSES OF THE VICTIMS

The denial of feeling manifested in emotional withdrawal and the blunting of feeling (psychic numbing, psychological closing off—Lifton, 1967) of different degrees is widely reported by the survivors as having enabled them to cope with the unbearable pain and horror witnessed and experienced daily in the ghettos and concentration camps. Furthermore, there is often a closely associated cognitive construction that supports the defense against feelings.

In the process of catastrophic trauma as described by Krystal (1978) "the blocking of the ability to feel emotions and pain as well as other physical sensations . . . is experienced with relief in relation to the previous painful effects of anxiety and panic." In the unbearable conditions of the Nazi concentration camps, suicide was a logical reaction. Many killed themselves on the electrified fence or by passive surrender to the Muselman state (cf. footnote 1 in Chapter 21).

Denial and the maintenance of hope are closely associated and, however illusory, can be looked upon as serving a life-preserving function in such extreme conditions.

Leo Eitinger (1983), writing of his personal observation of denial in the concentration camps, describes how through such things as selection for work might the immediate danger of death be reduced; thus a complete denial of the initial phase was painfully modified "to a more differentiated degree of understanding and emotional assessment of the real possibilities to survive." This "awareness control" involved varying admixtures of denial, inspired hope with vigilance and awareness in accordance with the fluctuating dangers of the reality situation.

Refusal to accept the inevitability of one's death in the Nazi concentration camps was associated with other coping mechanisms and notably with reciprocal interpersonal relationships. Elsewhere, I have discussed the significance of these relationships formed in the concentration camps (Davidson, 1984, 1988).

Denial processes, hope, and the motivation to continue the struggle to survive were sustained by the mutual support, solidarity, and encouragement of friendships and group relations. When verbalized in the group interaction, denial and hope become more powerful through suggestion and mutual validation.

The utilization of professional and vocational skills by ghetto and concentration camp inmates (who were fortunate to have these opportunities) strikingly demonstrates the use of denial as a positive life-sustaining force. Prisoner doctors in the concentration camps were able to alleviate suffering and to give important, albeit limited, medical help to fellow inmates merely by augmenting denial (Eitinger, 1983). In the Warsaw Ghetto, a group of doctors scientifically collected and collated their observations on the process of starvation while themselves starving to death (Winick, 1979).

Rabbis have described how in Auschwitz and other camps they would concentrate on Halachic questions, rationally working out how they would in the future determine such questions as the marital status of survivors whose spouses had been selected and sent "to the left" (which meant certain death) without there being a witness to the actual death, as is required in normal life for the declaration of widowhood (Zimmels, 1975).

The degree and complexity of these protective processes vary considerably in accordance with the different Holocaust situations—the conditions and the particular individuals involved. Furthermore, because of the vast numbers and heterogeneity of the people involved, generalizations about psychological response should be looked at with reserve.

A striking description of denial processes in the face of catastrophic tragedy appears in the *Chronicle of the Lodz Ghetto, 1941–1944* (Dobroszychi, 1984) published on the fortieth anniversary of the liquidation of the Lodz Ghetto. Written on a daily basis in the Department of Archives of the Lodz Ghetto, it provides a unique account of a persecuted community caught in the Nazi vise. At the beginning of 1942, it was announced that 25,000 people were to be deported for "resettlement." Rapid actions followed, involving the surrounding of buildings by Jewish police, firemen, and gestapo representatives who collected all the inhabitants of several blocks and sorted them into two groups—those who were to remain and those to be deported. In commenting on these horrifying and tragic events a week later, the chronicler, Josef Zalkowitz, writes that it is worth noting the strange response of the population to these events. Despite the unquestioned fact that the actions caused a terrible shock, it was astonishing to realize how apathetically did those whose loved ones were taken react and how "normally" those who were not directly involved continued to carry on. One would have expected that such events would envelop the entire ghetto in mourning for a long time. Yet even before the action was over, the population was again completely preoccupied with everyday problems—getting bread, food, and so on—reverting immediately from any reaction to personal tragedy toward the "routine" daily life of the ghetto.

The use of avoidance and denial mechanisms by victims on entry to a concentration camp is described in the following personal account by an Israeli physician.

C.S.-M., a 23-year-old Czech student, after 1¼ years in a Gestapo prison for anti-Nazi political activities, was transferred with her group to Bergen-Belsen in November 1944. They arrived at night, and, when they awoke in the morning, "wild-eyed emaciated figures with shaven heads in rags" were hammering at the windows and doors of their wooden barrack telling them of the systematic mass killings in the death camps and that their parents and siblings had been sent to their deaths in Auschwitz where there were gas chambers and crematoria. She and her comrades refused to believe them and thought that they were mentally ill and their stories of Auschwitz delusions. They took turns in guarding the windows and doors so that "the crazy Belsen inmates could not get in and tell us such terrible stories and destroy our morale." Although she and her comrades had been isolated in prison and had no information of the Nazi genocidal activities, they had undergone systematic torture by the Gestapo and were fully aware of the brutality and murderousness of the Nazis. Nevertheless, their humanistic value system, derived from their upbringing in Masaryk's Czechoslovakia, made them unable to believe at first the tales of systematic mass murder.

DENIAL PROCESSES IN THE POST-HOLOCAUST YEARS

The struggle to adapt to the new reality after the Holocaust demanded maximal mobilization of the psychic energies of the survivors. The experiences of catastrophic trauma and loss could not be integrated into psychic functioning. Avoidance and denial mechanisms were thus of considerable coping value for the survivors. In fact, denial of various degrees, forms, and complexities seems to constitute the psychic mechanism most fundamentally and widely used in Western culture for dealing with the effects of traumatic experiences (especially when of catastrophic dimensions and when "man-made"). The new social frameworks in which the uprooted and traumatized survivors found themselves after the war demanded great efforts for adaptation. In fact, surprising quantities of energy seem to have been available in many of the survivors, especially those of the teenage and young-adult groups, in their determination to create new lives. This often resulted in the establishment of patterns of overactivity. This capacity for work, when associated with a tenacity of purpose and the determination to succeed, has resulted in considerable productivity with economic and occupational success. The tendency to be constantly active and self-driving seems to be closely linked with the mechanisms of avoidance and denial; an association that emphasizes the primarily adaptive direction of psychic functioning after massive trauma. Denial mechanisms and activity seem mutually reinforcing—as long as the individual can remain active, these mechanisms can be maintained as efficient defensive systems throughout the life span. The hunger for success and activity in some survivors has also been interpreted by psychodynamically oriented clinicians as serving omnipotent needs and attitudes as overcompensation for the impotence and helplessness experienced in the Holocaust.

It should also be remembered that activity in the concentration camps, after selection for various work situations of importance to the Nazis, in general enabled postponement of one's death. This sense of the significance of work in warding off the danger of death often continued thereafter into the normal working life and contributed to the anxiety experienced whenever the threat of loss of work arose. Limitation or loss of activity can thus seriously undermine the denial defenses with possible clinical consequences as discussed later.

THE SURVIVOR SYNDROME

In the early postwar years, many who later suffered from the clinical symptoms of the survivor syndrome were free of symptoms (Luchterhand, 1970). This apparently "symptom-free interval" is explained by several factors related to denial.

Undoubtedly, the need for adaptation to new conditions and to cope with many hardships during the early years after the war demanded maximal utilization of psychic energy. Furthermore, many of the survivors were preoccupied in the early months and sometimes years, with the process of physical recovery from malnutrition, disease, and injury.

What sustained the motivation to survive in the concentration camps and involved many in a constant search and expectation that they would suddenly reappear after the war was the hope that murdered family members were still alive. Denial played a central role in the maintenance of these hopes and the consequent avoidance of grief and mourning.

Sooner or later the bitter truth could not be denied—most survivors came to realize that they had no basis for the hope that their loved ones had survived. Depression and other symptoms of the survivor syndrome would then appear. In some cases, acceptance of the death of entire families proved overwhelming so that severe depression, accompanied by profound guilt and shame, often appeared, even to the extent of occasional suicidal acts. Although 40 years have passed, some few are still unable to accept that a particularly loved and idealized child or sibling is dead and continue in a more-or-less delusional elaboration of denial by fantasy, to believe that he or she is still alive somewhere and that reunion remains possible.

Probably a majority of the survivors have suffered from one or more of the traumatogenic anxiety and grief components of the survivor syndrome (Niederland, 1961; Trautman, 1971). The more intractable and "secondary" manifestations—personality disturbance, psychosomatic disorders, and chronic depression are of more severe psychopathological significance. The unusually rigid deniers tend to be more restricted in their emotional functioning, their interpersonal relationships, and the quality of family life, despite the fact that they are clinically symptom-free (Davidson, 1967; Lorenzer, 1968).

THE SURVIVOR AND SOCIETY

The great majority of the survivors did not become psychiatric patients, nor can they be categorized as belonging to the group of extreme deniers. However, in the struggle to adapt to the demands of reality on their emergence from the catastrophic trauma of the Holocaust, avoidance and denial mechanisms were central to their attempts "to forget" the agonizing memories of the recent past. To recall and recount them to others involved for many a traumatic reexperiencing that they wished to avoid.

Some were categorical about this. "I have given up enough of my life, and I don't want to take up any more by talking about it." Others were conflicted between the longing "to forget" and the commitment to remember and to bear witness—needs of equal importance. Recently a survivor summed up the dilemma with these words:

> They brought us to the lowest level of existence and were made to feel the
> deepest shame. Our shame is greater than that of those murderers who did it
> to us. Therefore we want to forget it . . . also not to forget it . . . to remember
> it at the same time. We go over this broken bridge of our lives and try not to
> look back.

The reluctance to talk about the traumata of the past and the long-ing desire to forget interacted with a general avoidance by society of the survivor's personal experiences of death and terror. This "occurrence avoidance"—avoidance of the realization that "this could have hap-pened to me"—is manifested as a shying away from confrontation with what the observer might have experienced had circumstances been dif-ferent (Shaw, 1972). In this way, avoidance and denial of the past are reinforced, and efforts toward social integration in the present encour-aged as a major life task.

Rappaport (1968) describes how his determination to write and publish his concentration camp experiences was weakened by the fear of appearing abnormal, and he reflects wryly that: "It is considered an attribute of normality to retain a resigned or acquiescent silence in the face of crime." Too little has been written of such survivor shame. The survivor here not only is tacitly encouraged to forget the past in the service of social acceptance but should he insist on telling about what happened to him, his traumatic experiences and their long-term effects are converted into psychiatric symptoms to be dealt with by an expert. However, because the experts also belong to the "denying society," they by and large tended to avoid their patients' Holocaust experiences—even in long-term psychotherapy or psychoanalysis.

As therapists to these survivors, we ourselves had difficulty as we empathized with and therefore experienced the extremes of emotion that had been their reality. Our own avoidance and denial resulted in characteristic social attitudes that contained split-off aspects of our own feelings. When we referred to survivors as heroes (ghetto or concentra-tion camp fighters or partisans) or to the dead as holy martyrs, we represented the shameful, vulnerable, and helpless aspects of the Holo-caust experience by glorification through "splitting off and denial through inversion." These undesirable aspects were expressed in jux-taposed attitudes of contempt by the Israeli youth in their slang ex-pressions in the 1940s and 1950s for the survivor–immigrants—"ga-luti," "gachaletznik" (disdainful terms relating to the European origins of the survivor), and "sabon" (soap). The denial and repudiation of their own vulnerability were seen in the disdainful Sabra self-image of mas-tery and invincibility.

Blaming the victims as in some way responsible for the Holocaust events (for not getting out before, or escaping or resisting) implies that "it couldn't happen to us." According to "defensive attribution" theory (Shaw & Skolnick, 1971), when disaster strikes beyond a certain level, observers insulate themselves from the realization of the possibility of a similar danger occurring to them by assigning responsibility to the victims. Blame, sometimes angrily directed against the survivors, was often derived from guilt at having "abandoned" their relatives and friends, guilt particularly important to Israelis who left Europe before the war. After the survivors began to receive reparations, certain cynical and vulgar, pragmatic attitudes of denial toward their experiences were seen in such provocative questions addressed to survivors with a concentration camp number tatooed on the forearm as: "How much did you get for that?"

Nonetheless, this social climate of denial, in which Israel dealt with the Holocaust experience in such a matter-of-fact way can, however, be seen as having been sociotherapeutic for the rapid resettlement and adaptation of the hundreds of thousands of survivors who poured into Israel in the early years of the state. The personal need to build new lives and new families paralleled central needs of the state—the building of the new state enabled them to achieve new identities.

THE BREAKDOWN OF DENIAL

The large survivor group who were teenagers and young adults during the Holocaust has enabled us to study throughout the life span the struggle "to live with" the traumata of the past over the 40 years since the Holocaust. For long periods, and especially during the years of maximal activity demanded by work and family, memories of the traumatic experiences were "held off" by avoidance and denial mechanisms, and, to a greater or lesser degree, "walled off" and encapsulated from the rest of psychic functioning. Vulnerability, always present though often quiescent for long periods, would be revealed in the face of specific stresses and life events, or during the late "midlife" or aging periods in the life span, manifested as the flooding of consciousness by warded-off traumatic memories and postponed mourning.

The specific vulnerabilities commonly encountered related to:

1. The sudden confrontation with a stimulus in everyday life that triggered traumatic memories.
2. Severe illness, especially when associated with physical wasting (recalling the concentration camp emaciation); certain medical procedures with instruments, treatments, and operations, and even hospitalization itself arousing fears of incarceration, hu-

miliation, torture, and the like (Edelstein, 1982). This was decision-making in relation to life-threatening illness.

3. War, terrorist activities, and accidents involving sudden confrontation with death.
4. Death of family members or friends arousing grief and uncompleted mourning for Holocaust losses.
5. Loss of activity due to illness, accident or age, and the like.
6. A great variety of life events can have specific significance for individual survivors according to their unique individual experiences and their meaning. Joyful life events signifying personal and family achievement and family events such as bar-mitzvahs and weddings can arouse guilt and sorrowful awareness of family losses with consequent depressive moods. Anniversaries of significant dates during the war can have a similar effect.
7. During the later "mid-life" and aging periods particular vulnerability to these stressful and other life events is evident with greater possibility of the breakdown of denial (Antonovsky, Moaz, Dowty, & Wijsenbeck, 1971).

At those periods of life, the achievement of occupational goals, material success, and the support and upbringing of children, and the like may make continued maximal working activity unnecessary. Children leaving home and the separation and distancing involved are often particularly stressful for survivors (Shavit, 1979). Furthermore, the urge to reflect on the past and to review one's life as is typical of the later stages of the life span, frequently confronts survivors with the avoided and unworked-through traumatic experiences and losses of the past:

8. The laborious reconstruction of meaning through the creation of new lives, families, and identities has been a lifelong task for the survivors of the Holocaust. Thus, disappointments in family life, in marriage, and with children can undermine the tenuous framework of meaning rebuilt with such effort.
9. The aging process itself is more than one of physical weakening—it can be particularly traumatic for the survivor, bringing with it diminution in support, lessened personal activity, and decreased gratification and meaning.
10. The existential climate of the past decade, with its mood of increasing disillusionment, disappointment in society, and continued injustice daunting the postwar hopes for a new world, all contributed to doubt and the development of depressive thinking in survivors as they reconsider the significance and validity of their lives and their survival.

The breakdown of denial can result from such specific issues and life events arousing "undigested" traumatic memories, especially poignant after the midlife period. Clinical decompensation, taking the form of acute anxiety associated with flashbacks and/or depressive states characterized by memories of Holocaust losses incompletely mourned, is frequent. The severity of "breakdown" was proportional to the degree of denial involved. The most severe clinical states (often intractable paranoid depressions) were seen in those whose denial defenses were especially strong and rigid. These survivors had claimed to be entirely symptom-free and to have emerged unscathed from the traumas of the past. Individuals who had used lesser degrees of denial reacted with milder symptoms of the survivor syndrome or an exacerbation of these. It is important to stress that the majority of the survivors have not clinically decompensated in the face of stressful life events and during the later phases of their life span (Davidson, 1983).

As it would for anybody, the threat of the breakdown of denial presents for many survivors new opportunities for the emotional processing of the avoided traumatic events of the past. There is thus always this "double-edged" aspect in the life span of the individual who has experienced the extremes of emotional life.

Stressful life events bring the risk of decompensation into symptoms but also the possibility of reaching a new level of personal integration. Those survivors whose personality structures are characterized by flexibility in their denial defenses and plasticity in development since the traumatic period often embark on a late "working-through" of traumatic experiences and losses with consequent major progress toward resolution. Static clinical diagnosis obscures the fact that the lives of many survivors, when looked at longitudinally, reveal recurrent dynamic interaction involving the progressive reduction of denial.

The supportive medium of interpersonal relationships has been a vital factor for many. Most important has been the quality of the marital relationship and the parenting experience, but pairing friendships, social groups with fellow survivors, and even communal and ideological activity have also often been of significance for many. These supportive and developmental frameworks have enabled direct and indirect "working-through" of the traumata and losses of the past. When denial crumbles, delayed "working-through" can also be achieved through such creative activity as the writing of autobiographies or expressing aspects of avoided traumatic experiences through poetry, prose, and painting. Recently, the changing climate of society, bringing with it the new interest in survivor experiences, has reduced the necessity to avoid and deny things previously reinforced by social process. Time itself has been a healing balm. For many survivors, the current era is enough distant from the actual events, the initial traumas, that for the first time they can tell their story. Often it appears that survivors must balance the safety of silence against the fear that no one will know their story and that the future of others will not be instructed by the survivor's past. The silence within many of the survivors families about the survivor's Holocaust experiences, which may also include pre-Holocaust life and childhood, often involved the children in avoidance, denial, and related defensive processes.

The importance of enabling the survivor to reduce his or her guilt by fulfilling his or her commitment to remember and to tell the world cannot be overestimated. The mental health community is presented with an important challenge. Many aging survivors "attacked by memories" (Danieli, 1981; Krystal, 1981) have no words to describe meaningfully their experiences and to express their grief, rage, and shame. The creation of an empathic bond of trust, sincerity, and solidarity can enable them to give expression to traumatic memories and affects denied and inaccessible for so long. Bridges can thus be created between the denied and split-off, unarticulated world of Holocaust trauma, as well as the avoided pre-Holocaust life, with its "enduring repository" of good memories as a source of psychic strength in the struggle toward integration (Peskin & Livson, 1981). This can be a life-enhancing process for the aging survivor.

Now that society is ready to listen, and the survivors ready to talk, a new process of integration can begin. What was once a mélange of split-off attitudes derived from trauma-induced denial enhanced by repetition compulsion (Rosenman, 1982) now presents new possibilities for self-definition. Two generations after the Holocaust, at the other end of their life span, survivors find new roles in a changing world. Psychotherapy, with its tradition of open discussion, can further the goal of personal integration by allowing collective discourse to provide consensual validation for the lives and experiences of those who can teach us so much. When personal denial and social denial can be overcome by such processes, then truly has psychotherapy been transmuted and transcended into a new form of healing.

REFERENCES

Antonovsky, A., Maoz, B., Dowty, N., & Wijsenbeck, H. (1971). Twenty-five years later: A limited study of the sequelae of the concentration camp experience. *Social Psychiatry, 6,* 186–193.

Carmi, T. (1977). Anatomy of a war. *Jerusalem Quarterly, 3,* 102.

Danieli, Y. (1981). On the achievement of integration in aging survivors of the Holocaust. *Journal of Geriatric Psychiatry, 14,* 191–210.

Davidson, S. (1967). The psychiatric disturbances of Holocaust survivors. *Israeli Annals of Psychiatry, 5,* 96–98.

Davidson, S. (1983). The psychosocial aspects of Holocaust trauma in the life cycle of survivor refugees and their families. In Ron Baker (Ed.), *The psychosocial problems of refugees* (pp. 21–31). London: Bondway House.

Davidson, S. (1984). Human reciprocity among the Jewish prisoners in the Nazi concentration camps. In *The Nazi concentration camps.* Jerusalem: Yad Vashem.

Davidson, S. (1988). Group formation and its significance in the Nazi concentration camps. *Israeli Journal of Psychiatry.*

Dobroszycki, L. (Ed.). (1984). *The chronicle of the Lodz Ghetto.* New Haven and London: Yale University Press.

Edelstein, E. (1982). Reactivation of concentration camp experiences as a result of hospitalization. In N. A. Milgram (Ed.), *Stress and Anxiety, 8,* Hemisphere.

Eitinger, L. (1983). Denial in concentration camps: Some personal observations on the positive and negative functions of denial in extreme life situations. In S. Breznitz (Ed.), *The denial of stress.* New York: International Universities Press.

Krystal, H. (1978). Trauma and affects. *Psa. S. Child., 33,* 81–116.

Krystal, H. (1981). Integration and self-healing in post-traumatic states. *Journal of Geriatric Psychiatry, 14,* 165–189.

Lifton, R. J. (1967). Death in life.

Lorenzer, A. (1968). Some observations on the latency of symptoms in patients suffering from persecution sequelae. *International Journal of Psycho-Analysis, 49,* 316.

Luchterhand, E. (1970). Early and late effects of imprisonment in Nazi concentration camps. *Social Psychiatry, 5,* 102–110.

Niederland, W. G. (1961). The problem of the survivor. *Journal of Hillside Hospital, 10,* 233.

Peskin, H., & Livson, N. (1981). Uses of the past in adult psychological health. In *Present and past in middle life* (pp. 153–181). New York: Academic.

Rappaport, E. (1968). Beyond traumatic neurosis. *International Journal of Psycho-Analysis, 49,* 719.

Rosenman, S. (1982). Compassion versus contempt toward Holocaust victims: Difficulties in attaining an adaptive identity in an annihilative world. *International Journal of Psychiatry and Related Sciences, 19,* 39–73.

Shavit, H. (1979). The empty nest as a transitional period for the mother. Unpublished master's thesis, School of Social Work, Haifa University.

Shaw, J. I. (1972). Reactions to victims and defendants of varying degrees of attractiveness. *Psychonomic Science, 27,* 329–330.

Shaw, J. I., & Skolnick, P. (1971). Attribution of responsibility for a happy accident. *Journal of Personal and Social Psychology, 18,* 380–383.

Trautman. (1971). Violence and victims in Nazi concentration camps and the psychopathology of the survivors. In *Psychic Traumatization,* International Psychiatric Clinics, *8.* Boston: Little, Brown.

Winick, M. (Ed.). (1979). *Hunger disease.* Chichester: Wiley.

Zimmels, H. J. (1975). *The echo of the Nazi holocaust in rabbinic literature.* Marla Publications.

Index

321

Date Due